ONCOGENES AND THE MOLECULAR ORIGINS OF CANCER

COLD SPRING HARBOR MONOGRAPH SERIES

The Lactose Operon
The Bacteriophage Lambda
The Molecular Biology of Tumour Viruses
Ribosomes
RNA Phages
RNA Polymerase
The Operon
The Single-Stranded DNA Phages
Transfer RNA:
  Structure, Properties, and Recognition
  Biological Aspects
Molecular Biology of Tumor Viruses, Second Edition:
  DNA Tumor Viruses
  RNA Tumor Viruses
The Molecular Biology of the Yeast Saccharomyces:
  Life Cycle and Inheritance
  Metabolism and Gene Expression
Mitochondrial Genes
Lambda II
Nucleases
Gene Function in Prokaryotes
Microbial Development
The Nematode *Caenorhabditis elegans*
Oncogenes and the Molecular Origins of Cancer

ONCOGENES AND THE MOLECULAR ORIGINS OF CANCER

Edited by

Robert A. Weinberg
Massachusetts Institute of Technology
and Member, Whitehead Institute for
Biomedical Research

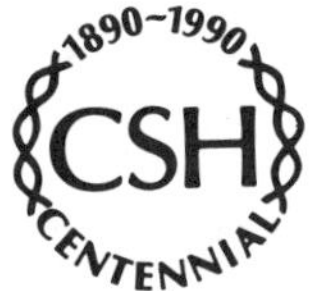

COLD SPRING HARBOR LABORATORY PRESS
1989

ONCOGENES AND THE MOLECULAR ORIGINS OF CANCER
Monograph 18

Printed in the United States of America
Book design by Emily Harste

Library of Congress Cataloging-in-Publication Data

Oncogenes and the molecular origins of cancer/edited by Robert A. Weinberg.
p. cm.—(Cold Spring Harbor monograph series; 18)
Includes bibliographical references.
ISBN 0-87969-336-3 (cloth)
0-87969-340-1 (pbk.)
1. Oncogenes. 2. Oncogenesis. 3. Pathology, Molecular.
I. Weinberg, Robert A. (Robert Allan), 1942– . II. Cold Spring Harbor Laboratory Press. III. Series.
RC268.42.0526 1989
616.99′4071—dc20 89-23927
CIP

Paperback edition:

Cover: Three-dimensional structure of human *ras* oncoprotein in its switch "on" (nonhydrolyzable GTP analog-bound) state. The backbone of the protein is represented by a seven-stranded ribbon and the GTP analog by a dot-surfaced space-filing model. Courtesy of Michael V. Milburn and Sung-Hou Kim (Department of Chemistry and Lawrence Berkeley Laboratory, University of California, Berkeley).

Back cover: Courtesy of Julian P. Heath (Baylor College of Medicine).

All Cold Spring Harbor Laboratory Press publications may be ordered directly from Cold Spring Harbor Laboratory, Box 100, Cold Spring Harbor, New York 11724. (Phone: 1-800-843-4388.) In New York (516) 367-8325.

This book is dedicated to the memory of George Khoury—schoolmate, colleague, dear friend—who did so very much to further the study of oncogenes and viral carcinogenesis and was snatched away from family, friends, and colleagues in mid-life by the disease he sought so hard to understand.

Preface

Like individual careers, scientific fields have their days of wine and roses. These periods may last for a few short years or for a generation. Before these periods of intense productivity, little is known or understood in the field; by the end of the periods, a large corpus of information becomes conceptualized, principles are codified, and all becomes engraved in stone. Once the big problems are worked out, the adventurous souls flee for greener pastures, leaving behind a core of diehards to flesh out the details.

These dynamics create a problem for those intent on producing a book like the present one, a book that purports to describe a field of research. Timing is crucial. Written too early, such a book becomes a compendium of wild speculations and pooled ignorance. Appearing too late, the volume acquires archival value, a grim phrase that connotes dusty shelves in little-used reference libraries. Then there is the other problem for those assembling a book like this one: For whom should it be written?

These issues led to some clear decisions concerning the timing and tone of this particular book. The field of oncogene research is a decade old. Many basic concepts are now well established, yet the field gives signs of flourishing for a long time to come, and solutions to many of its big problems still lie ahead of us. In the life of this field, 1989 would seem to represent a midpoint. The field still has the vitality and intrinsic interest to attract those who love challenging and important problems. Properly done, a book like this one can describe the ongoing dynamism of a field rather than act as a chronicle of battles fought and won years ago.

The intended readership of this volume is quite different from that served by many of its kind, indeed, different from most books in this series published by Cold Spring Harbor Laboratory Press. The present chapters are not written as a monograph for the expert deeply immersed in oncogene research. This book is not intended as a review or reference source of all the facts and ideas produced by this very fertile field of inquiry. The intent is much different: This book is designed as a recruiting pamphlet, a device to interest and excite those outside the field. New blood and new thinking are required to attack the many big problems that still remain.

The authors have written their chapters with the intent of expressing basic concepts and thus have tried to avoid exhaustive, encyclopedic recounting of experimental results. This book is intended as a statement of the ideas that shape current research in this rapidly moving field. The intended audience includes undergraduate and graduate students in biology, medical students, physicians familiar with the basics of molecular biology, and research scientists involved in other areas of biology. Serving such a broad constituency represents an ambitious goal for a multi-authored anthology like this one. The editor hopes very much that we have gone at least part way in realizing what we set out to do. We have been assisted in this undertaking by the staff of Cold Spring Harbor Laboratory Press: John Inglis, Executive Director of Publications; Nancy Ford, Managing Director of Publications; Patricia Barker, production editor; and Mary Cozza, editorial assistant.

R.A. Weinberg

Contents

ONCOGENES AND THE MOLECULAR ORIGINS OF CANCER

Introduction

Robert A. Weinberg
Department of Biology
Massachusetts Institute of Technology and Whitehead
Institute for Biomedical Research Cambridge, Massachusetts 02142

Contemporary oncogene research traces its roots to several distinct lines of work on tumor viruses. The papovaviruses, polyoma and SV40, and the Rous sarcoma retrovirus provided the seminal observations that launched this field by showing that cultured cells infected by these viruses acquire many of the phenotypes of cancer cells, including tumorigenicity. The importance of these observations is hard to overestimate. By infecting cells growing in monolayer culture, an investigator could recapitulate a process that hitherto was thought to occur only in the matrix of a living tissue. With one blow, the process of malignant transformation was demystified.

Equally profound were the insights that this provided into the molecular basis of the observed transformation. The genomes of these viruses encompass only 10^{-6} of the DNA content of the cell. It soon became apparent that this small amount of genetic information sufficed to orchestrate malignant transformation, being involved in its initiation and maintenance in virus-transformed cells. Indeed, the transforming functions could be ascribed to a subset of the genetic sequences of these various viral genomes.

Malignant transformation could now be understood in terms of a small number of genetic regulators working within the cell to control cell growth. The field of oncogene research represents a playing out of this theme in endless variations. An important chapter in this saga was ushered in by the discovery that the viral oncogene associated with the genome of Rous sarcoma virus derives from a normal cellular gene. This led to the model, vindicated in a dozen ways, that the cellular genome harbors a variety of genes that can be converted into oncogenes by specific types of genetic change. Intervention by infecting tumor viruses in the process of tumorigenesis was now seen to be unnecessary. The molecular details of the changes that activate the cell's endogenous genes are often observed in human tumor genomes and involve point mutation, chromosomal translocation, gene truncation, and amplification. In one sense, these genetic changes represent details that elaborate on the central notion that the cell genome carries among its various genes the seeds of neoplasia and of the organism's destruction.

The next chapters in this saga are still being played out, but now in the arenas of cell physiology and protein biochemistry. Although hundreds of research papers have reported on the transforming powers of oncogenes, the biochemical mechanisms used to achieve these changes are still, with rare exception, quite obscure. Workers in this field will spend the coming decade studying the biochemistry of oncogene proteins and signaling pathways. Those adept at molecular cloning, who played such an important role in oncogene research over the past decade, will yield center stage to the biochemists.

At the level of cell physiology, we already have clues about the roles of oncogenes and antecedent proto-oncogenes. Not unexpectedly, they appear to serve as elements in signaling pathways that begin with mitogenic growth factors and, via numerous intermediate signal-transducing steps, end in the complex biological responses of a cell committing itself to growth or differentiation. A goal of contemporary oncogene research is a description of the wiring diagram of the cell—the circuitry that makes the big decisions about growth and quiescence. The field is robust and growing, and promises to provide insights into other areas of biology including development, neuronal signaling, and human genetics. The pages that follow lay it out in all its splendor.

1

An Historical Overview of Oncogenes

Harold Varmus
Departments of Microbiology and Immunology and Biochemistry and Biophysics
University of California Medical Center
San Francisco, California 94143-0502

Oncogenes and the Molecular Origins of Cancer.

I. INTRODUCTION

Medical science has been comfortable for at least a few decades with the general idea that cancer represents a fundamental disorder of cellular growth control, a disorder that arises in rare cells after birth through changes in genes or their expression, gives those cells a growth advantage over surrounding cells, and is inherited by daughter cells like a stable genetic trait. By these properties, cancer differs from the other large categories of disease to which vertebrates fall prey—infections that destroy tissues, degenerative disorders of aging, and inherited genetic deficiencies—even though cancer also can be caused by infection, occurs more often with advancing age, and sometimes depends on inherited mutations.

What has been much less clear until the past decade is the identity of the genes affected in a cancer cell and the nature of the changes. Many hypotheses have been advanced to account for the origins of cancer: e.g., that cancers result from genes introduced into somatic cells by viruses; that cancers depend on activation of viral genes that preexist in our germ lines as a consequence of ancient infections; that cancers arise upon inappropriate expression of cellular genes that are beneficial in other cell types, especially embryonic cells; and that cancers are caused by mutations (physical changes) in an important subset of our genes. The hypothetical viral or cellular genes that influence carcinogenesis have been proposed to control nuclear events (DNA replication and transcription), metabolic pathways, or cell-surface interactions that regulate growth.

Evaluation of such possibilities has depended heavily on the development of potent technologies in molecular biology (for the isolation, characterization, and expression of eukaryotic genes), cell biology (for the study of the molecular basis of growth control), and somatic cell and viral genetics (for functional tests of individual genes). The approaches fostered by these methods have produced some unifying conclusions about the molecular basis of cancer that provide a frame of reference for the chapters that follow:

1. Eukaryotic genomes are endowed with a substantial list of genes (presently numbering between 50 and 100) that may participate in neoplasia as a consequence of mutations.
2. Most of these genes, generally referred to as proto-oncogenes, have fundamental roles in the governance of cell growth or differentiation, have been highly conserved during evolution, and can be partitioned into gene families on the basis of their sequence, their function, or both.
3. The mutations that convert proto-oncogenes to active oncogenes range from subtle changes in sequence (e.g., single nucleotide substitutions) to gross rearrangements (insertions, deletions, gene amplifications, or chromosomal translocations); they may be induced by a variety of

chemical, physical, or viral reagents; they may affect the level of gene expression or the nature of the gene product, or both; and they appear to act in a dominant fashion.

4. Other cancer-inducing mutations appear to behave in a recessive fashion by inactivating genes now known as "tumor suppressor genes"; only a few such genes have been isolated thus far.
5. Many viruses (most DNA viruses and some retroviruses) contain one or a few genes that can induce neoplastic change in animals or in cells grown in culture, but retroviral oncogenes have the particularly useful property of being derived directly from cellular proto-oncogenes.
6. Combinations of oncogenes are generally required to convert a normal cell to a tumor cell. Viral oncogenes or cellular oncogenes may act at different points in a growth regulatory network in which the products of several proto-oncogenes and other proteins normally interact.

The purpose of this chapter is to trace the origins of these now generally accepted principles of oncogenetics. What were the early observations about cancer that suggested that most cancers are genetic diseases of somatic cells? What were the crucial experiments that demonstrated the existence of cellular proto-oncogenes and showed that mutations of them might be important in many kinds of cancer? How were the protein products of proto-oncogenes and oncogenes identified, analyzed for functional properties, and grouped in families?

II. CANCER AS A GENETIC DISEASE

A. The Neoplastic Phenotype

Clinical observation of cancer patients and pathological examination of tumors have long favored the premise that cancers result from permanent changes that unleash cells from their usual restraints to growth. Histologically, cancer cells can often be recognized as derivatives of certain cell lineages on the basis of their initial location, retention of differentiated functions, morphology, or intercellular arrangements. However, the expansion of cell number, the invasion of surrounding stroma and vessels, the relocation at ectopic sites (metastases), the atypical appearance of cells, and the high frequency of mitotic figures indicate fundamental alterations in control of cell growth, shape, and function. Cancers behave clinically as though they are irreversible disorders, curable only through elimination of cells in which pathological changes have occurred. Although there are rare instances of apparently spontaneous remissions of cancer, such as might be attributed to an effective immune response or reversion of epigenetic phenomena, the vast majority of cancers advance inexorably and even progress to more malignant states, as would be expected for genetically altered cells competing for dominance (Foulds 1951; Nowell 1976).

It is generally difficult to grow cancer cells, particularly human cancer cells, under laboratory conditions. Therefore, much of what is known about the characteristics of cultivated cancer cells has been learned from cells experimentally converted from normal (or quasi-normal) states to neoplastic phenotypes by a variety of carcinogens; this process is usually referred to as transformation (or neoplastic transformation) of cultured cells. Both naturally occurring cancer cells and transformed cells exhibit properties in culture that echo the behavior of cancers encountered clinically. The cells usually differ morphologically from their normal counterparts, appearing more refractile and rounded, with an absence of actin cables. They exhibit a loss of growth control, demonstrated by relative independence from growth factors and by a tendency to overgrow a confluent monolayer. The cells are also less adherent (due to reduction of the large extracellular glycoprotein, fibronectin, or its receptors [Hynes 1987]) and more likely to form colonies when suspended in semisolid media and deprived of the anchorage most normal cells require for growth. Other metabolic alterations can be observed as well, such as an enhanced rate of sugar transport and depressed level of cAMP. To meet the most stringent criterion for neoplastic transformation, the cells must form tumors when reintroduced into susceptible animals. (For a fuller discussion of the transformed phenotype, see Hanafusa et al. 1977; Tooze 1980; Feramisco et al. 1985.)

B. Environmental Causes of Cancer

Several kinds of observations—both epidemiological and experimental—support the general idea that most cancers arise from prolonged exposure to physical and chemical agents with mutagenic potential.

1. Epidemiology

The annals of oncology are replete with correlations between cancer and life style—habits, diet, occupation, location—that implicate a variety of factors in carcinogenesis (Hiatt et al. 1977). The time-honored anecdote is Percival Pott's perception that scrotal cancers were common among London's chimney sweeps, but other examples abound: bladder carcinomas among factory workers exposed to radium, aromatic amines, and nitrosoamines; myeloid leukemias among radiologists exposed to X-rays; lung, laryngeal, and oral cancers among tobacco smokers; mesotheliomas among workers exposed to asbestos; skin cancers among sailors with protracted exposure to sunlight (UV irradiation); and many others.

Comparisons of cancer rates in migratory and indigenous populations show that racial and geographic origins are less important in determining cancer statistics than is the environment in which a person lives most of his life (Hiatt et al. 1977; Cairns 1981). Incidences often differ severalfold between nations with very different dietary and other habits, implicating environmental factors in the etiology of many common cancers. The rate of occurrence of most tumors as a function of age predicts a requirement for as many as five or six steps in carcinogenesis (Armitage and Doll 1954; Peto et al. 1975). It is not known for any human cancer whether all of these steps may be mediated by a single causative factor, but in several types of cancers, multiple factors are likely to be involved.

2. *Identification of Carcinogenic Agents*

Attempts to induce cancers in animals with substances suspected from epidemiological study to have carcinogenic activity led to the first reproducible models of carcinogenesis. In the most instructive of these studies (Berenblum 1975), aromatic hydrocarbons present in coal tars were shown to act as initiators of skin cancers in mice. Tumors appeared more frequently and after shorter latency if exposure to the initiation factor was followed by application of a second substance, called a tumor promoter. The most commonly used promoter was croton oil, whose active ingredients proved to be phorbol esters, growth stimulating compounds that are now known to bind and activate protein kinase C (see Chapter 4). This so-called "two-stage" experimental model for carcinogenesis permitted identification of many initiators and promoters, several of which proved to be useful for transformation of cultured cells (Heidelberger 1975), for studies of growth control, and for tests of the metabolic steps often required to convert chemicals into active carcinogens (Miller and Miller 1977). Other means were necessary, however, to define the effects of these agents on specific genes in molecular terms (see Chapter 5 and Section III.D.4 below).

A major advance in our understanding of the causation of cancer resulted from attempts to ask whether such carcinogenic substances (identified either on epidemiological grounds or through cancer induction in animals) were also mutagenic. Simple genetic screening tests have been devised in which, for example, chemicals are assayed for their ability to revert bacterial auxotrophs to prototrophy (Ames 1979). Usually such tests incorporate exposure of the chemical to mammalian liver microsomes to permit metabolic changes that might be essential for carcinogenic or mutagenic activity. The outcome of testing large numbers of agents can be summarized simply: Over 90% of carcinogens are mutagens. These findings fostered the idea that cancer is commonly a disease caused by somatic mutations, intensified interest in the genetic targets for oncogenic mutations, and provided a more practical way than animal testing to screen many compounds for potential carcinogenic activity.

C. Early Assessments of the Neoplastic Genotype

1. Dominance Versus Recessivity: Somatic Cell Hybrids

Some of the earliest assessments of the genetic changes responsible for cancerous change emerged from the formation of hybrid somatic cells in culture. The products of fusion of normal cells with tumor (or transformed) cells can be identified by the expression of genetic markers contributed by each of the parental cell types, and the characteristics of the hybrid cells can be used to determine whether the neoplastic trait is dominant or recessive (Chapter 11). Although such experiments are jeopardized by variations in chromosome number during propagation of the hybrid lines, the most common conclusion is that cancer-causing alleles are recessive to normal alleles (Stanbridge et al. 1982; see Chapter 11): Most hybrid cells appear normal by some measure of transformation (e.g., tumorigenic potential) and often revert to the transformed phenotype as chromosomes are lost during cell passage. It is still unclear how to reconcile this sort of experiment with current ideas about dominant oncogenes and tumor suppressor genes discussed throughout this volume.

2. Karyological Clues

The development of staining and spreading techniques for the microscopic examination of metaphase chromosomes permitted the first physical definition of genetic alterations in cancer cells. Most tumor cells show abnormal karyotypes, usually with elevated numbers of chromosomes and rearranged chromosomes, known as marker chromosomes. The karyotype serves as a "fingerprint" of a tumor cell, setting it apart from normal cells in the same individual and supporting the claim, also made from analysis of X-linked markers in tumors in females (Fialkow 1972; Wolman and Horland 1975), that tumors are composed of clonal or semiclonal cell populations. (This idea has subsequently been further documented in certain types of tumors by analysis of immunoglobulin gene rearrangements [Klein 1981, 1983] or proto-oncogene mutations [Varmus 1984].)

Some types of cancers are regularly associated with certain chromosomal changes. The first to be identified was the apparently truncated version of chromosome 22, known as the Philadelphia chromosome (Ph^1), in the advanced phase of chronic myeloid leukemia (Nowell and Hungerford 1960). Ph^1 is now known to result from a translocation between chromosomes 9 and 22, denoted t(9;22)(q34;q11), which replaces a large portion of the long arm of chromosome 22 with a small terminal piece of chromosome 9 (Heisterkamp et al. 1983; Groffen et al. 1984). A large number of other translocations have subsequently been identified in a variety of human and experimental cancers (Mitelman 1985); prominent among these are three translocations found in Burkitt's lymphoma, a B-cell tumor usually associated with Epstein-Barr virus (EBV), a human herpesvirus

(Klein 1983). The regularity of these rearrangements suggests that they are not random consequences of cellular malfunction, but instead genetic lesions that may make specific contributions to neoplasia (see Chapter 13 and Section III.D.2).

Studies of tumor cell karyotypes also first unveiled the possibility that genes might be amplified during carcinogenesis. Two kinds of chromosomal abnormalities, homogeneously staining regions (HSRs) and double minute chromosomes (DMs), were first recognized as emblems of gene amplification during investigations of drug resistance (Cowell 1982; Schimke 1984). Subsequently, both HSRs and DMs have been found sporadically in several types of tumors and with great regularity in a few types (e.g., neuroblastomas and small cell lung carcinomas; Chapter 13).

D. Inherited Mutations Predisposing to Cancer

For over 100 years, there has been evidence for inherited predispositions to cancer (Ponder 1980; Hansen and Cavenee 1987; see Chapter 11). Such evidence comes both from large families with a slightly higher than expected incidence of all types of cancers (e.g., Skolnick et al. 1981) and from families in which some members have a great likelihood and even a virtual certainty of developing cancer, often cancer of a single type. Among these stronger and thus better-studied predispositions, some result from genetic disorders that increase the effective mutation rate for all genes and hence indirectly contribute to cancer by augmenting the frequency of oncogenic mutations. Others predispose to restricted types of tumors as a result of inherited mutations at loci believed to be implicated in growth control.

1. In a number of autosomal recessive diseases—Fanconi's anemia, Bloom's syndrome, and the several forms of xeroderma pigmentosum—normal defenses against mutational change are impaired, producing an increased incidence of certain kinds of tumors (Cleaver 1980; German 1974; Ponder 1980). For example, a defect in excision repair of UV-induced DNA lesions in xeroderma pigmentosum appears to be responsible for frequent skin carcinomas that follow exposure to sunlight. In Bloom's syndrome, the high incidence of cancers in internal organs has been attributed to abnormalities of DNA ligase I (Chan et al. 1987; Willis and Lindahl 1987). Syndromes of this type argue strongly for the idea that somatic mutations produce cancers. However, the kinds of mutations and the tissues involved may vary greatly among these disorders (Cairns 1981).
2. Strong predispositions to certain types of tumors, especially retinoblastoma (RB), Wilms' tumor (WT), endocrine tumors, colonic polyps and carcinomas, and neurofibromatosis, appear from clinical observations to be inherited as autosomal dominant traits. However, it is now

believed that tumorigenesis depends on somatic mutation of the second copy of the affected gene; thus, the mutations behave in a recessive fashion at the cellular level (see Chapter 11 and Section III.E). In some cases of RB or WT, overt chromosomal deletions regularly affecting the same domain (e.g., band 14 on the long arm of chromosome 13 [13q14] in RB, 11p13 in WT) have focused attention on parts of the genome where the affected genes presumably reside.

III. DISCOVERIES OF ONCOGENES AND PROTO-ONCOGENES

A. Definitions

For the purposes of this book, an oncogene is a viral or cellular gene that can induce one or more characteristics of neoplastic transformation when introduced, either alone or in combination with another gene, into an appropriate cell type. Normal cellular genes that can be converted to active oncogenes by mutation are called proto-oncogenes.

Less rigorous criteria, e.g., recurrent mutations of a gene in several tumors of a single type, have also been used to argue for that gene's role in oncogenesis; such claims should be approached with caution in the absence of more direct experiments. Evidence for oncogenic function may be difficult to obtain with genes that work in concert, but not alone, to produce an oncogenic phenotype and with genes that are active in cell types difficult to grow and evaluate in cell culture. In such settings, it may be helpful to evaluate the gene's oncogenic potential in the intact animal, either by use of virus vectors or by creation of transgenic mice. Finally, current definitions of oncogenes apply to dominantly acting genes and do not accommodate genes that behave in a recessive fashion and are involved in neoplastic transformation only when they fail to function; such genes are referred to here as "tumor suppressor genes" and may counter the effects of conventional oncogenes (see below and Chapter 11).

B. Oncogenes of DNA Tumor Viruses

Two small DNA viruses, polyomavirus and simian virus 40 (SV40), the most closely studied members of the papovavirus group, first nurtured the idea that addition of one or a few genes to a cell could drastically alter cell behavior (Tooze 1980; see Chapter 8). Once it was appreciated, early in the 1960s, that viruses with genomes consisting of only about 5000 bp could cause tumors in animals and induce equivalent changes in cultured cell lines, it seemed highly likely that the apparatus necessary for such changes could be analyzed in detail, both genetically and biochemically.

Mutants isolated about 20 years ago offered the first strong evidence for the idea that specific viral genes could be directly implicated in the initiation of the transformed state. Members of one class of mutants, *tsA* mutants of polyomavirus and SV40, are deficient at an elevated (nonpermissive) temperature in a function (the *A* gene) required early in the virus life cycle (Tegtmeyer and Ozer 1971; Butel 1986). Such mutants are unable to initiate transformation at the nonpermissive temperature (Fried 1965), and many are unable to maintain all aspects of the transformed phenotype when the temperature is shifted up after infection. Another class of mutants, the *hr-t* mutants of polyomavirus, are unable to transform cells under any conditions, and their growth is restricted to certain types of cells (Benjamin 1970). The existence of these two classes of mutants suggested that more than one viral gene might be involved in transformation by polyomavirus (see Chapter 8). Direct demonstration that viral DNA remains linked to host DNA in transformed cells strongly suggested that persistence of viral genes is required to maintain the altered phenotype (Sambrook et al. 1968); the cells retain and express genes used early in the virus life cycle, consistent with the behavior of *tsA* mutants.

Other DNA viruses, especially the adenoviruses, the papillomaviruses, and a few of the herpesviruses (EBV, in particular), have subsequently been the source of additional viral oncogenes (Table 1) (see Chapters 8–10). On the other hand, the large genomes of herpes and pox viruses have usually frustrated efforts to assign oncogenic functions to single genes. In recent years, refined molecular dissection of the regions of DNA tumor virus genomes implicated in transformation has contributed heavily to some current themes in oncogenetics discussed later in this volume. DNA tumor viruses have demonstrated (1) cooperation between two oncogenes during transformation (e.g., the middle and large T antigen genes of polyomavirus [Rassoulzadegan et al. 1982] or the E1A and E1B genes of adenoviruses [Elsen et al. 1983]); (2) the multifunctional properties of a protein encoded by a single oncogene (e.g., the large T antigen of SV40 [Butel 1986]); and (3) the interactions between proteins encoded by viral and cellular genes (e.g., complexes formed between SV40 T antigen and p53 [Lane and Crawford 1979], between polyoma middle T antigen and the c-*src* protein [Courtneidge and Smith 1983]), and between several DNA tumor virus proteins and the product of the retinoblastoma gene [Green 1989]).

C. Retroviruses and Their Oncogenes

The RNA tumor viruses, now known as retroviruses, were among the first recognized oncogenic agents of any kind: Viruses of this type were identified as filterable leukemogenic and sarcomagenic factors in chickens nearly 80 years ago (Rous 1911; Gross 1970). An intensive attack on the oncogenic mechanisms employed by these viruses, however, began contemporaneously with study of the papovaviruses, stimulated by the de-

Table 1 Oncogenes of DNA tumor viruses

Virus	Gene	Protein	Location	Function
Polyomavirus	A	large T	nucleus	binds DNA
	hr-t	middle T	PM	complexes with c-*src* protein
		small t	cyto	?
SV40	A	large T	nucleus/PM	binds DNA, p53, and RB gene product
		small t	cyto	?
Bovine papillomavirus	E5	44 a.a.	?	?
	E6		?	?
Adenoviruses	E1A	289 a.a., 243 a.a.	nucleus	transcriptional regulators; bind RB gene product
	E1B	53–58 kD, 15 kD	nucleus (?)	?
Epstein-Barr virus	EBNA1–4	several	nucleus	?
	LMP	44 kD	PM	?

(EBNA) Epstein-Barr nuclear antigen; (LMP) latent membrane protein; (PM) plasma membrane; (RB) retinoblastoma. See Chapters 8–10 for greater detail.

velopment of assays for transformation of cultured cells and biochemical methods for analysis of viral genomes and proteins (for review, see Weiss et al. 1982). It was through this area of experimental oncology that investigators first came in direct contact with cellular genes that could be implicated in neoplasia.

1. General Properties of Retroviruses

Although retroviruses are the source of many of the oncogenes discussed in this volume, no chapter is explicitly devoted to them. Thus, a few words of introduction are appropriate here (for fuller discussions, see Weiss et al. 1982, 1985; Varmus 1983, 1988; Varmus and Brown 1989). Retroviral genomes are composed of two identical single strands of RNA, 5–10 kb in length, capable of encoding 1–10 polypeptides. Generally, three coding regions are present: *gag* for the major structural proteins of the viral nucleocapsid, *pol* for enzymes found in virus particles, and *env* for envelope glycoproteins. During the course of infection, viral genes are converted to a double-stranded DNA form by the virus-coded enzyme, reverse transcriptase, and the DNA is covalently linked to host DNA by a specialized mechanism mediated by a virus-coded integration protein. Viral genes are then expressed through host mechanisms for RNA synthesis, processing, and translation, using the integrated DNA (the provirus) as a stable repository of viral genetic information.

By virtue of genomic size and stable inheritance of viral genes within host chromosomes, retroviruses show some resemblance to SV40 and other DNA viruses as experimental carcinogens, but the retroviruses have proved to have several advantages:

1. Most DNA viruses transform only foreign host cells, cells in which they fail to grow, and stably alter only a small percentage of infected cells. However, many retroviruses can transform their natural host cells and other cells in which they replicate; moreover, they can do so in virtually every infected cell.
2. The oncogenes of DNA tumor viruses are required for replication as well as for transformation, but the retroviral genes implicated in transformation are dispensable for replication, thereby simplifying the analysis of oncogenic functions.
3. The origins of the DNA virus oncogenes remain as mysterious as those of any other animal virus genes, but the oncogenes of retroviruses (called v-*onc*s) (Table 2) are clearly derived from normal cellular genes (c-*onc*s). (As will soon be evident, the c-*onc*s are one set of the larger class of genes known as proto-oncogenes.)
4. Many retroviruses do not carry viral oncogenes and fail to transform cells in culture, but they are nevertheless able to cause tumors in animals, usually after a long latent period. The oncogenic mechanisms

Table 2 Retroviral oncogenes (v-*oncs*)

Prototype virus[a]	v-*onc*	Species of origin	Protein product[b] location	Protein product[b] biochemical property	Major disease(s)
RSV	*src*	chicken	PM	PK-Tyr	sarcoma
Y73/ESV	*yes*	chicken	PM	PK-Tyr	sarcoma
FuSV/PRCII	*fps*[c]	chicken	C/PM	PK-Tyr	sarcoma
UR2	*ros*	chicken	TM	PK-Tyr	sarcoma
CT10	*crk*	chicken	(?)	activates PK-Tyr	sarcoma
MH2[d]	*mil*[e]	chicken	C	PK-Ser/Thr	sarcoma
MC29	*myc*	chicken	N	DB	carcinoma, endothelioma, myeloid leukemia
S13	*sea*	chicken	TM	PK-Tyr	erythroleukemia
ASV17	*jun*	chicken	N	TR, DB	sarcoma
AMV	*myb*	chicken	N	DB	myeloid leukemia
E26[d]	*ets*	chicken	?	?	erythroleukemia
AEV-H	*erbB*	chicken	TM	PK-Tyr	erythroleukemia, sarcoma
AEV-ES[d]	*erbA*	chicken	N	TR, DB	erythroleukemia
SKV77	*ski*	chicken	N	?	
REV-T	*rel*	turkey	N/C	?	immature B-cell lymphoma
Ab-MLV	*abl*	mouse	C/PM	PK-Tyr	pre-B-cell lymphoma

Mo-MSV	*mos*	mouse	C	PK-Ser/Thr	sarcoma
MSV-3611	*raf*[e]	mouse	C	PK-Ser/Thr	sarcoma
Ha-MSV	Ha-*ras*	rat	PM	G binding	sarcoma, erythroleukemia
Ki-MSV	Ki-*ras*	rat	PM	G binding	sarcoma, erythroleukemia
FBJ-MSV	*fos*	mouse	N	TR	osteosarcoma
ST-FeSV	*fes*[c]	cat	C/PM	PK-Tyr	sarcoma
SM-FeSV	*fms*	cat	TM	PK-Tyr	sarcoma
GR-FeSV[f]	*fgr*	cat	PM	PK-Tyr	sarcoma
SSV	*sis*	wooly monkey	S	R binding	sarcoma
HZ4-ReSV	*kit*	cat	TM	PK-Tyr	sarcoma

Further description and bibliography can be found elsewhere (Bishop and Varmus 1985; Varmus and Bishop 1986; Kahn and Graf 1987).

[a]Abbreviations: (RSV) Rous sarcoma virus; (Y73) Yamaguchi 73 sarcoma virus; (FuSV) Fujinami sarcoma virus; (MC29) myelocytomatosis-29 virus; (MH2) Mill Hill-2 virus; (AMV) avian myeloblastosis virus; (AEV) avian erythroblastosis virus; (REV-T) reticulo-endotheliosis virus, strain T; (Mo-MSV) Moloney murine sarcoma virus; (Ab-MLV) Abelson murine leukemia virus; (Ha-MSV) Harvey murine sarcoma virus; (Ki-MSV) Kirsten murine sarcoma virus; (ST-, SM-, GR-) Snyder-Theilen, Susan McDonough, and Gardner-Rasheed feline sarcoma viruses; (SSV) simian sarcoma virus.

[b](PM) Plasma membrane-associated but not a transmembrane protein; (TM) transmembrane; (C) cytoplasmic; (N) nuclear; (S) secreted, (PK-Tyr) protein-tyrosine kinase; (PK-Ser/Thr) protein-serine/threonine kinase; (TR) transcriptional regulator; (DB) DNA binding; (G binding) GTP/GDP binding protein; (R binding) receptor binding.

[c]v-*fps* and v-*fes* are derived from the same cognate c-*onc*.

[d]These viruses carry a second oncogene contributing to oncogenesis: MH2, v-*myc*, E26, v-*myc*; AEV-ES4, v-*erb*B.

[e]v-*mil* (also known as v-*mht*) and v-*raf* are derived from the same cognate c-*onc*.

[f]Part of the mammalian-actin sequence is found in the genome of GR-FeSV.

used by such viruses include insertion of proviral DNA into chromosomes adjacent to a proto-oncogene, thereby perturbing its expression. These proviral insertion mutations also allow the identification of cellular proto-oncogenes (Section III.D.1.).

5. The small DNA tumor viruses and many retroviruses generally cause sarcomas (a relatively uncommon form of human cancer), but the large assortment of retroviruses also includes agents of various leukemias and carcinomas (Table 2).

2. *Rous Sarcoma Virus and the Discovery of c-*src

Many of the seminal experiments that established the principal facts about retroviral oncogenes were performed with Rous sarcoma virus (RSV), one of the first animal viruses to be isolated (Rous 1911) and one that remains unique among retroviruses because it carries all the genetic information required for both replication and efficient transformation. Two kinds of RSV mutants, isolated around 1970, provided powerful tools for genetic and biochemical analysis of transformation by this virus: (1) temperature-sensitive (*ts*) mutants that grow normally at 35 and 41°C, but neither initiate nor maintain the transformed phenotype at the higher (nonpermissive) temperature (Martin 1970); and (2) nonconditional, transformation-defective (*td*) mutants that replicate to wild-type levels but cannot transform cells as a result of an extensive deletion of genetic information (Vogt 1971; Martin and Duesberg 1972). The behavior of these mutants clearly dissociated the replication- and transformation-specific functions of RSV. Chemical and genetic analysis of wild-type and mutant RNA genomes indicated that the transforming region, called *src*, was partially or completely ensconced in a 2-kb region near the 3′ end of viral RNA (Wang et al. 1975).

The *td* deletion mutants, in particular, were crucial to the design of experiments that first revealed sequences related to retroviral oncogenes in cellular DNA. Complementary DNA (cDNA) unique to the *src* region of RSV genomic RNA was isolated by removing from a diverse population of RSV cDNAs those components that could hybridize to the RNA from a *td* mutant of RSV (Stehelin et al. 1976a). The *src*-specific cDNA was then shown to anneal to the DNA of all tested vertebrate animals, with efficiency of formation and stability of the duplexes directly related to the evolutionary distance between the DNA source and chickens, the natural host for RSV (Stehelin et al. 1976b). Subsequent studies established that the cellular sequences related to the RSV *src* gene were exons of a large cellular gene, now known as c-*src*, which has been extremely well conserved during evolution and can be isolated from organisms as diverse as flies, frogs, fish, birds, rodents, and man (Spector et al. 1978a; Parker et al. 1981; Shalloway et al. 1981; Shilo and Weinberg 1981; Simon et al. 1983; Takeya and Hanafusa 1983).

The experiments that led to the discovery of c-*src* were, in part, inspired by an earlier proposal, known as the virogene-oncogene hypothesis, which argued that silent oncogenes are present in normal cellular genomes as part of proviruses transmitted through the germ line ("endogenous proviruses") and that such genes could be transcriptionally activated by various carcinogenic agents (Todaro and Huebner 1972). Two central features of c-*src* were soon perceived to be at odds with this hypothesis: (1) c-*src* has the structural features of a normal cellular gene (Parker et al. 1981; Shalloway et al. 1981; Takeya and Hanafusa 1983) and is unlinked to any recognizable viral genes (Padgett et al. 1977) and (2) c-*src* is widely expressed in normal host tissues (Spector et al. 1978b), often at rather high levels, to produce a protein that differs in small but functionally important ways from that of viral *src* (v-*src*) (Takeya and Hanafusa 1983; Sefton and Hunter 1986). Taken in concert, these findings were more consistent with the proposal that c-*src* is a gene normally beneficial to the host, but which can be converted to an oncogene through capture (transduction) by a retrovirus. The process of transduction (models for which are described elsewhere: Varmus 1982; Bishop 1983; Swanstrom et al. 1983) introduces mutations within the gene and promotes efficient expression under the control of viral regulatory sequences (see Section III.C.4).

3. *Other Retroviral Oncogenes*

The *src* paradigm fostered belief that other highly oncogenic retroviruses also carry genes transduced from normal cellular chromosomes. These other viruses, however, are all deficient in one or more genes needed for replication and must be propagated together with helper viruses; thus, no mutants analogous to *td* RSVs could provide a secure genetic basis for preparation of viral oncogene-specific probes. Nevertheless, several retroviruses were found to contain sequences closely related to single-copy, highly conserved cellular DNA (for reviews, see Bishop and Varmus 1982, 1985; Bishop 1983, 1985). With the advent of molecular cloning, it was feasible to define the boundaries of the transduced sequences within viral genomes, to establish the precise relationship between viral oncogenes (v-*onc*s) and their cellular progenitors (c-*onc*s), and to demonstrate that the v-*onc*s encoded proteins with oncogenic activity.

At last count, 23 distinct cellular genes have been identified through their derivative v-*onc*s in retroviral genomes (Table 2). Several of these have been transduced several times, by infection of a single animal species or by infection of different species with different retroviruses. Some retroviruses even contain v-*onc*s derived from two separate, unlinked, and functionally disparate cellular loci. The structural dissection of v- and c-*onc*s has set limits on mechanisms for transduction and oncogene activation and has suggested other ways to identify possible oncogenes (see Section III.D.1).

The use of retroviral oncogenes to isolate cellular homologs is the most venerable route to proto-oncogenes, and it has not lost its vitality as a source of interesting genes. New sporadic isolates of highly oncogenic retroviruses or old unstudied isolates frozen in storage for decades have both been gainfully employed in the recent past, bringing to attention genes such as *jun* (Maki et al. 1987), *sea* (Hayman et al. 1985), and *crk* (Mayer et al. 1988). However, it is generally less profitable to attempt to capture new oncogenes by passage of retroviruses lacking oncogenes through animal hosts. Although some viruses will transduce certain genes quite efficiently under such circumstances (Miles and Robinson 1983; Neil et al. 1984), especially if part of the oncogene is already present in the transducing virus (Hanafusa et al. 1977), transduction is generally a very rare event. Moreover, all the genes recovered after deliberate infection of animals in the recent past are genes that were previously isolated from oncogenic retroviruses.

4. *Implications of the Cellular Origins of Retroviral Oncogenes*

Many questions were raised by the discovery of c-*src* and other cellular progenitors of retroviral oncogenes. Three of these were particularly important and have guided much of the story that follows.

First, *how does a viral oncogene differ from its normal cellular progenitor?* It was reasonable to presume that viral oncogenes, capable of rapid transformation and tumorigenesis, must differ in fundamental ways from the highly conserved cellular genes from which they were derived. The most obvious difference is a *quantitative* one: Viral oncogenes are expressed under the influence of strong transcriptional signals provided by retroviral long terminal repeats (LTRs), the regulatory sequences present at the ends of proviral DNA, whereas c-*onc*s are expressed from their own, usually much less efficient promoters. *Qualitative* differences are also important: The coding sequences may incur a variety of mutations—terminal truncations, internal deletions, and point mutations—during or after viral transduction. As will be apparent in many chapters in this book, both qualitative and quantitative factors appear to be important in the generation of an oncogene, but to different extents for different genes.

Second, *can the cellular progenitors of retroviral oncogenes be activated to serve as oncogenes without a requirement for viral transduction?* In other words, do the c-*onc*s discovered through retrovirology play some role in cancer in their original chromosomal setting? As described in subsequent sections (III.D.1–4), this is often the case, regardless of the methods used to search for cellular oncogenes. Furthermore, such searches sometimes uncover genes that have never surfaced in the form of retroviral oncogenes. The mutations that activate cellular genes produce qualitative or quantitative effects that often simulate the consequences of viral transduction. Thus, genetic rearrangements, due to DNA insertions, chromosomal translocations, and gene amplifications, generally have a quantitative effect on gene expression, whereas the primary effects of base substitutions are usually qualitative, altering the biochemical properties of a gene product.

Third, *what are the normal functions of the progenitors of retroviral oncogenes?* The extraordinary degree of conservation of c-*src* and other c-*oncs* throughout metazoan evolution and the involvement of mutant alleles of these genes in neoplasia strongly implied that proto-oncogenes control crucial steps in cell growth and development. Such controls would presumably be perturbed by the mutations that rendered the genes into oncogenes. As the final sections of this chapter will relate, the protein products of proto-oncogenes function in many cellular compartments, performing a variety of biochemical tasks in the pathways that lead from extracellular signals to transcriptional controls within the nucleus.

D. Discoveries of Cellular Oncogenes

Several strategies have been employed to identify cellular genes that contribute to oncogenesis in their native chromosomal setting (Varmus 1984). The first successful one originated with attempts to ask how retroviruses that lack their own oncogenes are nevertheless often capable of inducing tumors in animals.

1. Targets for Proviral Insertion Mutagenesis

The avian leukosis viruses (ALVs) are replication-proficient retroviruses that can cause a variety of diseases several weeks or months after infection—most commonly lymphoma in the Bursa of Fabricius (the B-cell forming organ of birds), but also erythroleukemia, nephroblastoma, anemia, and osteopetrosis—without the assistance of viral genes other than those required for replication (Gross 1970; Teich et al. 1982, 1985). These tumors (and others induced by retroviruses without oncogenes) are clonal or oligoclonal outgrowths of one or a few infected cells. Close examination of ALV proviral DNA in bursal lymphomas demonstrated that proviruses in different tumors appeared to be located at different positions within a single cellular locus. Moreover, some tumors contained novel species of RNA in which viral regulatory sequences were joined to cellular sequences presumed to come from exons adjacent to proviral integration sites, as might be expected if the proviruses were affecting expression of an adjacent gene (Neel et al. 1981; Payne et al. 1981). The use of molecular probes specific for the few available retroviral oncogenes then showed that a large majority of bursal lymphomas harbored ALV proviral DNA in the c-*myc* locus (Hayward et al. 1981), a gene first identified as the homolog of v-*myc*, the oncogene found in several strains of avian retroviruses that usually cause acute myeloid leukemias (Roussel et al. 1979; Sheiness and Bishop 1979; Sheiness et al. 1980). The interpretation of these and further related findings was that infection by ALV introduced viral DNA, more or less at random, into the chromosomes of a large number of bursal cells; that the occasional cell that acquired a provirus in the c-*myc* locus, in any of the several arrangements that augment expression of c-*myc* (Payne et al. 1982), acquired a growth advantage over neighboring cells; and that additional mutations—in the adjacent provirus (Fung et al. 1981; Payne et al. 1981), in c-*myc* itself (Westaway et al. 1984), or in other genes—were likely to contribute to neoplastic growth.

Altered expression of a c-*onc* gene by proviral insertion occurs in highly repetitive patterns in other cell lineages after infection by ALV or other retroviruses without oncogenes (Table 3). In addition, several retroviruses cause insertion mutations of previously unknown genes, thereby offering an opportunity to isolate novel proto-oncogenes by cloning cellular DNA

Table 3 Proto-oncogenes affected by insertion mutations

Gene	Insertion mutagen[a]	Tumor type	Species
c-*myc*	ALV, CSV, RPV	B-cell lymphoma	chicken
	Mo-MLV, MCF-MLV	T-cell lymphoma	rat, mouse
	FeLV	T-cell lymphoma	cat
c-*erbB*	ALV	erythroblastosis	chicken
c-*fms*	MLV	T-cell leukemia	mice
c-Ha-*ras*	MAV	nephroblastoma	chicken
	MLV	T-cell lymphoma	mouse
c-*mos*	IAP	plasmacytoma	mouse
c-*myb*	Mo-MLV	plasmacytoid lymphosarcoma	mouse
	ALV	B-cell lymphoma	chicken
int-1	MMTV	mammary carcinoma	mouse
int-2	MMTV	mammary carcinoma	mouse
int-3	MMTV	mammary carcinoma	mouse
int-4	MMTV	mammary carcinoma	mouse
pim-1	MCF-MLV, Mo-MLV	T-cell lymphoma	mouse
pvt/mis	Mo-MLV	T-cell lymphoma	mouse
lck	Mo-MLV	T-cell lymphoma	mouse
p53[b]	Mo-MLV	erythroleukemia	mouse
IL-2 gene[c]	GaLV	T-cell lymphoma	gibbon
IL-3 gene[c]	IAP	T-cell lymphoma	mouse

For references, see Nusse and Berns (1988).

[a]Abbreviations: (ALV) avian leukosis virus; (CLV) chicken syncytial virus; (RPV) ring-necked pheasant virus; (MAV) myeloblastosis-associated virus; (Mo-MLV) Moloney murine leukemia virus; (FeLV) feline leukemia virus; (IAP), intracisternal A particle; (MMTV) mouse mammary tumor virus; (MCF-MLV) mink cell focus-forming murine leukemia virus.

[b]These mutations may be recessive.

[c]Affected in only a single tumor or cell line.

adjacent to proviral DNA (Table 3). The first examples, *int-1* and *int-2* (Nusse and Varmus 1982; Peters et al. 1983), emerged from the study of the mouse mammary tumor virus (MMTV), but the proviral tagging strategy has now been used to isolate several other putative oncogenes from various kinds of retrovirus-induced tumors (Table 3; Nusse and Berns 1988).

As early as 1982, it was evident that not all oncogenic retroviruses without v-*onc* genes induced tumors through insertion mutations. A few of these, e.g., the human T-cell and bovine leukemia viruses, now appear to depend on unusual viral regulatory genes for oncogenic activity. These genes are believed to induce tumors, at least in part, by *trans*-activating unidentified cellular genes that promote growth of lymphoid cells (Chen et al. 1986).

2. *Translocated Genes*

The demonstration that retroviruses could affect the behavior of c-*onc* genes by insertion mutation fueled optimism about explaining the significance of genomic rearrangements commonly encountered in the karyotypes of cancer cells by identifying the altered genes. Investigation was initially focused on two kinds of chromosomal translocations: the various translocations that join one of three immunoglobulin loci (Ig) to a common chromosome in B-cell tumors of rodents and man, and Ph^1 in human myeloid leukemias (see Section II.C.2).

Molecular immunologists had recognized for some years that rearranged Ig heavy-chain loci in mouse plasmacytomas were often positioned next to an unfamiliar region of the mouse genome. A clear connection was established between these local juxtapositions and the frequently observed chromosomal translocations, particularly t(12;15), when the region adjacent to the IgH gene (located on chromosome 12) was identified as part of the mouse c-*myc* locus (normally found on chromosome 15) (Shen-Ong et al. 1982). Similar deductions were made about the translocations common to human B-cell lines derived from patients with Burkitt's lymphoma: The c-*myc* gene on chromosome 8 was joined to the IgH locus on chromosome 14 or, less commonly, to one of the Ig light-chain loci on chromosome 2 or 22 (Dalla-Favera et al. 1982; Taub et al. 1982, 1984; Battey et al. 1983). Although the precise effects of these realignments on expression of c-*myc* are still matters of dispute, it is generally accepted that the translocations perturb control of c-*myc* and potentiate oncogenic growth of B cells (Leder et al. 1984).

The genetic implications of Ph^1 were clarified by the discoveries that the c-*abl* gene resides near the tip of 9q, that it is moved to chromosome 22 during the construction of Ph^1, and that sequences within its large first intron are joined to a restricted region of a hitherto unknown gene on chromosome 22, now called *bcr* (Groffen et al. 1984). As a consequence, a hybrid *bcr-abl* protein with oncogenic potential is produced (Konopka et al. 1984).

Recognition that previously identified c-*oncs*, such as c-*myc* and c-*abl*, are directly affected by some of the best known translocations in tumor cells has spurred efforts to make accurate chromosomal assignments for proto-oncogenes, in hopes that the assignments would connect other known genes with other known translocations (Hecht 1988), or to identify new genes located at translocation breakpoints. In the absence of a simple procedure for isolating breakpoint regions, those searching for new proto-oncogenes rearranged by translocations have concentrated initially on those B- and T-cell lymphomas in which one partner in the translocation process has been identified as an Ig or T-cell-receptor (TCR) locus, and this search has already produced a few new candidate proto-oncogenes (see Table 1 in Chapter 13). The frequent involvement of Ig and TCR loci argues that the translocation mechanism may be an aberrant form of the mechanism normally used to rearrange Ig or TCR genes in normal B and T cells.

3. Amplified Genes

It was established in the 1970s that some genes encoding enzymes sensitive to growth-inhibiting drugs could undergo dramatic expansion of copy number and that amplified genes were manifest in the karyotype as DMs or HSRs in cells selected for drug resistance (Cowell 1982; Schimke 1984). Sporadic findings of modest degrees of amplification of known c-*onc* genes in some commonly studied tumor cell lines inspired a wider and often successful search for amplified proto-oncogenes in other cell lines with more obvious karyological signs of amplification (see Table 2 in Chapter 13). The most provocative findings were obtained with both cell lines and fresh tumor material from certain types of tumors that frequently displayed DMs or HSRs (especially neuroblastoma [NB] of childhood and small cell lung carcinoma [SCLC]). Because of the increased numbers of copies of the amplified genes (usually in the range of 20–50, but sometimes extending into the hundreds), novel amplified genes were detected in DNA from such tumors by molecular hybridization with c-*onc* probes on the basis of partial sequence identity. In this way, the N-*myc* and L-*myc* genes were discovered in NB and SCLC cell lines, respectively (Kohl et al. 1983; Schwab et al. 1983; Nau et al. 1985). Work with these two diseases established that the same proto-oncogene was very often amplified and hence overexpressed in the tumors, and that amplification sometimes correlates with the biological behavior of the tumor cell and with the prognosis of the patient (see Chapter 13).

4. Oncogenes Identified by Gene Transfer Methods

Cellular genes were first implicated in oncogenesis by virtue of genomic rearrangements—insertion mutations, translocations, and amplification—

but the evidence was mostly circumstantial: Among tumors of a certain type, unusual genetic events reproducibly affected one gene, often a gene already known to be a progenitor or a relative of a retroviral oncogene, and altered the level of production and sometimes the composition of the gene product. However strong and doubtless influential, such arguments lacked the force of a direct functional test of oncogenicity.

Functional tests for the isolation of oncogenes are based on the idea that transfer of a gene in the form of naked DNA from a transformed to a nontransformed cell can change the phenotype of the recipient cell to resemble that of the donor cell. In this sense, the approach finds its historical antecedents in early experiments showing that DNA is the repository of genetic information, and its more immediate precedents in experiments demonstrating that retroviral genes, both for replication and

Table 4 Oncogenes identified in gene transfer assays

Gene	Tumor (examples)
c-Ha-*ras*	bladder carcinoma
	NMU-induced mammary carcinoma
	lung carcinoma
c-Ki-*ras*	colon carcinoma
	lung carcinoma
	pancreatic carcinoma
	myeloid leukemia
	myelodysplasia
N-*ras*	myeloid leukemia
	myelodysplasia
	neuroblastoma
	melanoma
	fibrosarcoma
	lung sarcoma
c-*mos*	plasmacytoma (mouse)
c-*ros*[a]	mammary carcinoma cell line
c-*raf*[a]	
neu/*erbB2*	ENU-induced neuroblastoma (rat)
met	MNNG-induced transformant of osteosarcoma line
dbl[a]	B-cell lymphoma
hst/K-*fgf*[a]	gastric carcinoma, Kaposi's sarcoma
mas[a]	mammary carcinoma cell line
ret[a]	reticulum cell carcinoma
trk	pancreatic carcinoma

All are human in origin, unless indicated otherwise. References can be found in Varmus (1984 and 1987).

[a]In these instances, transforming activity was generated by rearrangements occurring after extraction of DNA from the tumor or cell line.

transformation, are in a DNA form that can function in new cells (Hill and Hillova 1972). The functional tests, moreover, unlike tests for structural alterations in DNA, make no assumptions about the nature of the genetic lesions and are thus as likely to detect oncogenes with point mutations as those with gross rearrangements.

The explicit strategy that first demonstrated the usefulness of this approach was to prepare DNA (or chromatin) from chemically transformed rodent cells, such as methylcholanthrene-transformed cells from a line established from a C3H mouse, and to show that it could induce transformation of the established mouse fibroblast cell line, NIH-3T3 (Shih et al. 1979). When applied to human tumor cell lines and primary tumors, such procedures have generally revealed transforming genes in 10–30% of samples (Table 4). Although the presence of highly repeated human sequences in the transformed mouse cells and cotransfer of human sequences with the oncogenic activity in secondary DNA tranformations provided good evidence that human DNA was responsible for the changes, identification of the oncogene was initially difficult. In 1982, two approaches—hybridization with probes for known c-*onc*s and molecular cloning of transformed NIH-3T3 cell DNA linked to human repeat sequences—revealed the same result: The transformed cells had acquired human Ki-*ras* and Ha-*ras* genes (Der et al. 1982; Parada et al. 1982; Santos et al. 1982), the human homologs of the progenitors of the oncogenes of Kirsten and Harvey sarcoma viruses. Soon thereafter, molecular cloning of transforming DNA from a human neuroblastoma identified a third member of the *ras* gene family, called N-*ras* (Shimizu et al. 1983). Comparison of the nucleotide sequences of normal human *ras* alleles and the putative transforming genes was equally dramatic: A single nucleotide change (in codon 12 in the first instance [Tabin et al. 1982; Santos et al. 1982], but often in codons 13 and 61 as well as 12 in other alleles studied later) appeared to explain conversion of a proto-oncogene to a cellular oncogene (see Varmus 1984; Barbacid 1987; Chapter 5).

Mutant alleles of three *ras* loci (Ha-, Ki-, and N-*ras*) account for the vast majority of transforming genes detected with the NIH-3T3 cell assay, using DNA from spontaneous human tumors or from tumors chemically induced in animals. Nevertheless, mutant forms of several other genes, some known c-*onc*s and some novel, have been isolated through this assay (Table 4). The mutations are sometimes base substitutions, as in the *ras* gene precedents, but sometimes rearrangements, and the latter, in particular, have often occurred during experimental manipulation of the DNA, rather than as lesions in the original tumors. Several variations of the assay have been recommended to make it sensitive to oncogenes that might not be detected under standard conditions. These changes include the use of other recipient lines, assays for tumor formation in animals rather than transformation in cell culture, and attempts to activate DNA from normal cells by adding strong promoter elements prior to DNA transfer.

5. *Detection of Proto-oncogenes through Structural or Functional Similarities to Known Proto-oncogenes*

As the repertoire of well-characterized genes and proteins expanded during the past decade, many genes were recognized to be close relatives of known proto-oncogenes and thus possible proto-oncogenes, even though they have not been encountered in mutant form in naturally occurring tumors. To advance the claim that a relative of a proto-oncogene might be a proto-oncogene as well, candidate genes have been tested for oncogenic effects after they have been mutated or efficiently expressed (e.g., in the context of a retroviral vector). In this way, for example, genes encoding known growth factors (epidermal growth factor [EGF], fibroblast growth factor, or granulocyte-macrophage colony-stimulating factor) have been shown to mediate transformation in culture or to induce tumors in animals (e.g., Lang et al. 1985 and Chapter 2).

E. Isolation of Genes That Normally Suppress Tumorigenesis

Around 1970, statistical analyses of two cancers, retinoblastoma (RB) and Wilms' tumor (WT), that often occur in a familial pattern inspired a "two-hit hypothesis." According to this proposal, one of the two genetic lesions required for development of these tumors was inherited and thus present constitutionally (i.e., in all somatic cells) in familial cases (Knudson 1971). In a few particularly informative cases, karyological studies revealed visible deletions in characteristic chromosomal regions (see Chapter 11). Such deletions strongly suggested that the inherited "hit" produced a loss-of-function (or recessive) mutation of a gene located within the regions common to all the observed deletions (13q14 for RB, 11p13 for WT). The presumption that the second (acquired) hit would eliminate the other functional copy of the relevant gene was confirmed by the use of restriction fragment length polymorphisms (RFLPs). Comparison of DNA from normal and tumor tissue indicated that constitutional heterozygosity of the appropriate chromosomes was lost during tumorigenesis by nondisjunction, somatic recombination, or other mechanisms (Cavenee et al. 1983; Hansen and Cavenee 1987), favoring the idea that recessive mutations had occurred in genes that normally suppress tumorigenesis.

Although an imposing list of chromosomal assignments for potential tumor suppressor genes can now be assembled (see Table 2 in Chapter 11 and Klein 1987), we remain largely in the dark about the nature of such genes. There are no simple functional tests for the normal alleles of the affected genes, so attempts at gene isolation have taken as their starting points the assignments of such genes to chromosomal positions through observed deletions (in RB and WT) and through mapping of the RFLP probes that demonstrate loss of heterozygosity. At the present degree of resolution of the human gene map, such assignments may still be hundreds or thousands of kilobases from the gene of interest.

The first claim to isolation of a recessive oncogene was staked in 1986, when a human DNA clone from the region of 13q14 was found to detect deletions in RBs and in osteosarcomas (Friend et al. 1986; Lee et al. 1987). (Osteosarcomas are relatively rare tumors often associated with RB and believed to be dependent on the same genetic lesions.) Aberrant or absent transcripts from the gene detected by this probe in several tumors (Fung et al. 1987; Lee et al. 1987) provided further support for the conclusion that the locus is the correct one. Finally, expression of a cDNA clone in retinoblastoma and osteosarcoma cell lines appears to reverse their oncogenicity (Huang et al. 1988).

Chromosomal walking procedures may eventually allow isolation of fragments from the WT locus, since analysis of deletion mutants has placed the gene between two cloned genes that are probably less than 1000 kb apart (Compton et al. 1988). However, new techniques will probably be required to isolate loci subject to recessive mutations in disorders unaccompanied by informative karyotypic changes.

IV. CHARACTERIZATION OF ONCOGENES AND PROTO-ONCOGENES

The discoveries of viral and cellular oncogenes have dramatically affected experimental approaches to the physiological basis of cancer. Rather than attempt to catalog the many ways in which cancer cells differ from their normal counterparts, it is now possible to determine the biochemical functions of proteins encoded by precisely those genes known to initiate neoplastic change. To ask how oncogenes transform cells (and what proto-oncogenes do in normal cells), several disciplines have been essential: molecular genetics for introducing various forms of a gene of interest into appropriate cells; cell biology for assaying the consequences of gene transfer; immunology for developing antisera that permit characterization of oncogenic proteins; and biochemistry for seeking the relevant activities of those proteins.

A. Molecular Oncogenetics

Molecular genetics—especially the in vitro manipulation of cloned genes and their reintroduction into cells—has provided the leverage for addressing many central questions in contemporary oncology: What are the effects of one or a combination of oncogenes upon a cell? What are the changes that convert a proto-oncogene to an oncogene? Where are the functional sites in protein products of such genes? What are the proteins with which the products of oncogenes and proto-oncogenes interact?

The biological effects of naturally occurring oncogenes and proto-oncogenes, or of mutant alleles engineered in vitro, can best be appreciated by returning them to cells, a goal that is now generally achieved in one of three ways: (1) by direct introduction of the genes in the form of DNA, using the calcium-phosphate-mediated DNA transformation procedure, electroporation, protoplast fusion, or microinjection; (2) by infection of cultured cells or animals with virus vectors, usually constructed with retroviral components, to carry the gene(s) of interest; and most recently, (3) by production of transgenic mice (Palmiter and Brinster 1984). Such mice are made by microinjection of DNA into fertilized mouse eggs; they transmit newly implanted genes through the germ line, express those genes in accord with the tissue specificity of adjacent transcriptional machinery, and sometimes develop tumors at a characteristic time and place, providing especially attractive experimental models for carcinogenesis (Cory and Adams 1988; Hanahan 1988).

Strategies that examine the reversion of oncogenic activation are also important, since they help define portions of oncoproteins that are essential for neoplastic activity and since they might identify cellular genes whose proteins interact with oncoproteins in functionally significant ways. Such strategies may be based on classic somatic cell genetics, to seek naturally occurring or induced mutations that produce conditional or nonconditional reversion of the transformed state, or they may employ site-directed mutagenic procedures, to examine the functional importance of defined regions of a protein. The latter method will become increasingly useful as the products of oncogenes and proto-oncogenes are subjected to high-resolution analysis of structure, a feat that has been successful thus far only with *ras* proteins (de Vos et al. 1988; Chapter 5).

To decipher the functions of proto-oncogenes (or tumor suppressor genes) by genetic procedures, it is necessary to produce cells or organisms that are homozygous for mutant alleles. One widely used strategy depends on the identification of homologs of proto-oncogenes in organisms, such as *Drosophila* or yeast, that are more malleable genetically than birds or mammals. A substantial number of *Drosophila* genes encoding proteins related to vertebrate oncoproteins have now been isolated (Table 5) (Shilo 1987): At least two of them—*wingless*, the homolog of the *int-1* proto-oncogene, and *dorsal*, the homolog of c-*rel*—were already known to be essential for early developmental events, thereby confirming the prediction that proto-oncogenes are important for normal growth or differentiation. The *ras* genes are the only proto-oncogenes for which close relatives have been found in yeast; the results of genetic and biochemical studies of yeast *RAS* genes are discussed in Chapter 5. In the near future, it may be possible to study homozygous recessive mutations in mammals, as well as in simpler metazoans. Homologous recombination between DNA introduced into embryonic mouse stem cells and resident genes allows the isolation of mutant cell lines from which mutant mice may ultimately be derived; such mutant lines have already been obtained using the *int-2* proto-oncogene as a target (Mansour et al. 1988).

Table 5 Genes in *Drosophila melanogaster* related to vertebrate proto-oncogenes

Locus	Chromosomal position	Proposed biochemical function	Mutants isolated
ras-1	62B	GTPase	–
ras-2	64B	GTPase	–
ras-3	85D	GTPase	–
abl	73B	PK-Tyr	+
src-1	64B	PK-Tyr	–
src-2	29A	PK-Tyr	–
fps	85D	PK-Tyr	–
myb	13F	DNA binding	–
erbB/faint little ball	57F	PK-Tyr receptor	+
int-1/wingless	28A	morphogen	+
rel/dorsal		?	+
sevenless	10A	PK-Tyr receptor	+
insulin receptor	93E	PK-Tyr receptor	–
torso	43D	PK-Tyr receptor	+
raf/l(1)*polehole*	2F	PK-Ser/Thr	+

For references, see Shilo (1987).

B. Making Antibodies against Oncoproteins

The protein products of oncogenes and proto-oncogenes are often present in small amounts relative to other proteins in a cell and hence difficult to identify and characterize. The crucial experimental tools used to circumvent this problem have been antibodies raised in various ways. The first antisera that recognized an oncoprotein, the SV40 T antigen, the product of the viral *A* gene, were obtained from animals bearing SV40-induced tumor cells (Tooze 1980; Chapter 8). In such animals, there is often systemic evidence of an immune response: tumor regression or resistance to subsequent transplantations. To demonstrate that the response was directed, at least in part, against a viral gene product, immunofluorescent techniques were used to show that the antisera detected antigens in virus-infected cells (mainly in the nucleus), but not in uninfected cells. The specificity was confirmed and the apparent molecular weight of the protein was determined when the sera were used to immunoprecipitate radiolabeled proteins from virus-infected and control cells, the precipitates were fractionated by electrophoresis in polyacrylamide gels, and mutations in the *A* gene were found to affect the mobility of the protein.

These fundamental procedures were in place for SV40 and a few other DNA tumor viruses by the early 1970s, but it was not until 1977 that any retroviral oncoproteins were detected. Again the pioneering experiments were performed with RSV. After many failed efforts to obtain antisera against the protein product of v-*src*, success was achieved by infecting rabbits (an unusual host for RSV, but a potent immune responder). Rabbits that developed RSV-induced tumors, especially tumors that later regressed, produced antibodies that recognized the ~60-kD product of v-*src* (Brugge and Erikson 1977). (According to conventions established for retroviral proteins, the 60-kD phosphoprotein encoded by v-*src* is designated $pp60^{v\text{-}src}$.)

Although products of a few other retroviral oncogenes and their cognate c-*oncs* were first identified through similar strategies (e.g., the $p21^{ras}$ proteins [Shih et al. 1979]), several retroviral oncoproteins could be characterized with antisera raised against viral structural proteins (Bishop and Varmus 1982, 1985). This is so because transduction of host proto-oncogenes often fuses their open reading frames with viral structural genes, yielding hybrid proteins recognized by easily procured antiviral antibodies.

There are now a number of improved methods for generating antisera directed against the protein products of any gene that has been molecularly cloned, including oncogenes and proto-oncogenes. Planted in plasmid or virus vectors, the gene may be expressed at high levels after introduction into a variety of cells (bacteria, yeast, insect, or mammalian cells); partially purified protein can then be used to induce antibodies appropriate for identifying the natural product of the gene. Alternatively, the nucleotide sequence of the gene can be used to predict the amino acid sequence of the protein, and synthetic peptides, linked to carrier protein, can serve as effective immunogens. In numerous instances described in this volume, either of these two strategies has produced the antibodies crucial to the study of oncoproteins.

C. Biochemical Properties of Oncoproteins

Three experimental approaches have been especially revealing about the biochemical properties of proteins encoded by oncogenes and proto-oncogenes: nucleotide sequencing of cloned genes to deduce the primary sequence of oncoproteins; the use of antibodies in combination with protein biochemistry and cell fractionation procedures to determine the size, cellular location, and chemical modifications of encoded proteins; and tests of proteins (e.g., for enzymatic or binding activities) to seek biochemical properties that might explain the biological consequences of oncogene expression. By these criteria, most of the known oncogenes and proto-oncogenes have been grouped into functional families.

1. Protein Kinases

The protein encoded by the RSV *src* gene, $pp60^{v\text{-}src}$, was the first product of an oncogene to be assigned a provocative biochemical function, the ability to phosphorylate proteins (Collett and Erikson 1978; Levinson et al. 1978). It was also among the first to be localized at the periphery of the cell, the plasma membrane (Willingham et al. 1979; Courtneidge et al. 1980; Rohrschreider 1980), far from the nucleus where oncoproteins had traditionally been expected to reside.

To discover the protein kinase activity of *src* protein, two groups of investigators, stimulated by different rationales, added [γ-^{32}P]ATP to immunoprecipitates formed with pp60$^{v\text{-}src}$ and antisera from tumor-bearing rabbits; labeled phosphate was transferred to the heavy chain of rabbit immunoglobulins (Collett and Erikson 1978; Levinson et al. 1978). The protein kinase activity that resides in pp60$^{v\text{-}src}$ could be demonstrated in this way because the heavy chain in the rabbit anti-*src* antibodies proved to be good substrates for the kinase. This procedure, now known as the immune complex kinase assay, has permitted many proteins to be tested for kinase activity without prior purification. Among these are the protein product of the c-*src* proto-oncogene, pp60$^{c\text{-}src}$, and the products of many other retroviral oncogenes and their cellular progenitors (Chapter 6).

A second important and surprising development was the recognition that protein kinase activities associated with oncoproteins may phosphorylate tyrosine (Eckhart et al. 1979; Smith et al. 1979; Hunter and Sefton 1980; Witte et al. 1980). Prior to this discovery, all protein phosphorylation was thought to occur on serine and threonine residues; in most cell types only about 0.1–1% of phosphoaminoacid is phosphotyrosine (Hunter and Cooper 1985). Nevertheless, animal cells are well-endowed with protein tyrosine kinases (Hanks et al. 1988). From the study of retroviral oncogenes alone, it has become evident that at least ten such kinases existed, some of them transmembrane proteins and others, like pp60^{src}, plasma-membrane-affiliated proteins without transmembranous or extracellular domains (see Table 2 in Chapter 6).

The family of protein tyrosine kinases has been expanded by at least two other perceptions. (1) Many transmembrane receptors for secreted polypeptide growth factors exhibit protein tyrosine kinase activities in their cytoplasmic domains. This point was made most dramatically by the discoveries that the proto-oncogenes, c-*erbB* and c-*fms*, encode the protein tyrosine kinase receptors for known growth factors, EGF (Downward et al. 1984) and colony-stimulating factor-1 (CSF-1) (Sherr et al. 1985). (2) Protein tyrosine kinases have highly conserved sequence motifs that are strongly predictive of catalytic activity (Hanks et al. 1988). On this basis, genes fortuitously cloned or cloned during explicit searches for novel protein tyrosine kinases have been added to the still-growing roster of kinase-encoding genes (see Table 3 in Chapter 6).

Major efforts have been directed toward the identification of the functionally significant targets for protein tyrosine kinases (Radke and Martin 1979; Hunter and Cooper 1985). Two-dimensional electrophoresis of phosphorylated proteins, deliberate testing of individual proteins for phosphotyrosine, and antiphosphotyrosine antibodies have all been employed in this quest. Although many proteins, several of which are well-characterized, are now known to contain phosphotyrosine in cells transformed by v-*src* or related oncogenes, or in cells stimulated with ligands for receptor-kinases, no protein is yet known to be a physiologically relevant target.

2. *Growth Factors*

Endocrinology has taught us that circulating factors (hormones) can have profound effects on cell growth, and the search for mitogenic substances in serum has identified a number of polypeptide growth factors. The idea that transformation might be due, at least in part, to such extracellular components first took firm hold with reports that factors produced by transformed or tumor cells are capable of inducing transformation transiently in cultured cells (DeLarco and Todaro 1978; Sporn and Roberts 1985). Unregulated production of growth factors or production of mutant growth factors might affect the producer cell itself (autocrine stimulation), adjacent cells (paracrine), or distant cells (endocrine).

Speculations of this sort achieved great currency in 1983 when it was recognized that the normal progenitor of the v-*sis* oncogene from simian sarcoma virus (SSV) encodes the B chain of the platelet-derived growth factor (PDGF). This came about when enough PDGF was prepared to allow partial amino acid sequencing and comparison with the sequence of v-*sis* protein, as deduced from the cloned provirus of SSV (Doolittle et al. 1983; Waterfield et al. 1983).

Subsequently, a number of other secretory polypeptides have been strongly or weakly implicated as oncoproteins (see Table 1 in Chapter 2). Some of these were first discovered as products of oncogenes and perceived to be secretory proteins through sequence analysis or protein biochemistry, whereas others were first recognized as growth or differentiation factors that have been subsequently tested for oncogenic activities. For both types, the mechanisms by which secretory proteins contribute to transformation is still largely a matter of debate (Chapter 2).

3. *Signal Transducers*

Early biochemical studies of the *ras* proteins, p21, demonstrated their capacity to bind guanosine nucleotides (GDP and GTP) and their location at the plasma membrane (Shih et al. 1980; Barbacid 1987). Once the *ras* oncogenes and proto-oncogenes were expressed in *Escherichia coli*, it was possible to show that normal p21 proteins exhibited GTPase activity, but the oncogenic p21 proteins had considerably lower levels of activity (Gibbs et al. 1984; Sweet et al. 1984). A more than coincidental similarity to G proteins, multicomponent factors with GDP/GTP-binding-and GTPase activities, was assured when the first sequences of the α subunits of G proteins were found to be strikingly related to the known sequences of p21 proteins (Hurley et al. 1984; see Chapter 4). Some of the best-known G proteins transduce signals from transmembrane receptors for catecholamines to activate adenylate cyclase, stimulating production of cAMP and consequent activation of the cAMP-dependent protein kinase. Although *ras* proteins of *Saccharomyces cerevisiae* also appear to activate adenylate cyclase (Broek et al. 1985), *ras* proteins in mammalian cells have yet to be placed within any known signal transmission pathway. The recent discovery of a cytoplasmic protein that stimulates the GTPase activity of normal *ras* proteins may provide a portal to the relevant pathway (Trahey and McCormick 1987; McCormick 1989).

Recognition of the relationship between *ras* and G proteins has inspired a wider search for other *ras*-related genes, and several have been found, some intentionally and some by chance (Chapter 5). It is not yet known whether these genes (or the genes encoding G factors) can participate in neoplastic change, although at least one of them, *rap1*, can act as an anti-*ras* tumor suppressor gene when overexpressed (Kitayama et al. 1989).

4. *Transcription Factors*

It was an early presumption in molecular oncology that transforming proteins would function in the nucleus, where DNA replication and RNA synthesis occur, and the first studies of an oncoprotein, SV40 T antigen, offered support for that presumption. Over the years, however, the protein products of most oncogenes have been located in the cytoplasm, the plasma membrane, or even the extracellular space. Moreover, it has proven easier to assign biochemical functions to most of the nonnuclear oncoproteins than to those several oncoproteins that reside in the nucleus. Even for the oncogenic products of DNA tumor virus genes with well-defined functions in the virus life cycle, attribution of their oncogenic activity to a known biochemical activity has been difficult (Chapters 8–10).

The impasse in the study of what have come to be called "nuclear oncogenes" has recently been alleviated by rapid advances in the study of eukaryotic transcription factors and by the happy discovery of an informative avian retroviral oncogene, called v-*jun* (Maki et al. 1987). Translation of the nucleotide sequence of v-*jun* revealed substantial amino acid similarity to the yeast transcriptional factor encoded by the *GCN4* gene (Vogt et al. 1987). The GCN4 protein and the mammalian transcription factor, AP-1, were known to bind the same short DNA sequence (Struhl 1987); c-*jun* has now been shown to encode the major component of AP-1 (Bohmann et al. 1987), a 39-kD protein that regularly associates with nuclear proteins encoded by c-*fos* and v-*fos* (Rauscher et al. 1988).

Other signs also point to a major role for nuclear oncogenes in transcriptional control: (1) The transforming potential of the adenovirus E1A gene has been genetically linked to transcriptional regulation, predominantly repression (Lillie et al. 1986). (2) A region of c-*myc* protein shows sequence similarity to some of the mammalian transcription factors (Landschulz et al. 1988). (3) The v-*erbA* protein is a close relative of the glucocorticoid and other steroid hormone receptors, ligand-dependent transcriptional activators (Evans 1988); c-*erbA* products have recently been identified as receptors for thyroid hormones (Sap et al. 1986). These developments are discussed in greater detail in Chapter 7.

D. Where Oncoproteins Meddle in Growth Control

As many of the subsequent chapters in this volume demonstrate, there is ample evidence to suggest that oncogenes either alter the level of activity in one or more of the known metabolic pathways implicated in growth control or supercede regulation by a pathway, with the common consequence of uncontrolled growth. At least three potentially intersecting pathways are likely to be involved and resurface repeatedly in this book:

1. *Tyrosine phosphorylation* of proteins occurs as a consequence of binding extracellular growth factors to transmembrane receptors or as a consequence of activation of other kinases lacking extracellular domains. Although phosphotyrosine comprises a small fraction of phosphoamino acid in animal cells, many protein tyrosine kinases have been identified (Hunter and Cooper 1985; Hanks et al. 1988; also see Chapters 3 and 6), and a large number of proteins appear to contain phosphotyrosine. It is likely that the biochemical functions of several of these target proteins will prove to be regulated by tyrosine phosphorylation. Several oncoproteins appear to affect this pathway as ligands for receptor-kinases, as kinases, and possibly as targets for kinases.
2. *Phosphatidylinositol metabolism* is strongly influenced by the activities of several species of phospholipase C, which hydrolyzes phosphatidylinositides, leading to production of diacylglycerol and inositol triphosphate. Diacylglycerol, in turn, stimulates protein kinase C, and inositol triphosphate signals release of internal stores of calcium, thereby activating calcium-dependent kinases and other enzymes (Berridge and Irvine 1984; Chapter 4). Phosphorylation of phosphatidylinositols at various sites on the sugar ring by specific phosphatidylinositol kinases also appears to figure in this regulatory pathway, and such kinases have been described in association with oncogenic protein kinases (e.g., Courtneidge and Heber 1987; Kaplan et al. 1987). Substances such as phorbol esters (TPA) that activate protein kinase C can mimic the actions of the pathway, and several oncogenes have been claimed to augment the pathway's activity (Chapter 4).
3. *cAMP* is synthesized by adenylate cyclase under the control of G

proteins, which, in turn, respond to signals from a variety of membrane receptors (Gottesman and Fleischmann 1986; Chapter 4). cAMP concentrations determine the activity of the cAMP-dependent protein kinase, and the resulting phosphorylations of serine and threonine can affect the biochemical properties of several target proteins. As analogs of classic G proteins, *ras* proteins have been implicated in control of cAMP levels (Chapter 5), but other oncoproteins may perturb the function of this pathway by less direct means.

E. Interactions between Proteins Implicated in Oncogenesis

The discoveries summarized here imply that the protein products of oncogenes meddle in growth control at many different points in a complex regulatory network, a network that depends on several kinds of signaling: protein-protein interactions, small secondary messengers, and protein-nucleic acid interactions. It is reasonable to predict that interactions occurring during oncogenesis will sometimes involve one protein encoded by a viral or cellular oncogene and another encoded by a proto-oncogene (or a tumor suppressor gene) and that interactions occurring during normal growth control will sometimes involve the products of two proto-oncogenes. During the past few years, such predictions have been fulfilled, usually in surprising and mechanistically revealing ways:

1. Attempts to identify the source of the protein tyrosine kinase activity associated with the middle T antigen of polyomavirus led to the discovery that this DNA tumor virus oncoprotein forms a complex with c-*src* protein (Courtneidge and Smith 1983), thereby augmenting the specific activity of the c-*src*-encoded kinase (Bolen et al. 1984). This phenomenon is presumably the basis for the oncogenicity of middle T antigen (Chapter 8); it also illustrates a novel means for activation (and detection) of proto-oncogenes and implies that middle T antigen may mimic the action of a normal cellular protein.
2. The cellular homolog of the newly discovered retroviral oncogene, v-*jun*, encodes the transcription factor, AP-1 (see above, Section III.C.4 and Chapter 7). Yet more recently, the c-*jun*/AP-1 protein was recognized to be the protein previously called p39, known for many years to be complexed with c- and v-*fos* proteins (Rauscher et al. 1988). It now appears likely that c-*fos* protein (and the products of *fos*-related genes [Cohen and Curran 1988]) modulate the action of AP-1 through such interactions.
3. The oncoproteins of several DNA tumor viruses—the E1A proteins of adenoviruses (Whyte et al. 1988), the large T antigens of SV40 (DeCaprio et al. 1988) and other papovaviruses (Dyson et al. 1989), and the E7 protein of human papillomavirus (Dyson et al. 1989)—have

been discovered to bind to the protein product of the retinoblastoma susceptibility gene, probably through closely related blocks of amino acid sequences believed to be responsible for the transforming activity of these several viral proteins. Since the retinoblastoma gene product likely acts as a tumor suppressor (see Section III.D above and Chapter 11), the DNA tumor virus proteins may be interfering with a mechanism that normally constrains cell growth.

4. A 53-kD protein, known as p53, was shown several years ago to associate with the large T antigen of SV40 (Lane and Crawford 1979) and with the large E1B protein of adenoviruses (Sarnow et al. 1982). Cloning of the gene that encodes p53 (called *p53*) led to tests that documented transforming effects of p53 in the absence of DNA tumor virus oncogenes (Parada et al. 1984). Despite these initial suggestions that *p53* was a classic proto-oncogene, more recent work argues that *p53* may be a tumor suppressor gene and that transforming alleles may act as dominant negative mutants (Finlay et al. 1989).

V. SUMMARY AND PERSPECTIVE

The foregoing account makes plain the multiplicity of ways in which genes relevant to oncogenesis may be discovered and the various molecular

Table 6 Mechanisms of activation of proto-oncogenes

Mechanism	Genetic and biochemical consequences	Examples
Transduction	insertion of exons of a proto-oncogene into a retrovirus genome, usually with truncations or internal mutations of coding sequences, causing efficient production of an abnormal protein	v-*src*
Point mutation	altered sequence and biochemical function of protein product	c-Ha-*ras*
Insertion mutation	augmented production of mRNA and protein, via promoter or enhancer in LTR; sometimes accompanied by truncation, fusion, or point mutation of coding sequences	c-*myc*, *int-1*
Amplification	augmented production of mRNA and protein via increased gene dosage	N-*myc*
Chromosomal translocation	altered regulation of expression, sometimes with creation of hybrid proteins	c-*myc*, *abl-bcr*
Protein-protein interaction	stabilization and altered biochemical function	$pp60^{c\text{-}src}$ and middle T Ag

mechanisms by which such genes may be activated to participate in oncogenic conversion (Table 6). This information has revolutionized the study of cancer, brought together investigators from initially disparate fields, and prompted strong clinical interest in the diagnostic and prognostic applications of tests for common mutations of proto-oncogenes (see Chapter 13).

Although the roster of proto-oncogenes is large and can be categorized in instructive ways, it is still not possible to be specific either about the number and kinds of oncogenes required to convert a particular cell into a cancer cell or about biochemical events that are crucial for transformation. One message seems clear: Oncogenesis is a distorted form of growth control, employing mutant forms of proteins that normally interact in a complex regulatory network to drive excessive rounds of cell division. The obvious challenge is to learn how this happens. What are the specific targets for the action of an oncogenic protein? What regulatory apparatus is superceded? What countervailing forces might be harnessed to ameliorate the effects of an oncogene? We approach such questions with the hope that, as we come closer to a full description of the biochemistry of cell transformation, we will come closer to rational therapeutics for cancer.

REFERENCES

Ames, B.N. 1979. Identifying environmental chemicals causing mutations and cancer. *Science* **204:** 587–593.

Armitage, P. and R. Doll. 1954. The age distribution of cancer and a multistage theory of cancer. *Br. J. Cancer* **8:** 1–12.

Barbacid, M. 1987. *ras* Genes. *Annu. Rev. Biochem.* **56:** 779–827.

Battey, J., C. Moulding, R. Taub, W. Murphy, T. Stewart, H. Potter, G. Lenoir and P. Leder. 1983. The human c-*myc* oncogene: Structural consequences of translocation into the IgH locus in Burkitt lymphoma. *Cell* **34:** 779–787.

Benjamin, T. 1970. Host-range mutants of polyoma virus. *Proc. Natl. Acad. Sci.* **67:** 394–399.

Berenblum, I. 1975. Sequential aspects of chemical carcinogenesis: Skin. In *Cancer: Etiology* (ed. F.F. Becker), vol. 1, pp. 323–344. Plenum Press, New York.

Berridge, M.J. and R.F. Irvine. 1984. Inositol trisphosphate, a novel second messenger in cellular signal transduction. *Nature* **312:** 315–321.

Bishop, J.M. 1983. Cellular oncogenes and retroviruses. *Annu. Rev. Biochem.* **52:** 301–354.

———. 1985. Viral oncogenes. *Cell* **42:** 23–38.

Bishop, J.M. and H.E. Varmus. 1982. Functions and origins of retroviral transforming genes. In *Molecular biology of tumor viruses*, 2nd edition: *RNA tumor viruses* (ed. R. Weiss et al.), pp. 999–1108. Cold Spring Harbor Laboratory, Cold Spring Harbor, New York.

———. 1985. Functions and origins of retroviral transforming genes. In *Molecular biology of tumor viruses,* 2nd edition: *RNA tumor viruses, 2/Supplements and appendixes* (ed. R. Weiss et al.), pp. 249–356. Cold Spring Harbor Laboratory, Cold Spring Harbor, New York.

Bohmann, D., T.J. Bos, A. Admon, T. Nishimura, P.K. Vogt, and R. Tjian. 1987. Human proto-oncogene c-*jun* encodes a DNA binding protein with structural and functional properties of transcription factor AP-1. *Science* **238:** 1386–1392.

Bolen, J.B., C.J. Thiele, M.A. Israel, W. Yonemoto, L.A. Lipsich, and J.S. Brugge. 1984. Enhancement of cellular *src* gene product associated tyrosylkinase activity following polyoma virus infection and transformation. *Cell* **38:** 767–777.

Broek, D., N. Samiy, O. Fasano, A. Fujiyama, F. Tamanoi, J. Northup, and M. Wigler. 1985. Differential activation of yeast adenylate cyclase by wild-type and mutant *RAS* proteins. *Cell* **41:** 763–769.

Brugge, J.S. and R.L. Erikson. 1977. Identification of a transformation-specific antigen induced by an avian sarcoma virus. *Nature* **269:** 346–348.

Butel, J.S. 1986. SV40 large T-antigen: Dual oncogene. *Cancer Surv.* **5:** 343–365.

Cairns, J. 1981. The origins of human cancers. *Nature* **289:** 353–357.

Cavenee, W.K., T.P. Dryja, R.A. Phillips, W.F. Benedict, R. Godbout, B.L. Gallie, A.L. Murphee, L.C. Strong, and R. White. 1983. Expression of recessive alleles by chromosomal mechanisms in retinoblastoma. *Nature* **305:** 779–784.

Chan, J.Y.H., F.F. Becker, J. German, and J.H. Ray. 1987. Altered DNA ligase I activity in Bloom's syndrome. *Nature* **325:** 357–359.

Chen, I.S.Y., W. Wachsman, J.D. Rosenblatt, and A.J. Cann. 1986. The role of the X gene in HTLV-associated malignancy. *Cancer Surv.* **5:** 329–342.

Cleaver, J.E. 1980. DNA damage, repair systems and human hypersensitivity diseases. *J. Environ. Pathol. Toxicol.* **3:** 53–68.

Cohen, D.R. and T. Curran. 1988. *fra*-1: A serum-inducible, cellular immediate-early gene that encodes a *fos*-related antigen. *Mol. Cell. Biol.* **8:** 2063–2069.

Collett, M.S. and R.L. Erikson. 1978. Protein kinase activity associated with the avian sarcoma virus *src* gene product. *Proc. Natl. Acad. Sci.* **75:** 2021–2024.

Compton, D.A., M.M. Weil, C. Jones, V.M. Riccardi, L.C. Strong, and G.F. Saunders. 1988. Long range physical map of the Wilms' tumor-aniridia region on human chromosome 11. *Cell* **55:** 827–836.

Cory, S. and J. Adams. 1988. Transgenic mice and oncogenesis. *Annu. Rev. Immunol.* **6:** 25–48.

Courtneidge, S.A. and A. Heber. 1987. An 81 kd protein complexed with middle T antigen and pp60$^{c\text{-}src}$: A possible phosphatidylinositol kinase. *Cell* **50:** 1031–1037.

Courtneidge, S.A. and A.E. Smith. 1983. Polyoma virus transforming protein associates with the product of the c-*src* cellular gene. *Nature* **303:** 435–439.

Courtneidge, S.A., A.D. Levinson, and J.M. Bishop. 1980. The protein encoded by the transforming gene of avian sarcoma virus (pp60^{src}) and a homologous protein in normal cells (pp60$^{\text{proto-}src}$) are associated with the plasma membrane. *Proc. Natl. Acad. Sci.* **77:** 3783–3787.

Cowell, J.K. 1982. Double minutes and homogeneously staining regions: Gene amplification in mammalian cells. *Annu. Rev. Genet.* **16:** 21–59.

Dalla-Favera, R., M. Bregni, J. Erickson, D. Patterson, R.C. Gallo, and C.M. Croce. 1982. Human c-*myc onc* gene is located on the region of chromosome 8 that is translocated in Burkitt lymphoma cells. *Proc. Natl. Acad. Sci.* **79:** 7824–7827.

DeCaprio, J.A., J.W. Ludlow, J. Figge, J.-Y. Shew, C.-M. Huang, W.-H. Lee, E. Marsilio, E. Paucha, and D.M. Livingston. 1988. SV40 large tumor antigen forms a specific complex with the product of the retinoblastoma susceptibility gene. *Cell* **54:** 275–283.

Delarco, J.E., and G.J. Todaro. 1978. Growth factors from murine sarcoma virus-transformed cells. *Proc. Natl. Acad. Sci.* **75:** 4001–4005.

Der, C.J., T.G. Krontiris, and G.M. Cooper. 1982. Transforming genes of human bladder and lung carcinoma cell lines are homologous to the *ras* genes of Harvey and Kirsten sarcoma viruses. *Proc. Natl. Acad. Sci.* **79:** 3637–3640.

de Vos, A.M., L. Tong, M.V. Milburn, P.M. Matias, J. Jancarik, S. Noguchi, S. Nishimura, K. Miura, E. Ohtsuka, and S.-H. Kim. 1988. Three-dimensional structure of an oncogene protein: Catalytic domain of human c-Ha-*ras* p21. *Science* **239:** 888–893.

Doolittle, R.F., M.W. Hunkapiller, L.E. Hood, S.G. Deuare, K.G. Robbins, A. Aaronson, and H.N. Antoniades. 1983. Simian sarcoma virus oncogene v-*sis* is derived from the gene encoding a platelet-derived growth factor. *Science* **221:** 275–277.

Downward, J., Y. Yarden, E. Mayes, G. Scrace, N. Totty, P. Stockwell, A. Ullrich, J. Schlessinger, and M. Waterfield. 1984. Close similarity of epidermal growth factor receptor and v-*erb* B oncogene protein sequences. *Nature* **307:** 521–527.

Dyson, N., P.M. Howley, K. Munger, and E. Harlow. 1989. The human papilloma virus-16 E7 oncoprotein is able to bind to the retinoblastoma gene product. *Science* **243:** 934–937.

Eckhart, W., M.A. Hutchinson, and T. Hunter. 1979. An activity phosphorylating tyrosine in polyoma T antigen immunoprecipitates. *Cell* **18:** 925–933.

Elsen, P.V.D., A. Houweling, and A. Van der Eb. 1983. Expression of region E1b of human adenoviruses in the absence of region E1b is not sufficient for complete transformation. *Virology* **128:** 377–390.

Evans, R.M. 1988. The steroid and thyroid hormone receptor superfamily. *Science* **240:** 889–895.

Feramisco, J., B. Ozanne, and C. Stiles, eds. 1985. *Cancer cells: Growth factors and transformation*, volume 3. Cold Spring Harbor Laboratory, Cold Spring Harbor, New York.

Fialkow, P.J. 1972. Use of genetic markers to study cellular origin and development of tumors in human females. *Adv. Cancer Res.* **15:** 191–226.

Finlay, C.A., P.W. Hinds, and A.J. Levine. 1989. The p53 proto-oncogene can act as a suppressor of transformation. *Cell* **57:** 1083–1093.

Foulds, L. 1951. Tumor progession: A review. *Cancer Res.* **14:** 327–345.

Fried, M. 1965. Cell-transforming ability of a temperature-sensitive mutant of polyoma virus. *Proc. Natl. Acad. Sci.* **53:** 486–491.

Friend, S.H., R. Bernards, S. Rogelj, R.A. Weinberg, J.M. Rapoport, D.M. Albert, and T.P. Dryja. 1986. A human DNA segment with properties of the gene that predisposes to retinoblastoma and osteosarcoma. *Nature* **323:** 643–646.

Fung, Y.-K.T, A.M. Fadley, L.B. Crittenden, and H.J. Kung. 1981. On the mechanism of retrovirus-induced avian lymphoid leukosis: Deletion and integration of the proviruses. *Proc. Natl. Acad. Sci.* **78:** 3418–3422.

Fung, Y.-K.T., A.L. Murphee, A. T'Ang, J. Qian, S.H. Hinrichs, and W.F. Benedict. 1987. Structural evidence for the authenticity of the human retinoblastoma gene. *Science* **236:** 1657–1661.

German, J. 1974. Bloom's syndrome: The prototype of human genetic disorders predisposing to chromosomal instability and cancer. In *Chromosomes and cancer* (ed. J. German), pp. 601–617. John Wiley and Sons, New York.

Gibbs, J.B., I.S. Sigal, M. Poe, and E.M. Scolnick. 1984. Intrinsic GTPase activity distinguishes normal and oncogenic *ras* p21 molecules. *Proc. Natl. Acad. Sci.* **81:** 5704–5708.

Gottesman, M.M. and R.D. Fleischmann. 1986. The role of cAMP in regulating tumour cell growth. *Cancer Surv.* **5:** 291–308.

Green, M. R. 1989. When the products of oncogenes and anti-oncogenes meet. *Cell* **56:** 1–3.

Groffen, J., J.R. Stephenson, N. Heisterkamp, A. de Klein, C.R. Bartram, and G. Grosveld. 1984. Philadelphia chromosomal breakpoints are clustered within a limited region, bcr, on chromosome 22. *Cell* **36:** 93–99.

Gross, L. 1970. *Oncogenic viruses*, 3rd edition. Pergamon Press, New York.

Hanafusa, H., C.C. Halpern, D.L. Buchhagen, and S. Kawai. 1977. Recovery of avian sarcoma virus from tumors induced by transformation-defective mutants. *J. Exp. Med.* **146:** 1735–1747.

Hanahan, D. 1988. Dissecting multistep tumorigenesis in transgenic mice. *Annu. Rev. Genet.* **22:** 479–519.

Hanks, S.K., A.M. Quinn, and T. Hunter. 1988. The protein kinase family: Conserved features and deduced phylogeny of the catalytic domains. *Science* **241:** 42–52.

Hansen, M.F. and W.K. Cavenee. 1987. Genetics of cancer predisposition. *Cancer Res.* **47:** 5518–5528.

Hayman, M.J., G. Kitchener, P.K. Vogt, and H. Beug. 1985. The putative transforming protein of S13 avian erythroblastosis virus is a transmembrane glycoprotein with an associated protein kinase activity. *Proc. Natl. Acad. Sci.* **82:** 8237–8241.

Hayward, W.S., B.G. Neel, and S.M. Astrin. 1981. Activation of a cellular *onc* gene by promoter insertion in ALV-induced lymphoid leukosis. *Nature* **290:** 475–480.

Hecht, F. 1988. Appendix D. Oncogene location update. *Cancer Genet. Cytogenet.* **31:** 142–145.

Heidelberger, C. 1975. Chemical carcinogenesis. *Annu. Rev. Biochem.* **44:** 79–121.

Heisterkamp, N., J.R. Stephenson, J. Groffen, P.F. Hansen, A. de Klein, C.R. Bartram, and G. Grosveld. 1983. Localization of the c-*abl* oncogene adjacent to a translocation break point in chronic myelocytic leukaemia. *Nature* **306:** 239–242.

Hiatt, H.H., J.D. Watson, and J.A. Winsten, eds. 1977. *Origins of human cancer, Book A.* Cold Spring Harbor Laboratory, Cold Spring Harbor, New York.

Hill, M. and J. Hillova. 1972. Recovery of the temperature-sensitive mutant of Rous sarcoma virus from chicken cells exposed to DNA extracted from hamster cells transformed by the mutant. *Virology* **49:** 309–313.

Huang, H-J.S., J-K. Yee, J-Y. Shew, P-L. Chen, R. Bookstein, T. Friedmann, E.Y-H. Lee, and W-H. Lee. 1988. Suppression of the neoplastic phenotype by replacement of the RB gene in human cancer cells. *Science* **242:** 1563–1566.

Hunter, T. and J.A. Cooper. 1985. Protein-tyrosine kinases. *Annu. Rev. Biochem.* **54:** 897–930.

Hunter, T. and B.M. Sefton. 1980. Transforming gene product of Rous sarcoma virus phosphorylates tyrosine. *Proc. Natl. Acad. Sci.* **77:** 1311-1315.

Hurley, J., M. Simon, D. Teplow, J. Robishaw, and A. Gilman. 1984. Homologies between signal transducing G proteins and ras gene products. *Science* **226:** 860–862.

Hynes, R.O. 1987. Integrins: A family of cell surface receptors. *Cell* **48:** 549–554.

Kahn, P. and R. Graf. 1987. *Growth factors and oncogenes.* Springer Verlag, New York.

Kaplan, D.R., M. Whitman, B. Schaffhausen, D.C. Pallas, M. White, L. Cantley, and T.M. Roberts. 1987. Common elements in growth factor stimulation and oncogenic transformation: 85 kd phosphoprotein and phosphatidylinositol kinase activity. *Cell* **50:** 1021–1029.

Kitayama, H., Y. Sugimoto, T. Matsuzaki, Y. Ikawa, and M. Noda. 1989. A *ras*-related gene with transformation suppressor activity. *Cell* **56:** 77–84.

Klein, G. 1981. The role of gene dosage and genetic transpositions in carcinogenesis. *Nature* **294:** 313–318.

———. 1983. Specific chromosomal translocations and the genesis of B cell derived tumors in mice and men. *Cell* **32:** 311–315.

———. 1987. The approaching era of the tumor suppressor genes. *Science* **238:** 1539–1545.

Knudson, A.G. 1971. Mutation and cancer: Statistical study of retinoblastoma. *Proc. Natl. Acad. Sci.* **68:** 820–823.

Kohl, N.E., N. Kanda, R.R. Schreck, G. Bruns, S.A. Latt, F. Gilbert, and F.W. Alt. 1983. Transposition and amplification of oncogene-related sequences in human neuroblastomas. *Cell* **35:** 359–367.

Konopka, J.B., S.M. Watanabe, and O.N. Witte. 1984. An alteration of the human c-*abl* protein in K562 leukemia cells unmasks associated tyrosine kinase activity. *Cell* **37:** 1035–1042.

Landschulz, W.H., P.F. Johnson, E.Y. Adashi, B.J. Graves, and S. L. McKnight. 1988. Isolation of a recombinant copy of the gene encoding C/EBP. *Genes Dev.* **2:** 786–800.

Lane, D.P. and L.V. Crawford. 1979. T antigen is bound to a host protein in SV40-transformed cells. *Nature* **278:** 261–263.

Lang, R.A., D. Metcalf, N.M. Gough, A.R. Dunn, and T.J. Gonda. 1985. Expression of a hemopoietic growth factor cDNA in a factor-dependent cell line results in autonomous growth and tumorigenicity. *Cell* **43:** 531–542.

Leder, P., J. Battey, G. Lenoir, C. Moulding, W. Murphy, H. Potter, T. Stewart, and R. Taub. 1984. Translocations among antibody genes in human cancer. *Science* **22:** 765–771.

Lee, W.-H., R. Bookstein, F. Hong, L.-J. Young, J.-Y. Shew, and E.Y.-H.P. Lee. 1987. Human retinoblastoma susceptibility gene: Cloning, identification, and sequence. *Science* **235:** 1394–1399.

Levinson, A.D., H. Oppermann, L. Levintow, H.E. Varmus, and J.M. Bishop. 1978. Evidence that the transforming gene of avian sarcoma virus encodes a protein kinase associated with a phosphoprotein. *Cell* **15:** 561–572.

Lillie, J.W., M. Green, and M.R. Green. 1986. An adenovirus E1a protein region required for transformation and transcriptional repression. *Cell* **46:** 1043–1051.

Maki, T., T.J. Bos, C. Davis, M. Starbuck, and P.K. Vogt. 1987. Avian sarcoma virus 17 carries the *jun* oncogene. *Proc. Natl. Acad. Sci.* **84:** 2848–2852.

Mansour, S.L., K.R. Thomas, and M.R. Capecchi. 1988. Disruption of the proto-oncogene *int*-2 in mouse embryo-derived stem cells: A general strategy for targeting mutations to non-selectable genes. *Nature* **336:** 348–352.

Martin, G.S. 1970. Rous sarcoma virus: A function required for the maintenance of the transformed state. *Nature* **227:** 1021–1023.

Martin, G.S. and P.H. Duesberg. 1972. The a subunit in the RNA of transforming avian tumor viruses. I. Occurrence in different virus strains. II. Spontaneous loss resulting in nontransforming variants. *Virology* **47:** 494–497.

Mayer, B.J., M. Hamaguchi, and H. Hanafusa. 1988. A novel viral oncogene with structural similarity to phospholipase C. *Nature* **332:** 272–275.

McCormick, F. 1989. *ras* GTPase activating protein: Signal transmitter and signal terminator. *Cell* **56:** 5–8.

Miles, B.D., and H.L. Robinson. 1983. High-frequency transduction of c-*erb*B in avian leukosis virus-induced erythroblastosis. *J. Virol.* **54:** 295–303.

Miller, J.A. and E.C. Miller. 1977. Ultimate chemical carcinogens as reactive mutagenic electrophiles. *Cold Spring Harbor Conf. Cell Proliferation* **4:** 605–628.

Mitelman, F. 1985. *Catalogue of chromosomal aberrations in cancer*. Alan R. Liss, New York.

Nau, M.M., B.J. Brooks, J. Battey, E. Sausville, A.F. Gazdar, I.R. Kirsch, O.W. McBride, V. Bertness, G.F. Hollis, and J.D. Minna. 1985. L-*myc*, a new *myc*-related gene amplified and expressed in human small cell lung cancer. *Nature* **318:** 69–73.

Neel, B.G., W.S. Hayward, H.L. Robinson, J. Fang, and S.M. Astrin. 1981. Avian leukosis virus-induced tumors have common proviral integration sites and synthesize discrete new RNAs: Oncogenesis by promoter insertion. *Cell* **23:** 323–334.

Neil, J.C., D. Hughes, R. McFarlene, N.M. Wilkie, D.E. Onions, G. Lees, and O. Jarrett. 1984. Transduction and rearrangement of the *myc* gene by feline leukemia virus in naturally occurring T-cell lymphomas. *Nature* **308:** 814–820.

Nowell, P.C. 1976. The clonal evolution of tumor cell populations. *Science* **194:** 23–28.

Nowell, P.C. and D.A Hungerford. 1960. A minute chromosome in human chronic granulocytic leukemia. *Science* **132:** 1497.

Nusse, R. and A. Berns. 1988. Cellular oncogene activation by insertion of retroviral DNA. Genes identified by provirus tagging. In *Cellular oncogene activation* (ed. G. Klein), pp. 95–119. Marcel Dekker, New York.

Nusse, R. and H.E. Varmus. 1982. Many tumors induced by the mouse mammary tumor virus contain a provirus integrated in the same region of the host genome. *Cell* **31:** 99–109.

Padgett, T.G., E. Stubblefield, and H.E. Varmus. 1977. Chicken macrochromosomes contain an endogenous provirus and microchromosomes contain sequences related to the transforming gene of ASV. *Cell* **10:** 649–657.

Palmiter, R.D. and R.L. Brinster. 1984. Transgenic mice. *Cell* **41:** 343–345.

Parada, L.F., H. Land, R.A. Weinberg, D. Wolf, and V. Rotter. 1984. Cooperation between gene encoding p53 tumour antigen and *ras* in cellular transformation. *Nature* **312:** 649–651.

Parada, L.F., C.J. Tabin, C. Shih, and R.A. Weinberg. 1982. Human EJ bladder carcinoma oncogene is homologue of Harvey sarcoma virus ras gene. *Nature* **297:** 474–478.

Parker, R.C., H.E. Varmus, and J.M. Bishop. 1981. Cellular homologue (c-*src*) of the transforming gene of Rous sarcoma virus-isolation, mapping, and transcriptional analysis of *src* and flanking regions. *Proc. Natl. Acad. Sci.* **78:** 5842–5846.

Payne, G.S., J.M. Bishop, and H.E. Varmus. 1982. Multiple arrangements of virus DNA and an activated host oncogene in bursal lymphomas. *Nature* **295:** 209–214.

Payne, G.S., S.A. Courtneidge, L.B. Crittenden, A.M. Fadly, J.M. Bishop, and H.E. Varmus. 1981. Analysis of avian leukosis virus DNA and RNA in bursal tumors: Viral gene expression is not required for maintenance of the tumor state. *Cell* **23:** 311–322.

Peters, G., S. Brookes, R. Smith, and C. Dickson. 1983. Tumorigenesis by mouse mammary tumor virus: Evidence for a common region for provirus integration in mammary tumors. *Cell* **33:** 369–377.

Peto, R., F.J.C. Roe, P.N. Lee, L. Levy, and J. Clack. 1975. Cancer and aging in mice and men. *Br. J. Cancer* **32:** 411–426.

Ponder, B.A.J. 1980. Genetics and cancer. *Biochim. Biophys. Acta* **605:** 369–410.

Radke, K. and G.S. Martin. 1979. Transformation by Rous sarcoma virus: Effects of *src* gene expression on the synthesis and phosphorylation of cellular polypeptides. *Proc. Natl. Acad. Sci.* **76:** 5212–5216.

Rassoulzadegan, M., A. Cowie, A. Carr, N. Glaichenhous, and R. Kamen. 1982. The roles of individual polyoma virus early proteins in oncogenic transformation. *Nature* **300:** 713–718.

Rauscher, F.J., III, D.R. Cohen, T. Curran, T.J. Bos, P.K. Vogt, D. Bohmann, R. Tijan, and B.R. Franza, Jr. 1988. Fos-associated protein p39 is the product of the *jun* proto-oncogene. *Science* **240:** 1010–1016.

Rohrschneider, L. 1980. Adhesion plaques of Rous sarcoma virus-transformed cells contain the *src* gene product. *Proc. Natl. Acad. Sci.* **77:** 3514–3518.

Rous, P. 1911. Transmission of a malignant new growth by means of a cell-free filtrate. *J. Am. Med. Assoc.* **56:** 198.

Roussel, M., S. Saule, C. Lagrou, C. Rommens, H. Beug, T. Graf, and D. Stehelin. 1979. Three new types of viral oncogene of cellular origin specific for haematopoietic cell transformation. *Nature* **281:** 452–455.

Sambrook, J., H. Westphal, P.R. Srinivasan, and R. Dulbecco. 1968. The integrated state of viral DNA in SV40-transformed cells. *Proc. Natl. Acad. Sci.* **60:** 1288–1295.

Santos, E., S.R. Tronick, S.A. Aaronson, S. Pulciani, and M. Barbacid. 1982. T24 human bladder carcinoma oncogene is an activated form of the normal human homologue of BALAB- and Harvey-MSV transforming genes. *Nature* **298:** 343–347.

Sap, J., A. Munoz, K. Damm, Y. Goldberg, J. Ghysdael, A. Leutz, H. Beug, and B. Vennstrom. 1986. The c-*erb*A protein is a high-affinity receptor for thyroid hormone. *Nature* **324:** 635–640.

Sarnow, P., Y.S. Ho, J. Williams, and A.J. Levine. 1982. Adenovirus E1b-58 kd tumor antigen and SV40 large tumor antigen are physically associated with the same 54 kd cellular protein in transformed cells. *Cell* **28:** 387–394.

Schimke, R.T. 1984. Gene amplification in cultured animal cells. *Cell* **37:** 705–713.

Schwab, M., K. Alitalo, K.-H. Klempnauer, H.E. Varmus, J.M. Bishop, F. Gilbert, G. Brodeur, M. Goldstein, and J. Trent. 1983. Amplified DNA with limited homology to *myc* cellular oncogene is shared by human neuroblastoma cell lines and a neuroblastoma tumour. *Nature* **305:** 245–247.

Sefton, B.M. and T. Hunter. 1986. From c-*src* to v-*src*, or the case of the missing C terminus. *Cancer Surv.* **5:** 159–172.

Shalloway, D., A.D. Zelenetz, and G.M. Cooper. 1981. Molecular cloning and characterization of the chicken gene homologous to the transforming gene of Rous sarcoma virus. *Cell* **24:** 531–542.

Sheiness, D. and J.M. Bishop. 1979. DNA and RNA from uninfected vertebrate cells contain nucleotide sequences related to the putative transforming gene of avian myelocytomatosis virus. *J. Virol.* **31:** 514–521.

Sheiness, D.K., S.H. Hughes, H.E. Varmus, E. Stubblefield, and J.M. Bishop. 1980. The vertebrate homolog of the putative transforming gene of avian myelocytomatosis virus: Characteristics of the DNA locus and its RNA transcript. *Virology* **105:** 415–424.

Shen-Ong, G.L., E.J. Keath, S.P. Piccoli, and M.D. Cole. 1982. Novel *myc* oncogene RNA from abortive immunoglobulin-gene recombination in mouse plasmacytomas. *Cell* **31:** 443–452.

Sherr, C.J., C.W. Rettenmier, R. Sacca, M.F. Roussel, A.T. Look, and E.R. Stanley. 1985. The c-*fms* proto-oncogene product is related to the receptor for the mononuclear phagocyte growth factor, CSF-1. *Cell* **41:** 665–676.

Shih, C., B.-Z. Shilo, M.P. Goldfarb, A. Dannenberg, and R.A. Weinberg. 1979. Passage of phenotypes of chemically transformed cells via transfection of DNA and chromatin. *Proc. Natl. Acad. Sci.* **76:** 5714–5718.

Shih, T.Y., A.G. Papageorge, P.E. Stokes, M.O. Weeks, and E.M. Scolnick. 1980. Guanine nucleotide-binding and autophosphorylating activities associated with the p21^{src} protein of Harvey murine sarcoma virus. *Nature* **287:** 686–691.

Shilo, B.-Z. 1987. Proto-oncogenes in *Drosophila melanogaster*. *Trends Genet.* **3:** 69–72.

Shilo, B.-Z. and R.A. Weinberg. 1981. DNA sequences homologous to vertebrate oncogenes are conserved in *Drosophila melanogaster*. *Proc. Natl. Acad. Sci.* **78:** 6789–6792.

Shimizu, K., M. Goldfarb, Y. Suard, M. Perucho, Y. Li, T. Kamata, J. Feramisco, E. Stavnezer, J. Fogh, and M.H. Wigler. 1983. Three human transforming genes are related to the viral *ras* oncogenes. *Proc. Natl. Acad. Sci.* **80:** 2112–2116.

Simon, M.A., T.B. Kornberg, and J.M. Bishop. 1983. Three loci related to the *src* oncogene and tyrosine-specific protein kinase activity in *Drosophila*. *Nature* **302:** 837–839.

Skolnick, M., D.T. Bishop, D. Carmelli, E. Gardner, R. Hadley, S. Hasstedt, J.R. Hill, S. Hunt, J.L. Lyon, and C.R. Smart. 1981. A population-based assessment of familial cancer risk in Utah Mormon genealogies. In *Genes, chromosomes, and neoplasia* (ed. F.E. Arrighi et al.), pp. 477–500. Raven Press, New York.

Smith, A.E., R. Smith, B.E. Griffin, and M. Fried. 1979. Protein kinase activity associated with polyoma virus middle T antigen *in vitro*. *Cell* **18:** 915–924.

Spector, D.H., H.E. Varmus, and J.M. Bishop. 1978a. Nucleotide sequences related to the transforming gene of avian sarcoma virus are present in the DNA of uninfected vertebrates. *Proc. Natl. Acad. Sci.* **75:** 4102–4106.

Spector, D.H., K. Smith, T. Padgett, P. McCombe, D. Roulland-Dussoix, C. Moscovici, H.E. Varmus, and J.M. Bishop. 1978b. Uninfected avian cells contain RNA related to the transforming gene of avian sarcoma viruses. *Cell* **13:** 371–379.

Sporn, M.B. and A. B. Roberts. 1985. Autocrine growth factors and cancer. *Nature* **313:** 745–747.

Stanbridge, E.J., C.J. Der, C.J. Doersen, R.Y. Nishimi, D.M. Peehl, B.E. Weissman, and J. Wilkinson. 1982. Human cell hybrids: Analysis of transformation and tumorigenicity. *Science* **215:** 252–259.

Stehelin, D., R.V. Guntaka, H.E. Varmus, and J.M. Bishop. 1976a. Purification of DNA complementary to nucleotide sequences required for neoplastic transformation of fibroblasts by avian sarcoma viruses. *J. Mol. Biol.* **101:** 349–365.

Stehelin, D., H.E. Varmus, J.M. Bishop, and P.K. Vogt. 1976b. DNA related to the transforming gene(s) of avian sarcoma viruses is present in normal avian DNA. *Nature* **260:** 170–173.

Struhl, K. 1987. The DNA-binding domains of the *jun* oncoprotein and the yeast GCN4 transcriptional activator protein are functionally homologous. *Cell* **50:** 841–846.

Swanstrom, R., R.C. Parker, H.E. Varmus, and J.M. Bishop. 1983. Transduction of a cellular oncogene—The genesis of Rous sarcoma virus. *Proc. Natl. Acad. Sci.* **80:** 2519–2523.

Sweet, R.W., S. Yokiyama, T. Kamata, J.R. Feramisco, M. Rosenberg, and M. Gross. 1984. The product of *ras* is a GTPase and the T24 oncogenic mutant is deficient in this activity. *Nature* **311:** 273–275.

Tabin, C.J., S.M. Bradley, C.I. Bargmann, R.A. Weinberg, A.G. Papageorge, E.M. Scolnick, R. Dhar, D.R. Lowy, and E.H. Chang. 1982. Mechanism of activation of a human oncogene. *Nature* **300:** 143–149.

Takeya, T. and H. Hanafusa. 1983. Structure and sequence of the cellular gene homologous to the RSV *src* gene and the mechanism for generating the transforming virus. *Cell* **32:** 881–890.

Taub, R., K. Kelly, J. Battey, S. Latt, G.M. Lenoir, U. Tantravahi, Z. Tu, and P. Leder. 1984. A novel alteration in the structure of an activated c-*myc* gene in a variant t(2;8) Burkitt lymphoma. *Cell* **37:** 511–520.

Taub, R., I. Kirsch, C. Morton, G. Lenoir, D. Swan, S. Tronick, S. Aaronson, and P. Leder. 1982. Translocation of the c-*myc* gene into the immunoglobulin heavy chain locus in human Burkitt lymphoma and murine plasmacytoma cells. *Proc. Natl. Acad. Sci.* **79:** 7837–7841.

Teich, N., J. Wyke, and P. Kaplan. 1985. Pathogenesis of retrovirus-induced disease. In *Molecular biology of tumor viruses*, 2nd edition: *RNA tumor viruses 2/Supplement and appendixes*. (ed. R. Weiss et al.), pp. 187–248. Cold Spring Harbor Laboratory, Cold Spring Harbor, New York.

Teich, N., J. Wyke, T. Mak, A. Bernstein, and W. Hardy. 1982. Pathogenesis of retrovirus-induced disease. In *Molecular biology of tumor viruses*, 2nd edition: *RNA tumor viruses* (ed. R. Weiss et al.), pp. 785–998. Cold Spring Harbor Laboratory, Cold Spring Harbor, New York.

Tegtmeyer, P. and H. Ozer. 1971. Temperature sensitive mutants of simian virus 40. Infection of permissive cells. *J. Virol.* **8:** 516–524.

Todaro, G.J. and R.J. Huebner. 1972. The viral oncogene hypothesis: New evidence. *Proc. Natl. Acad. Sci.* **69:** 1009–1015.

Tooze, J., ed. 1980. *Molecular biology of tumor viruses*, 2nd edition. *DNA tumor viruses*, part 2, pp. 61-338. Cold Spring Harbor Laboratory, Cold Spring Harbor, New York.

Trahey, M. and F. McCormick. 1987. A cytoplasmic protein regulates GTPase of normal N-*ras* p21, but does not affect oncogenic mutants. *Science* **238:** 542–545.

Varmus, H.E. 1982. Form and function of retroviral proviruses. *Science* **216:** 812–820.

———. 1983. Retroviruses. In *Transposable mobile genetic elements* (ed. J. Shapiro), pp. 411–503. Academic Press, New York.

———. 1984. The molecular genetics of cellular oncogenes. *Annu. Rev. Genet.* **18:** 553.

———. 1987. Cellular and viral oncogenes. In *Molecular basis of blood diseases* (ed. G. Stamatoyannopoulos et al.), pp. 271–346. W.B. Saunders, Philadelphia.

———. 1988. Retroviruses. *Science* **240:** 1427–1435.

Varmus, H.E. and J.M. Bishop. 1986. Introduction. *Cancer Surv.* **5:** 153–158.

Varmus, H.E. and P.O. Brown. 1989. Retroviruses. In *Mobile DNA* (ed. M. Howe and D. Berg), pp. 53–108. American Society for Microbiology Publications, Washington, D.C.

Vogt, P.K. 1971. Spontaneous segregation of nontransforming viruses from cloned sarcoma viruses. *Virology* **46:** 939–946.

Vogt, P.K., T.J. Bos, and R.F. Doolittle. 1987. Homology between the DNA-binding domain of the GCN4 regulatory protein of yeast and the carboxyl-terminal region of a protein coded for by the oncogene *jun*. *Proc. Natl. Acad. Sci.* **84:** 3316–3319.

Wang, H.-C.R. and J.T. Parsons. 1989. Deletions and insertions within an amino terminal domain of pp60$^{v\text{-}src}$ inactivate transformation and modulate membrane stability. *J. Virol.* **63:** 291–302.

Wang, L.-H., P. Duesberg, K. Beemon, and P.K. Vogt. 1975. Mapping RNase T_1-resistant oligonucleotides of avian tumor viruses RNAs: Sarcoma-specific oligonucleotides are near the poly(A) end and oligonucleotides common to sarcoma and transformation-defective viruses are at the poly(A) end. *J. Virol.* **16:** 1051–1070.

Waterfield, M.D., T. Scrace, N. Whittle, P. Stroobant, A. Johnsson, A. Wasteson, B. Westermark, C.-H. Heldin, J. Huang, and T. Deuel. 1983. Platelet-derived growth factor is structurally related to the putative transforming protein p28^{sis} of simian sarcoma virus. *Nature* **304:** 35–39.

Weiss, R., N. Teich, H. Varmus, and J. Coffin, eds. 1982 and 1985. *Molecular biology of tumor viruses*, 2nd edition. *RNA tumor viruses.* Cold Spring Harbor Laboratory, Cold Spring Harbor, New York.

Westaway, D., G. Payne, and H.E. Varmus. 1984. Deletion and base substitutions in provirally mutated c-*myc* alleles may contribute to the progression of B cell tumors. *Proc. Natl. Acad. Sci.* **81:** 843–847.

Whyte, P., K.J. Buchkovich, J.M. Horowitz, S.H. Friend, M. Raybuck, R.A. Weinberg, and E. Harlow. 1988. Association between an oncogene and an antioncogene: The adenovirus E1A proteins bind to the retinoblastoma gene product. *Nature* **334:** 124–129.

Willingham, M.C., C. Jay, and I. Pastan. 1979. Localization of the ASV *src* gene product to the plasma membrane of transformed cells by electron microscopic immunocytochemistry. *Cell* **18:** 125–134.

Willis, A.E. and T. Lindahl. 1987. DNA ligase I deficiency in Bloom's syndrome. *Nature* **325:** 355–357.

Witte, O.N., A. Dusgupta, and D. Baltimore. 1980. Abelson murine leukaemia virus protein is phosphorylated *in vitro* to form phosphotyrosine. *Nature* **283:** 826–831.

Wolman, S.R. and A.A. Horland. 1975. Genetics of tumor cells. In *Cancer: Biology of tumors* (ed. F.F. Becker) vol. 3, pp. 155–198. Plenum Press, New York.

2

Growth Factors and Oncogenes

Robert A. Weinberg
Department of Biology
Massachusetts Institute of Technology
and Whitehead Institute for Biomedical Research
Cambridge, Massachusetts 02142

I. INTRODUCTION

Cells within a normal tissue undertake programs of growth and differentiation on the basis of signals received from other cells in the tissue or organism. This network of intercellular signaling represents the basis for establishing and maintaining normal tissue architecture. Many of the signals passing between cells appear to be carried by growth factors (GFs), which can influence cell growth in a positive or negative way. Growth factors are released in carefully measured amounts by some cells and are conveyed via several mechanisms to target cells. They are bound to specific receptors displayed by these target cells. This binding in turn triggers a complex signal transduction cascade that ultimately affects the cell's decision to grow or to remain quiescent. Included in this cascade is the transduction of signals across the plasma membrane, the alteration of cytoplasmic proteins and low-molecular-weight "second-messenger" molecules, and finally, the transmission of signals to the nucleus where they affect the expression of critical genes involved in growth-controlling decisions.

The process of tumorigenesis represents a disruption of this complex signaling network. As a result, a cell may lose dependence on exogenous mitogenic growth factors and develop an autonomous mode of growth

Oncogenes and the Molecular Origins of Cancer.

control. Some oncogenes intervene in this process by enabling a cell to grow even in the absence of the mitogenic growth factors that are usually required to trigger growth. Yet others may enable a cell to proliferate despite the presence of negative environmental signals that would normally act to inhibit cell growth. As described in this chapter, a number of discoveries over the past decade have provided many examples of the ways in which oncogenes directly affect a cell's dependence on or responsiveness to growth factors.

II. DISCOVERY AND CHARACTERIZATION OF GROWTH FACTORS

Growth factors were first encountered experimentally as components of complex biological mixtures having growth-stimulatory activity. Historically, the first of these to be described was nerve growth factor (NGF), which was detected as a factor that was released by mouse sarcoma cells and that stimulated growth of chick embryo nerve cells (Levi-Montalcini and Hamburger 1951). Perhaps the most widely studied of the GFs, epidermal growth factor (EGF), was discovered through its ability to stimulate premature eyelid opening and incisor eruption in newborn mice (Cohen 1962). Other work showed that brain homogenates contain activities stimulating growth of fibroblasts in culture. A similarly behaving factor was subsequently demonstrated in pituitary extracts. This factor was named fibroblast growth factor (FGF) after its target cells. Later, it was demonstrated that there are really two FGFs, one having an acidic (aFGF) and the other a basic (bFGF) isoelectric point (for review, see Thomas and Gimenez-Gallego 1987).

Parallel lines of work in a number of laboratories have uncovered a series of ostensibly distinct GFs, often named after the tissue or cell of origin. Only recently has it been shown that many of these share chemical properties and a common structure with one or another of the well-characterized FGFs. For example, endothelial cell GF, eye-derived GFII, brain-derived GF, and astroglial GF1 are all related and possibly identical with aFGF; chondrosarcoma-, cartilage-, and hepatoma-derived GFs share many properties with bFGF (Thomas and Gimenez-Gallego 1987). This shows that the biological assays used to detect GFs may reveal a number of factors whose true identity only emerges upon biochemical analysis. Thus, the number of distinct, novel GFs is often found to be far less than biological assays of factor activity would indicate.

The transforming growth factors (TGFs) have their own distinct history. They were originally discovered in the culture medium in which murine sarcoma virus-transformed cells had been grown (De Larco and Todaro 1978). Such *conditioned* medium was seen to confer morphological transformation and anchorage independence on certain target cells, notably rat kidney (NRK) cells. This established the principle that tumor cells may often release potent GFs into their environment. As discussed below, the role of the released GFs in maintaining the transformed state of these cells is complex and not completely understood.

The initially encountered transforming growth factor was at first thought to represent a single biochemical entity, but biochemical fractionation subsequently revealed that its activities derived from two distinct polypeptide species that act synergistically to induce transformation phenotypes in certain cells. The two components, termed TGF-α and TGF-β, were subsequently found to be totally unrelated to one another in structure (Roberts et al. 1981; Anzano et al. 1983). Once released, each TGF adsorbs to the surface of a cell via a distinct receptor and acts on the cell through a distinct signaling pathway. The synthesis and release of these two GFs and perhaps others are coordinately activated by certain oncogenes, including *ras*, *mos*, *src*, and SV40 large T.

TGF-α was found to compete with EGF for binding to cells. The binding of both occurs specifically to the EGF receptors that are displayed on the surface of many types of cells. Such competition for binding to a common receptor suggested possible structural homology between TGF-α and EGF. This suspicion was confirmed by isolation and analysis of TGF-α, which showed that it indeed shares distant evolutionary relatedness with EGF and has a virtually equal affinity for binding to EGF receptors (Marquardt et al. 1983). There are apparently no other cell-surface receptors that specifically bind TGF-α. This raises the issue of why vertebrates have evolved two similarly acting and thus redundant GFs. An answer may ultimately derive from the observation that the synthesis of the two is regulated in quite different ways. For example, EGF can be found in mouse submaxillary glands; its production there can affect development of mammary tumors, suggesting an endocrine secretion designed to elicit responses at distant sites in the organism (Kurachi et al. 1985). In contrast, TGF-α seems to be released by single cells and may act in a *paracrine* manner to affect behavior of closely apposed neighbors or cell layers.

TGF-β also seems to act over short distances, but beyond this fact shares little in common with TGF-α. The initially described TGF-β binds to three distinct cell-surface proteins displayed by many cell types (Cheifetz et al. 1986). These TGF-β-binding proteins have been identified through their ability to bind radiolabeled TGF-β. Such high-affinity binding is consistent with the role of these proteins as receptors for transducing TGF-β-induced signals into the cell, but this remains unproven. These putative receptors have no similarity to the EGF receptor. Although none has been isolated, it appears that these receptors, unlike the EGF receptor, do not employ tyrosine kinases to inform the cell of encounter with ligand. Accordingly, the biochemical basis of TGF-β receptor-mediated signal transduction remains obscure.

TGF-β has recently been shown to be represented by at least three distinct molecular species in mammals, and these may have differential affinities for binding to the three putative receptors. Once again, the physiological rationale for multiple similar GFs is unclear. These TGF-βs are related in turn to a variety of other factors including inhibin, a protein that inhibits the secretion of pituitary follicle-stimulating hormone, and müllerian inhibiting substance, which causes regression of the rudiments of the female reproductive tract during male development. An equally distant TGF-β homolog is found in the frog oocyte and early embryo, being involved there in mesoderm induction. Yet another related protein is the product of the decapentaplegic gene of *Drosophila* (for review, see Massague 1987).

In mammals, the effects of the TGF-β are varied and complex. TGF-β is found in blood platelets and thus is apparently involved in wound healing. It stimulates anchorage-independent growth in rat NRK cells and is mitogenic for mouse AKR-2B cells. In contrast, as described later, TGF-β can also act as a potent growth-inhibitory compound for a wide variety of cell types. These effects indicate its complex role in regulating a variety of physiological processes.

The many seemingly paradoxical effects of TGF-β underscore the point that GFs do not act simply as agents conveying proliferative signals to cells. This is emphasized further by study of another class of GFs that regulate stem cell populations involved in hematopoiesis (Metcalf 1985). These GFs are often termed "colony-stimulating factors" (CSFs), reflecting the fact that some of their targets are hematopoietic stem cells that were initially studied through their ability to spawn discrete colonies in semisolid culture media. Hematopoietic stem cells participate in a number of distinct programmed changes in response to encounters with CSFs. They may be stimulated to proliferate, and resulting daughter cells may retain the phenotype of the parent or become committed to one or another pathway of endstage differentiation. In the absence of an appropriate CSF, stem cells may withdraw from the mitotic cycle and die within hours.

To cite an example, at least four distinct CSFs regulate stem cells of the myeloid lineage. M-CSF stimulates growth of murine macrophage colonies; G-CSF stimulates granulocyte progenitor cells; GM-CSF induces proliferation of the common, bipotential precursor to granulocytes and macrophages; and multi-CSF acts on a progenitor cell type located earlier in this lineage. This earlier, more primitive cell type can serve as a precursor to erythroid cells, megakaryocytes, and eosinophils as well as the granulocyte-macrophage stem cells described above. The regulation of the sizes of these various stem cell pools in response to physiological changes such as infection, wounding, low oxygen tension, or blood loss is mediated through the controlled release and targeted action of these and other CSFs.

The genes encoding these and other peptide growth factors have since been isolated by molecular cloning. Without exception, expression of the cloned genes results in production of factors having all the properties associated earlier with factors purified from biological fluids. This shows

Table 1 Some frequently studied growth factors

Acronym(s)	Name	Sources	Typical targets
EGF	epidermal GF	embryos submaxillary gland	epithelia
TGF-α	tumor GF-α	embryos oncogene-transformed cells	epithelia
PDGF-A, -B	platelet-derived GF	platelets, tumor cells	mesenchymal cells
aFGF	acidic fibroblast GF	brain, pituitary	mesenchymal cells
bFGF	basic fibroblast GF	brain, pituitary	mesenchymal cells
TGF-β 1, 2, 3	tumor GF-β	oncogene-transformed cells	wide spectrum
GM-CSF (CSF-2) (CSF-α)	granulocyte-macrophage colony-stimulating factor	T lymphocytes fibroblasts	mixed granulocyte-macrophage colonies
M-CSF (CSF-1)	macrophage colony-stimulating factor	fibroblasts	macrophages
G-CSF (CSFβ)	granulocyte colony-stimulating factor	monocytes	granulocytes
Multi-CSF (IL-3)	multipotential GF	T lymphocytes	multipotential progenitors
IGF-I, -II	insulin-like GF	extra-embryonic membranes, fetal serum	mesenchymal, epithelial cells
NGF	nerve growth factor	submaxillary gland	neuronal cells
TCGF (IL-2)	T-cell GF	T lymphocytes	B, T lymphocytes
IL-1	interleukin-1	leukemia cells	B, T lymphocytes, neutrophils
EPO	erythropoietin	kidney cells	erythroid precursors

that the pure factors indeed possess all the powers ascribed to them following their enrichment from complex biological mixtures (Table 1).

III. METABOLISM OF GROWTH FACTORS

The bulk of recent advances in understanding growth factor physiology has derived from observation of their effects on cultured cells. The study of corresponding effects on tissues or organisms has lagged, leaving unclear the role of many of these factors in normal organismic physiology. Thus, FGF, EGF, and platelet-derived growth factor (PDGF) have been intensively studied in tissue culture systems, but their functions in regulating normal tissue development and maintenance are still matters of speculation.

Most growth factors are normally present in intercellular fluids in very low concentrations and are deposited there only in response to specific stimuli. PDGF, normally sequestered in blood platelets, is released when these cells participate in clot formation, ostensibly to provoke tissue healing. It may also be released by an array of other cells, including macrophages, endothelial cells, and vascular smooth muscle cells in response to specific stimuli. bFGF is found in substantial amounts only within cells and may be released only upon cell damage. Yet other factors like erythropoietin may be released in tightly controlled amounts that regulate the levels of erythroid stem cells in the bone marrow and spleen. In general, however, the mechanisms governing GF production and release are poorly understood.

The pathways taken by GFs between cells are also poorly understood. Most GFs appear to act over very short intercellular distances, being present in nanomolar or lower concentrations for very short periods of time. Some, like the FGFs, may be deposited in and later released from the extracellular matrix. Others, like TGF-β, may be sequestered by complexing with other secreted proteins. These facts greatly complicate attempts to understand the metabolism of GFs once they are released into the extracellular space.

Understanding of GF function is further impeded by the fact that many factors induce disparate responses in different tissue contexts. Thus, EGF can induce proliferation of a number of epithelia including the skin, in which it induces both cellular proliferation and differentiation. It induces proliferation of dental epithelium but inhibits dental mesenchyme; in the stomach, EGF acts as a potent inhibitor of gastric secretion (for review, see Pimentel 1987). This variety of biological responses of target cells greatly complicates attempts at formulating simple schemes of GF action.

Much is known about the biochemistry of the interactions between GFs and their target cells. Once adsorbed to these cells, GF molecules might in principle affect these cells by a process involving internalization and subsequent direct interaction with intracellular substrates, but such a mechanism has never been documented. Instead, it seems that the critical confrontation between GF molecules and target cells occurs at the cell surface in the form of encounters with GF receptors that recognize and bind GF molecules with high specificity. Following the binding of a GF to the extracellular domain of its cognate receptor, the latter transduces signals across the plasma membrane and into the cell cytoplasm, thus informing the cell of an encounter with its GF ligand. The structure and function of GF receptors is described in the next chapter.

Because the intercellular signaling described here depends on both GFs and receptors, it is clear that these signals can be modulated at a number of critical regulatory steps: the decisions by one cell to synthesize, process, and release active GFs; the processes that convey these GFs through intercellular spaces; the synthesis and display of cognate receptors by the target cell; and the fine-tuned molecular mechanisms that modulate both GF-binding affinity to receptors and signal transmission by the receptor across the plasma membrane and through the cytoplasm of the target cell (Ross et al. 1986). Not unexpectedly, the ability of a GF to elicit effects from a cell is dependent absolutely on a display of appropriate receptors. For example, EGF, which normally has no effect on hematopoietic cells, becomes mitogenic following insertion of an EGF receptor gene into such cells (Pierce et al. 1988). This underscores the critical role of appropriate tissue-specific regulation of both GF release and receptor display in orchestrating intercellular signal networks.

IV. CELLULAR RESPONSES TO GROWTH FACTORS

As mentioned above, the biological literature describes the effects of GFs on a diversity of cell types. Rather than enumerate these, this section will focus exclusively on one well-studied model—the responses to GFs of cultured rodent fibroblasts grown in monolayer culture. The mitogenic factors present in the culture media generally used to grow these cells derive from admixed bovine serum; many of these serum factors originate from platelets that release GFs during the conversion of blood plasma to serum. Like the growth of most cultured cells, the proliferation of these fibroblasts ceases when the cells encounter insufficient mitogenic GFs in their growth medium. Such a quiescent state often occurs when these cells deplete essential factors from the medium, and it can be reversed by addition of fresh medium.

Culture medium containing serum represents a poorly defined and complex mixture of stimulatory and inhibitory growth factors. To resolve the serum components that are essential for in vitro growth, *defined media* have been created that are reconstituted by the addition of precise quantities of chemically well-defined constituents. For example, in addition to the salts and nutritive components of medium, rodent fibroblasts require at least three polypeptide mitogenic factors to grow in vitro: PDGF, EGF, and insulin (or insulin-like growth factor [IGF-I]). The response of quiescent serum-deprived fibroblasts to these factors includes the activation of a number of genes, entrance into the cell cycle, and, ultimately, DNA synthesis and cell division.

This requirement for a multiplicity of growth factors teaches several important lessons. It illustrates the fact that most cells do not undertake to grow on the basis of commands generated by an endogenous, spontaneously activated decision-making apparatus; instead, the commitment to grow is made in response to an array of extracellular signals, often, if not always, provided by the presence of GFs. Second, the signals required to grow are usually complex, involving several distinct GFs. Accordingly, the surfeit of one or another GF is usually insufficient to provoke the growth of a normal cell. Finally, because multiple, distinct GFs are required, it appears that their respective receptors release several qualitatively distinct types of biochemical signals within the cell. This suggests in turn that several distinct intracellular signaling pathways converge on the ultimate decision to grow or to remain quiescent.

The biological and biochemical effects of individual GFs are most readily studied when these factors are added to cells that have been deprived of them for a period of time. When rodent fibroblasts deplete GFs from their media or are starved of GFs by exposure to medium containing very low concentrations of serum, they enter a quiescent state termed G_0. Emergence from G_0, induced by addition of fresh serum or purified GFs, is accompanied by biochemical responses within seconds to minutes. Longer-term biological effects follow. The stimulated cells will enter the G_1 period of the cell cycle, a period in which the cells prepare for the DNA synthesis of the S period. The G_2 period follows and anticipates mitosis. Once cells have passed through mitosis, they must once again choose between the alternatives of quiescence or continued growth. In the continued presence of GFs, cells will go through a new round of the cell cycle. In their absence, cells will exit from the cell cycle into G_0, awaiting once again the GFs that will trigger reentry into a state of growth and division.

The multiple GFs involved in stimulating growth of these cells are required in a temporally well-defined order (Pledger et al. 1977). For example, the initial emergence of BALB/c-3T3 A31 cells from quiescence (G_0) is induced by *competence factors* such as PDGF or FGF. They are termed such because cells exposed to them subsequently develop a responsiveness (i.e., competence to respond) to a second set of GFs termed *progression factors*. Once cells have reached a state of competence, they no longer require the continued presence of competence factors like PDGF for maintenance of this state.

In the next step, sometimes termed progression, a combination of EGF and low concentrations of IGF-I is required to carry the competent 3T3 cells through as much as half of the 12-hour transition period between G_0 and the onset of S. Thereafter, these cells no longer require EGF but continue to depend on the IGF-I for continued progression to the S phase. This particular schedule and combination of required GFs may well represent an idiosyncracy of BALB/c-3T3 cells. Nonetheless, this scheme would appear to reflect in its outlines the growth regulation of many other cell types, each of which requires a particular constellation of GFs presented in a well-defined amount and order for its proliferation.

The biochemical bases of these complex series of steps from G_0 to S are poorly understood. The most intensively studied of these is the initial step provoked by PDGF. Within several minutes of exposure to this or similarly acting GFs, a hitherto quiescent cell will turn on expression of a bank of genes that may be larger than 100. These *immediate early* genes are transcribed without the need for concomitant protein synthesis and include actin, *fos*, JE, *jun*, and several dozen others that have been cloned but not yet characterized. The level of induction may correspond with 20–50-fold increases in expression and may peak within 15 minutes, after which some decline very rapidly (Cochran et al. 1983; Lau and Nathans 1985, 1987; Almendral et al. 1988). Other genes are subsequently induced with much slower kinetics: *myc* expression peaks only after several hours and then declines only slowly (see Chapter 7).

The mobilization of genes like actin can be viewed as necessary for the synthesis of the cellular building blocks needed to reconstitute and expand the cell in anticipation of DNA replication and cell division. But many of the other GF-responsive genes play a much more central role in cell growth: They are themselves pleiotropic regulators of growth. We know this because aberrant, deregulated forms of these inducible genes can function as oncogenes. *fos*, *jun*, and *myc* are examples; their encoded proteins function as regulators of expression of other genes. Yet other immediate early GF-induced genes appear to encode proteins that can also function as GFs (Anisowicz et al. 1987; Coffey et al. 1987; Paulson et al. 1987; Richmond et al. 1988; Rollins et al. 1988). By turning on genes specifying both transcription regulators and other growth factors, GFs like PDGF are able to activate ultimately a very large and diverse bank of responder genes. The expression of many of these genes would appear to be essential for the progression of the GF-stimulated cell into the cell cycle. This has been demonstrated directly only for the *fos* gene: Inhibition of *fos* expression with antisense RNA or antibodies blocks emergence from quiescence (Nishikura and Murray 1987; Riabowol et al. 1988).

V. CELLULAR TRANSFORMATION AND GROWTH FACTOR AUTONOMY

As described above, the growth of a cell is usually dependent on stimulation by several distinct growth factors. This dependence would appear to represent an essential element of the intercellular signaling network that ensures maintenance of appropriate cell numbers and types within a tissue and the associated maintenance of normal tissue architecture. By this logic, the ability of a cell to escape partially or completely from this dependence and to grow in an autonomous fashion underlies the process of tumorigenesis. Indeed, a number of experiments show that tumor cells lack dependence on one or more of the GFs whose presence is required by their normal counterparts for growth (Holley 1975).

As described in the sections that follow, such GF autonomy can be achieved through at least three distinct molecular mechanisms involving endogenous production of GFs by the tumor cell, alteration of the receptors responsible for recognizing GFs, and alteration of the signaling pathways normally activated by GF receptors. A separate strategy for deregulating growth is suggested by the existence of growth factors that have, perhaps paradoxically, an antimitogenic or growth-inhibitory effect on cells. Alterations displayed by certain tumor cells cause them to lose responsiveness to such antimitogenic factors and in this way to escape constraints normally imposed on their growth.

A. Growth Factor Autonomy: The Indirect Autocrine Pathway

The most direct route to GF autonomy comes from a mechanism in which the tumor cell synthesizes its own growth factors. As a consequence of this endogenous synthesis, the importation of growth factors from elsewhere is rendered unnecessary, and the tumor cell is able to stimulate its own growth. The involvement of this autostimulatory or autocrine-growth mechanism in neoplasia was first postulated by Sporn and Todaro (1980). Upon examination of the culture medium in which certain tumor cell lines had been growing, they found a growth-stimulatory activity that was not readily detectable in medium conditioned by nontransformed cells. This activity was also observed in medium conditioned by oncogene-transformed cells. They suggested that one mechanism of malignant transformation and oncogene action was the release by the transformed cell of specific growth factors, indeed, the TGFs described earlier. These TGFs could then stimulate the growth of the same cells that had just released them.

With such evidence in hand, the action of these oncogenes could be explained through their ability to encode secreted growth factors that in turn elicit a variety of transformation-specific phenotypes from the cell. However, detailed characterization of oncogenes like Ha-*ras* and *mos*, both of which induce TGF release, made it clear that these particular oncogenes encode the structures of nonsecreted, cytoplasmic proteins that are quite distinct from the TGFs. Accordingly, it appeared that the oncogene-induced secretion of these TGFs represents an indirect mechanism in which oncogene proteins are able to activate the expression of cellular growth factor genes, which in turn specify the secreted mitogenic TGFs.

This theme has been seen many times since these initial observations.

Certain oncogenes acting in a variety of cell types have been found to induce release of GFs, many of which are unrelated to the initially discovered TGFs. Of interest is the fact that these oncogenes encode cytoplasmic proteins. This suggests that these cytoplasmic oncogene proteins may act on a common regulatory pathway that triggers the expression of a number of genes, among them GF genes. One recent report showed that the Ha-*ras* and *mos* oncogenes can each trigger expression of at least four different GF genes: TGF-α, TGF-β, PDGF-A, and NGF (Jakowlew et al. 1988).

How can the oncogene-induced release of GFs be rationalized in terms of the physiology of the normal cell? One clue is provided by the observations that cells often respond to treatment by one GF by activating the expression of several GF genes (Anisowicz et al. 1987; Coffey et al. 1987; Paulson et al. 1987; Richmond et al. 1988; Rollins et al. 1988). For example, an encounter by a cell with TGF-β can result in the induction of its PDGF-B gene in one cell type; in another, the PDGF gene is inducible by a variety of GFs including EGF, TGF-α, bFGF, and even PDGF itself (Leof et al. 1986; Silver et al. 1989). Moreover, an encounter by the cell with TGF-α can result in activation of its own TGF-α genes (Coffey et al. 1987). Since cytoplasmic oncoproteins appear to represent deregulated versions of the signal transducers involved in the normal mitogenic pathway of the cell, it follows that they may mimic many elements of the mitogenic response, including the induction of certain GF genes. Of course, in the case of these oncoproteins, the induction of GF gene expression is constitutive and intense, differing markedly from the transient, highly regulated induction seen as part of the normal responses to mitogens.

A related question concerns the importance of oncogene-induced GF release to the transformation process: Do the transforming abilities of a *ras* or *mos* oncogene depend on an induced GF autocrine circuit, or does autocrine secretion represent a side pathway whose existence is not essential to the workings of these oncogenes? In the case of certain *ras*-transformed fibroblasts, the display of EGF receptors may enable these cells to respond to the TGF-α that they release. Nonetheless, the potential responsiveness of these cells to TGF-α hardly proves the essential role of autocrine circuits in maintaining the transformed state of these cells. This point is highlighted by the case of certain sublines of mouse NIH-3T3 cells, which release TGF-α in response to *ras* oncogenes but display virtually no EGF receptors. Although these cells are very sensitive to transformation by *ras* oncogenes, this sensitivity cannot be ascribed to the autocrine effects of the released TGF-α. It would appear in this instance that the *ras* oncogene is capable of transforming the cell through fully intracellular changes; the *ras*-induced secretion of the TGF-α is clearly gratuitous to the transformation process.

B. Growth Factor Autonomy: The Direct Autocrine Pathway

In the case of another class of oncogenes, the central importance of secreted growth factors for transformation is undisputed. The best-studied of these oncogenes is *sis*, originally discovered as the oncogene present in the genome of simian sarcoma virus. In 1983, analysis of the structure of the *sis* oncogene protein and of PDGF revealed the two proteins to be closely related in structure (Doolittle et al. 1983; Waterfield et al. 1983). This suggested that the transforming ability of the *sis* oncogene derives from its ability to encode and directly induce the production of PDGF or a PDGF-like molecule. Once released, this oncogene-encoded PDGF could then bind to the cell's PDGF receptors, which in turn would release a stream of stimulatory signals into the cell. These stimulatory signals would ultimately mediate the transforming effects of *sis*.

Unlike the autocrine action of an oncogene like *ras*, *sis* oncogene function does not depend on a complex regulatory pathway connecting an oncogene protein with a growth factor gene. Since the *sis* oncogene only encodes a PDGF-like protein, its transforming ability must derive exclusively from its ability to specify high, constitutive levels of PDGF production. Such constitutive production contrasts with the normal regulation of PDGF, which ensures that this factor is released in small, carefully rationed amounts. As expected, the *sis* oncogene is unable to transform cells that lack the PDGF receptor (Leal et al. 1985).

Although the essential role of PDGF in *sis*-mediated transformation is clear, an important mechanistic detail of the process remains in dispute: It is unclear where the *sis*-encoded PDGF encounters its receptor and triggers receptor firing. An obvious answer is that released PDGF present in the extracellular space binds to cell-surface PDGF receptors. Indeed, this scenario is supported by work showing that high concentrations of anti-PDGF antibody cause growth inhibition and reversion from transformation when applied to *sis*-transformed cells (Johnsson et al. 1985). Such antibody presumably can only neutralize soluble, extracellular PDGF, thereby preventing it from reaching and binding to its receptor. Analogous experiments have been performed and found to successfully revert transformation phenotypes of cells whose growth is driven by autocrine loops involving interleukin-1 (IL-1), IL-2, IL-3, IL-4k, IL-6, GM-CSF, CSF-1, TGF-α, and bombesin (for review, see Browder et al. 1989). In all these cases, the GF driving autocrine growth can be bound by antibody present in the growth medium. Therefore, these autocrine circuits must include an extracellular phase of secretion followed by readsorption to an appropriate cell-surface receptor.

Other work, once again on PDGF, yields a quite different conclusion by indicating that the autocrine circuit can be completed totally within the cell. Because both PDGF and its receptor pass through the same biosynthetic pathway from endoplasmic reticulum through the Golgi apparatus to the cell surface, it is plausible that productive receptor–ligand interactions occur long before these molecules reach the cell surface. Such intracellular encounters, presumably occurring in one or another secretory compartment, have been demonstrated for the *sis*-encoded PDGF-B. Indeed, the bulk of PDGF: PDGF-receptor binding seems to occur intracellularly. In contrast to the work using anti-GF antibodies, this indicates that an intracellular autocrine circuit is responsible for much of *sis*-mediated transformation (Keating and Williams 1988).

In addition to *sis*, several other oncogenes have been found that also appear to encode secreted proteins. Some of these oncogenes encode proteins that have strong structural homology with FGF. These include *hst*, an oncogene detected by transfection of human gastric carcinoma DNA; another closely related oncogene that may have become activated in the course of the transfection process; and a more distantly related oncogene, *fgf.5*, detected by virtue of its ability to stimulate cell growth in defined medium (Sakamoto et al. 1986; Delli-Bovi and Basilico 1987; Zhan et al. 1987, 1988). Apparently analogous processes are illustrated by two other oncogenes that become activated during tumorigenesis by mouse mammary tumor virus (MMTV). Activation of these oncogenes, termed *int-1* and *int-2*, is achieved through integration of MMTV proviruses into chromosomal sites that are adjacent to their respective proto-oncogenes. Here, the data supporting autocrine mechanisms are still indirect but highly suggestive: The *int*-1 gene product is a glycoprotein found in secretory compartments when the *int-1* gene is introduced into cultured cells; and the *int-2* gene product has been found to be related structurally to bFGF (Dickson and Peters 1987; Papkoff et al. 1987).

To date, these GF-encoding oncogenes have only been observed in a small number of naturally arising tumors. The structures of these particular oncogenes suggest a simple experimental method for constructing novel oncogenes by fusing high-efficiency transcriptional promoters with sequences encoding the structures of various GFs. In this fashion, oncogenes have been constructed utilizing the genes for PDGF, GM-CSF, IL-3, EGF, TGF-α, and bFGF and CSF-1 (Gazit et al. 1984; Lang et al. 1985; Hapel et al. 1986; Rosenthal et al. 1986; Finzi et al. 1987; Rettenmier et al. 1987; Stern et al. 1987; Watanabe et al. 1987; Rogelj et al. 1988).

Despite these experimental advances, the mechanism of autocrine transformation is incompletely understood. Transformation of a cell by an oncogene like *sis* does far more than simply alleviate the cell's normal requirement for exogenous PDGF. *sis*-transformed cells exhibit anchorage independence, refractility when viewed in the phase-contrast microscope, and other transformation-associated phenotypes. It would seem that the constitutive, intense stimulation of the PDGF receptor in these transformants drives the hyperactivity of central intracellular second-messenger pathways that may also be deregulated by a variety of other oncogenes. By activating these pathways, this autocrine stimulation by *sis* may relieve not only a normal requirement for PDGF but for other normally required factors as well.

Autocrine growth control has been depicted here as an aberration of normal cellular physiology. As argued earlier, the interdependence of different cell types mutually regulating each other's growth underlies normal tissue morphogenesis and maintenance of structure. In this sense, it would seem that the self-regulation of growth as exemplified by autocrine circuits is incompatible with normal physiology and indeed represents a first step toward the cell autonomy seen in the neoplastic state. However, there are clear indications that certain normal cell types also participate in autocrine growth regulation. Thus, placental trophoblasts secrete a PDGF-like factor, display PDGF receptors, and respond to exogenously added PDGF when grown in culture. A similar behavior is shown by smooth muscle cells from newborn rats (Heldin and Westermark 1986). Such data provide presumptive evidence that autocrine growth regulation is not limited to aberrantly growing neoplastic cells and that it may indeed play a role in regulating the normal proliferation of certain developmental lineages.

C. Growth Factor Autonomy Via Receptor Alteration

Virtually all cell types display a number of distinct GF receptor types on their surfaces, each able to bind and confer responsiveness to one or several GF ligands. These receptors are the subject of Chapter 3. Because receptors clearly play a central role in the physiology of GFs, they are mentioned here as well. Like the mechanisms leading to autocrine growth, aberrations in GF receptors can mediate GF autonomy; indeed, aberrant GF receptors can act as oncogene proteins. Thus, malfunctioning GF receptors may release growth-stimulatory signals into the cell even without any encounter with their ligand. Such constitutive, GF-independent signal emission can lead in turn to cell transformation.

An initial example of this mechanism was provided by studies of the structure of the EGF receptor. Examination of its amino acid sequence revealed near-identity with the protein encoded by the *erbB* oncogene, originally discovered as the transforming gene of avian erythroblastosis virus (Downward et al. 1984). More detailed analysis revealed that the *erbB* oncogene encodes a truncated version of the EGF receptor. This finding firmly established the principle that a growth factor receptor protein can function as an oncogene protein. By this logic, a GF receptor gene should be considered a proto-oncogene: Following appropriate genetic alteration, many, if not all, receptor genes may assume the functional properties of active oncogenes. Subsequent work has shown that the oncoproteins of the *fms* and *neu* oncogenes are also aberrantly structured receptor proteins; these proteins differ only subtly from their normal cell counterparts (Bargmann et al. 1986; Roussel et al. 1988; Woolford et al. 1988).

The connection between receptor and oncoprotein can be most easily rationalized in terms of the normal role of a GF receptor: Upon binding of a GF ligand to its extracellular domain, a receptor transduces a signal across the plasma membrane and emits an excitatory signal through its cytoplasmic domain. Alterations in the structure or amount of the receptor protein may uncouple signal emission from GF ligand binding. In this event, the receptor molecule may emit excitatory signals even without encountering its ligand. This creates a measure of GF autonomy, in that growth may ensue in the absence of GFs.

As detailed in Chapter 3, this uncoupling of signaling from ligand binding may be achieved through several different types of structural alteration of the receptor, including truncation of critical regulatory domains and subtle changes involving alteration of single amino acid residues. Other work has made it apparent that overexpression of structurally normal receptors may also create an oncogenic effect. For example, the EGF receptor is often overexpressed in glioblastomas; the related *neu/erbB2* protein is often overexpressed in mammary carcinomas. Such overexpression is often associated with an increase in the copy number of the GF receptor gene (Libermann et al. 1985; Slamon et al. 1987). The increased number of receptor molecules, which may often exceed by 50–100-fold the normal receptor complement, may act by conferring a hyperresponsiveness to low background levels of GF that are compatible with maintenance of normal tissue architecture. Alternatively, these increased receptors may amplify the low level of spontaneous background signaling that normal receptors emit even in the absence of ligand binding. In either case, the growth of cells is uncoupled from a normal dependency on ambient levels of GFs.

D. Growth Factor Autonomy and Intracellular Signal Transduction

Cells respond in seconds to minutes to encounters with mitogenic GFs (Chapter 4). Most immediate are changes in cytoplasmic metabolites, such as components of the phosphatidylinositol pathway. Almost as rapid are increases in cytosolic calcium achieved by release from cytoplasmic membrane stores or by opening of plasma membrane channels. The diacylglycerol resulting from breakdown of phosphatidylinositol metabolites may collaborate with cytoplasmic calcium ions to activate kinase C. In addition, the cytoplasm of the cell also undergoes a slower process of alkalinization due to alteration in the plasma membrane Na^+/H^+ antiporter.

The molecular mechanisms mediating these GF-induced changes in second-messenger levels are poorly understood. It would appear that growth factor receptors alter a set of regulatory proteins whose activities in turn govern second-messenger levels. Indeed, cytoplasmic proto-oncogene-encoded proteins like those of the *ras*, *src*, and *abl* genes are suspected to be involved as signal transducers responsible for the normal regulation of second-messenger pathways. Structurally altered forms of these proteins encoded by oncogenes may be able to activate these pathways, even in the absence of prior stimulation by receptors located upstream in a signaling pathway. Consequently, the normally required involvement of GF receptors and bound GFs becomes gratuitous. For example, a myeloid cell line has been developed that is nontumorigenic and dependent on GM-CSF for growth. When transformed by the *abl* oncogene, these cells lose GM-CSF dependence and acquire tumorigenicity. These tumor cells do not secrete GM-CSF, ruling out an autocrine transformation mechanism. It appears then that the *abl* oncoprotein can constitutively activate the same signaling pathways that are normally induced following encounter by these cells with GM-CSF (Cook et al. 1985; Kelly 1985; Wheeler et al. 1987).

The cytoplasmic changes represent only the immediate, proximal response to GFs created by signal-transducing proto-oncogene proteins. More distal steps in the response pathway are seen in the nucleus, where the expression of whole banks of genes is activated. As discussed earlier, some of these responder genes are proto-oncogenes that can assume oncogenic functions if mutated appropriately. Significantly, the genetic changes that create many of these "nuclear oncogenes" cause a deregulated, constitutive expression that uncouples their expression from cytoplasmic (and ultimately extracellular) signals. As an example, upon conversion to an oncogene, the expression of the *myc* gene, which is normally dependent on stimulation by agents like PDGF or EGF, may be driven by immunoglobulin or retrovirus control elements. The expression of *myc* thus becomes constitutive and uncoupled from normal physiological regulators such as GFs. The resulting *myc* oncogene functions as a powerful element for inducing neoplastic growth (see Chapters 7, 12, and 13). Once again, a measure of GF autonomy is achieved through the deregulation of a critical intracellular signal-transducing element.

E. Growth Factor Autonomy: Escape from Negative Regulators of Cell Growth

The GFs described in this chapter have been discussed in the context of their growth-promoting abilities, yet these and other GFs may have quite opposite effects on cell growth. Such antimitogenic effects may be achieved through direct growth-inhibitory effects on cells or, less directly, through an ability to induce differentiation, thereby creating nonproliferating end-stage cells. Such negative regulators include as examples TGF-β, certain interferons, hepatic proliferation inhibitor, fibroblast growth regulator, and a growth inhibitor of mammary cells (for review, see Wang and Hsu 1986).

The best-studied of these negative regulators is TGF-β. In the presence of PDGF and IGF, TGF-α and TGF-β can act synergistically to induce the anchorage-independent growth of NRK fibroblast cells. In many other contexts, TGF-β can act as a potent growth inhibitor, even when present in concentrations as low as 1 picomolar. Targets susceptible to inhibition include cell types as diverse as BSC-1 monkey kidney epithelial cells, human foreskin fibroblasts, keratinocytes, human megakaryocytes, and erythroid precursors (Moses et al. 1985).

Because TGF-β acts negatively on the growth of a variety of cell types, it would not appear to contribute to runaway neoplastic growth. However, as detailed elsewhere in this volume (Chapter 11), escape from negative growth control is a frequent mechanism underlying neoplastic transformation. Accordingly, mechanisms that would counteract the inhibitory influences of TGF-β on cell growth might represent important steps in the genesis of certain tumors.

Two such mechanisms have recently come to light. The first is seen in retinoblastoma tumors, which arise from primitive retinal precursor cells in the developing eye. In addition to the inactivation of retinoblastoma gene alleles seen in these tumor cells (Chapter 11), these cells are also seen to lack responsiveness to the growth-inhibitory effects of TGF-β. Such responsiveness is readily observed in normal retinoblasts and in a large variety of other cell types. The refractoriness to TGF-β inhibition displayed by retinoblastoma cells is due to absence of the TGF-β receptors that are displayed in substantial amounts by normal cells of the retinal lineage (Kimchi et al. 1987). By shedding these receptors, retinoblastoma cells would appear to escape the growth-inhibitory influences of TGF-β that is released in a paracrine manner from nearby tissue layers in the retina.

TGF-β may also regulate growth in an autocrine manner. Thus, a cell may constrain its own growth through its ability to secrete and respond to TGF-β. A breakdown of this circuit could serve to free the cell from self-imposed constraints on its growth. One illustration of this is provided by breast cancer cells, the growth of which is usually strongly inhibited by anti-estrogens. Such cells have been found to release TGF-β in response to these compounds; the released TGF-β then acts to shut down the growth of the cells that have just secreted it. Variant tumor cells whose growth is no longer inhibited by anti-estrogens have lost their ability to release TGF-β upon anti-estrogen treatment, although they remain TGF-β-sensitive (Knabbe et al. 1988). In this instance, an inhibitory autocrine circuit is interrupted through loss of the ability to secrete an autocrine growth-inhibitory factor.

A possibly related mechanism of escape from antimitogenic factors is suggested by experiments in which mouse embryo cultures are adapted to grow in vitro in a medium containing bovine serum. Generally, these cells will proliferate for a limited period of time before they senesce. Emerging from these senescent cultures are rare variants that have acquired an ability to proliferate indefinitely, i.e., they are immortalized. In contrast, when embryo cultures are grown in a defined, serum-free medium, they are able to grow indefinitely. Subsequent exposure to serum induces immediate senescence (Loo et al. 1987). This would suggest that serum contains growth inhibitory factor(s) to which cells must become adapted before they can become immortalized. Since immortalization is often seen as a precursor to full neoplastic transformation (see Chapter 12), this suggests that tumor cells frequently lose responsiveness to inhibitory factors in the course of their evolution to malignancy.

VI. SUMMARY AND CONCLUSIONS

The acquisition of growth factor autonomy appears to represent far more than a consequence of tumorigenesis; rather, it would seem to represent a driving, causal force in the process. This is indicated by the fact that in a number of cell types, loss of dependence on one or another mitogenic GF in vitro is accompanied by acquisition of tumorigenicity when such cells are assayed in vivo. Less well-studied are complementary mechanisms in which loss of responsiveness to inhibitory factors potentiates the tumorigenic qualities of a cell.

Loss of dependence on mitogenic factors can be achieved through at least three distinct mechanisms: (1) Cells may synthesize GFs to which they can respond, creating an autocrine stimulatory loop and obviating the need for GFs originating elsewhere in the tissue; (2) cell-surface receptors may undergo structural change or aberrant increase in number resulting in the release of gratuitous, factor-independent signals into the cells; (3) downstream signal-transducing elements in the cytoplasm and nucleus may undergo changes affecting their structure or concentration, resulting in a flux of growth-stimulatory signals even in the absence of encounters with GFs.

These mechanisms circumvent and subvert normal paracrine mechanisms that allow closely apposed, heterotypic cell layers to regulate each other's growth and normal autocrine mechanisms that may allow homogeneous cell populations to regulate their own growth. In the end, the study of GFs will provide insight into far more than the deregulated growth of neoplasia. GFs must govern a number of normal biological processes, including wound-healing and the morphogenesis of complex tissues that occurs during ontogeny. A complete understanding of the role of GFs in this latter process will require work extending well into the next century.

REFERENCES

Almendral, J. M., D. Sommer, H. MacDonald-Bravo, J. Burckhardt, J. Perera, and R. Bravo. 1988. Complexity of the early genetic response to growth factors in mouse fibroblasts. *Mol. Cell. Biol.* **8:** 2140–2148.

Anisowicz, A., L. Bardwell, and R. Sager. 1987. Constitutive overexpression of a growth-regulated gene in transformed Chinese hamster and human cells. *Proc. Natl. Acad. Sci.* **84:** 7188–7192.

Anzano, M.A., A.B. Roberts, J.M. Smith, M.B. Sporn, and J.E. De Larco. 1983. Sarcoma growth factor from conditioned medium of virally transformed cells is composed of both type-α and type-β transforming growth factors. *Proc. Natl. Acad. Sci.* **80:** 6264–6268.

Bargmann, C. I., M.-C. Hung, and R. A. Weinberg. 1986. Multiple independent activations of the c-*neu* oncogene by a point mutation altering the trans-membrane domain of p185. *Cell* **45:** 649–657.

Browder, T. M., J. S. Abrams, P. M. C. Wong, and A. W. Nienhuis. 1989. Mechanism of autocrine stimulation in hematopoietic cells producing Interleukin-3 after retrovirus-mediated gene transfer. *Mol. Cell. Biol.* **9:** 204–213.

Cheifetz, S., B. Like, and J. Massague. 1986. Cellular distribution of type I and type II receptors of transforming growth factor-β. *J. Biol. Chem.* **261:** 9972–9978.

Cochran, B., H. Reffel, and C. D. Stiles. 1983. Molecular cloning of gene sequences regulated by platelet-derived growth factor. *Cell* **33:** 939–947.

Coffey, F. J., R. Derynck, R. N. Wilcox, T. S. Bringman, A. S. Goustin, H. L. Moses, and M. R. Pittelkow. 1987. Production and auto-induction of transforming growth factor-α in human keratinocytes. *Nature* **328:** 817–820.

Cohen, S. 1962. Isolation of a submaxillary gland protein accelerating incisor eruption and eyelid opening in the newborn animal. *J. Biol. Chem.* **237:** 1555–1562.

Cook, W.D., D. Metcalf, N.A. Nicola, A.W. Burgess, and F. Walker. 1985. Malignant transformation of a growth factor-dependent myeloid cell line by Abelson virus without evidence of an autocrine mechanism. *Cell* **41:** 677–683.

De Larco, J. and G.J. Todaro. 1978. Growth factors from murine sarcoma virus-transformed cells. *Proc. Natl. Acad. Sci.* **75:** 4001–4005.

Delli-Bovi, P.A., A.M. Curatola, F.G. Kern, A. Greco, M. Ittmann, and C. Basilico. 1987. An oncogene isolated by transfection of Kaposi's sarcoma DNA encodes a growth factor that is a member of the FGF family. *Cell* **50:** 729–737.

Dickson, C. and G. Peters. 1987. Potential oncogene product related to growth factors. *Nature* **326:** 833.

Doolittle, R.F., M.W. Hunkapiller, L.E. Hood, S.G. De Vare, K.C. Robbins, S.A. Aaronson, and H.N. Antoniades. 1983. Simian sarcoma virus *onc* gene, v-*sis*, is derived from the gene (or genes) encoding a platelet-derived growth factor. *Science* **221:** 275–276.

Downward, J., Y. Yarden, E. Mayes, G. Scrace, N. Totty, P. Stockwell, A. Ullrich, J. Schlessinger, and M. D. Waterfield. 1984. Close similarity of epidermal growth factor receptor and v-*erb*B oncogene protein sequences. *Nature* **307:** 521–527.

Finzi, E., T. Fleming, O. Segatto, C.Y. Pennington, T.S. Bringman, R. Derynck, and S. Aaronson. 1987. The human transforming growth factor type-α coding sequence is not a direct-acting oncogene when overexpressed in NIH3T3 cells. *Proc. Natl. Acad. Sci.* **84:** 3733–3737.

Gazit, A., H. Igarashi, I.M. Chieu, A. Srinivasan, A. Yaniv, S.R. Tronick, K.C. Robbins, and S.A. Aaronson. 1984. Expression of the normal human *sis*/PDGF-2 coding sequence induces cellular transformation. *Cell* **39:** 89–97.

Hapel, A.G., G. Vande Woude, H.D. Campbell, I.G. Young, and T. Robins. 1986. Generation of an autocrine leukaemia using a retroviral vector carrying the interleukin-3 gene. *Lymphokine Res.* **5:** 249–254.

Heldin, C.-H. and B. Westermark. 1986. Role of PDGF-like growth factors in autocrine stimulation of growth of normal and transformed cells. In *Oncogenes and growth control* (ed. P. Kahn and T. Graf), p. 43–50. Springer Verlag, Heidelberg.

Holley, R. W. 1975. Control of growth of mammalian cells in cell culture. *Nature* **258:** 487–490.

Jakowlew, S.B., P. Kondaiah, K.C. Flanders, N.L. Thompson, P.J. Dillard, M.B. Sporn, and A.B. Roberts. 1988. Increased coordinate expression of growth factor mRNAs accompanies viral transformation of rodent cells. *Oncogene Res.* **2:** 135–148.

Johnsson, A., C. Betsholtz, C.-H. Heldin, and B. Westermark. 1985. Antibodies to platelet-derived growth factor inhibit acute transformation by simian sarcoma virus. *Nature* **317:** 438–440.

Keating, M. T. and L. T. Williams. 1988. Autocrine stimulation of intracellular PDGF receptors in v-*sis*-transformed cells. *Science* **239:** 914–915.

Kelly, K. 1985. Growth factors short-circuited. *Nature* **317:** 390.

Kimchi, A., X.-F. Wang, R.A. Weinberg, S. Cheifetz, and J. Massague. 1987. Absence of transforming growth factor-β receptors and growth inhibitory responses in retinoblastoma cells. *Science* **240:** 196–199.

Knabbe, C., M.E. Lippman, L.M. Wakefield, K.C. Flanders, A. Kasid, R. Derynck, and R.B. Dickson. 1988. Evidence that transforming growth factor-β is a hormonally regulated negative growth factor in human breast cancer cells. *Cell* **48:** 417–428.

Kurachi, H., S. Okamoto, and T. Oka. 1985. Evidence for the involvement of the submaxillary gland epidermal growth factor in mouse mammary tumorigenesis. *Proc. Natl. Acad. Sci.* **82:** 5940–5943.

Lang, R.A., D. Metcalf, N.M. Gough, A.R. Dunn, and T.J. Gonda. 1985. Expression of a hemopoietic growth factor cDNA in a factor-dependent cell line results in autonomous growth and tumorigenicity. *Cell* **43:** 531–542.

Lau, L. F. and D. Nathans. 1985. Identification of a set of genes expressed during the G_0/G_1 transition of cultured mouse cells. *EMBO J.* **4:** 3145–3151.

———. 1987. Expression of a set of growth-related immediate early genes in Balb/c3T3 cells: Coordinate regulation with c-*fos* or c-*myc*. *Proc. Natl. Acad. Sci.* **84:** 1182–1186.

Leal, F., L.T. Williams, K.C. Robbins, and S.A. Aaronson. 1985. Evidence that the v-*sis* gene product transforms by interaction with the receptor for platelet-derived growth factor. *Science* **230:** 327–330.

Leof, E.B., J.A. Proper, A.S. Goustin, G.D. Shipley, P.E. Di Couleto, and H.L. Moses. 1986. Induction of c-*sis* mRNA and activity similar to platelet-derived growth factor-like activity by transforming growth factor, type-β: A proposed model for indirect mitogenesis involving autocrine activity. *Proc. Natl. Acad. Sci.* **83:** 2453–2457.

Levi-Montalcini, R. and V. Hamburger. 1951. Selective growth stimulating effects of mouse sarcoma on the sensory and sympathetic nervous system of the chick embryo. *J. Exp. Zool.* **116:** 321–351.

Libermann, T.A., H.R. Nussbaum, N. Razon, R. Kris, I. Lax, M. Soreq, N. Whittle, M.D. Waterfield, A. Ullrich, and J. Schlessinger. 1985. Amplification, enhanced expression, and possible rearrangement of the EGF receptor gene in primary human brain tumors of glial origin. *Nature* **313:** 144-147.

Loo, D.T., J.I. Fuquay, C.I. Rawson, and D.W. Barnes. 1987. Extended culture of mouse embryo cells without senescence: Inhibition by serum. *Science* **236:** 200–202.

Marquardt, H., M.W. Hunkapiller, L.E. Hood, D.R. Twardzik, J.E. De Larco, J.R. Stephenson, and G.J. Todaro. 1983. Transforming growth factors produced by retrovirus-transformed rodent fibroblasts and human melanoma cells: Amino acid homology with epidermal growth factor. *Proc. Natl. Acad. Sci.* **80:** 4684–4688.

Massague, J. 1987. The TGF-β family of growth and differentiation factors. *Cell* **49:** 437–438.

Metcalf, D. 1985. The granulocyte-macrophage colony-stimulating factors. *Science* **229:** 16–22.

Moses, H.L., R.F. Tucker, E.B. Leof, R.J. Coffey, Jr., J. Halper, and G.D. Shipley. 1985. Type-β transforming growth factor is a growth stimulator and a growth inhibitor in cancer cells. In *Growth factors and transformation* (ed. J. Feramisco et al.), p. 65–71. Cold Spring Harbor Laboratory, Cold Spring Harbor, New York.

Nishikura, K. and J. M. Murray. 1987. Antisense RNA of proto-oncogene c-*fos* blocks renewed growth of quiescent 3T3 cells. *Mol. Cell. Biol.* **7:** 639–649.

Papkoff, J., A.M.C. Brown, and H.E. Varmus. 1987. The *int*-1 protooncogene products are glycoproteins that appear to enter the secretory pathway. *Mol. Cell. Biol.* **7:** 3978–3984.

Paulson, Y., A. Hammacher, C.H. Heldin, and B. Westermark. 1987. Possible positive autocrine feedback in the prereplicative phase of human fibroblasts. *Nature* **328:** 715–717.

Pierce, J.H., M. Ruggiero, T.P. Fleming, P.P. Di Fiore, J.S. Greenberg, L. Varticovski, J. Schlessinger, G. Rovera, and S.A. Aaronson. 1988. Signal transduction through the EGF receptor transfected in IL-3-dependent hematopoietic cells. *Science* **239:** 628–630.

Pimentel, E. 1987. *Hormones, growth factors and oncogenes*, pp. 111–140. CRC Press, Boca Raton.

Pledger, W.J., C.D. Stiles, H.N. Antoniades, and C.D. Scher. 1977. Induction of DNA synthesis in Balb/c3T3 cells by serum components: Reevaluation of the commitment process. *Proc. Natl. Acad. Sci.* **74:** 4481–4485.

Rettenmier, C.W., M.F. Roussel, R.A. Ashmun, P. Ralph, K. Price, and C.J. Sherr. 1987. Synthesis of membrane-bound colony stimulating factor (CSF-1) and down modulation of CSF-1 receptors in NIH3T3 cells transformed by cotransfection of the human CSF-1 and c-*fms* (CSF-1 receptor) genes. *Mol. Cell. Biol.* **7:** 2378–2387.

Riabowol, K.T., R.J. Vosatka, E.B. Ziff, N.J. Lamb, and J.R. Feramisco. 1988. Microinjection of *fos*-specific antibodies blocks DNA synthesis in fibroblast cells. *Mol. Cell. Biol.* **8:** 1670–1676.

Richmond, A., E. Balentien, H.G. Thomas, G. Flaggs, D.E. Barton, J. Spiess, R. Bordoni, U. Francke, and R. Derynck. 1988. Molecular characterization and chromosomal mapping of melanoma growth stimulatory activity, a growth factor structurally related to β-thyroglobulin. *EMBO J.* **7:** 2025–2033.

Roberts, A.B., M.A. Anzano, L.C. Lamb, J.M. Smith, and M.B. Sporn. 1981. New class of transforming growth factors potentiated by epidermal growth factor: Isolation from non-neoplastic tissues. *Proc. Natl. Acad. Sci.* **78:** 5339–5343.

Rogelj, S., R.A. Weinberg, P. Fanning, and M. Klagsbrun. 1988. Basic fibroblast growth factor fused to a signal peptide transforms cells. *Nature* **331:** 173–175.

Rollins, B.J., E.D. Morrison, and C.D. Stiles. 1988. Cloning and expression of JE, a gene inducible by platelet-derived growth factor and whose product has cytokine-like properties. *Proc. Natl. Acad. Sci.* **85:** 3738–3742.

Rosenthal, A., P.B. Lindquist, T.S. Bringman, D.V. Goeddel, and R. Derynck. 1986. Expression in rat fibroblasts of a human transforming growth factor-α cDNA results in transformation. *Cell* **46:** 301–309.

Ross, R., E.W. Raines, and D.F. Bowen-Pope. 1986. The biology of platelet-derived growth factor. *Cell* **46:** 155–159.

Roussel, M.F., J.R. Downing, C.W. Rettenmier, and C.J. Sherr. 1988. A point mutation is the extracellular domain of the human CSF-1 receptor (c-*fms* proto-oncogene product) activates its transforming potential. *Cell* **55:** 979-988.

Sakamoto, H., M. Mori, M. Taira, T. Yoshida, S. Matsukawa, K. Shimizu, M. Sekiguchi, M. Terada, and T. Sugimara. 1986. Transforming gene from human stomach cancers and a noncancerous portion of stomach mucosa. *Proc. Natl. Acad. Sci.* **83:** 3997–4001.

Silver, B.J., F.E. Jaffer, and H.E. Abboud. 1989. Platelet-derived growth factor synthesis in mesangial cells: Induction by multiple peptide mitogenes. *Proc. Natl. Acad. Sci.* **86:** 1056–1060.

Slamon, D.J., M. Clark, S.G. Wong, W.J. Levin, A. Ullrich, and W.L. McGuire. 1987.

Human breast cancer: Correlation of relapse and survival with amplification of HER-2/*neu* oncogene. *Science* **235:** 177–182.

Sporn, M.B. and G.J. Todaro. 1980. Autocrine secretion and malignant transformation of cells. *N. Engl. J. Med.* **308:** 878–880.

Stern, D.F., D.L. Hare, M.A. Cecchini, and R.A. Weinberg. 1987. Construction of a novel oncogene based on synthetic sequences encoding epidermal growth factor. *Science* **235:** 321–324.

Thomas, K.A. and G. Gimenez-Gallego. 1987. Fibroblast growth factors: Broad spectrum mitogens with potent angiogenic activity in oncogenes and growth factors. In *Oncogenes and growth factors* (ed. R. A. Bradshaw and S. Prentis), p. 149–156. Elsevier Science Publishers, Amsterdam.

Wang, J.L. and Y.M. Hsu. 1986. Negative regulators of cell growth. *Trends Biochem. Sci.* **11:** 24–26.

Watanabe, S., E. Lazar, and M.B. Sporn. 1987. Transformation of normal rat kidney (NRK) cells by an infectious retrovirus carrying a synthetic rat type α transforming growth factor gene. *Proc. Natl. Acad. Sci.* **84:** 1258–1262.

Waterfield, M.D., G.J. Scrace, N. Whittle, P Strooband, A. Johnson, A. Wasteson, B. Westermark, C.-H. Heldin, J.S. Huang, and T.F. Deuel. 1983. Platelet-derived growth factor is structurally related to the putative transforming protein $p28^{sis}$ of simian sarcoma virus. *Nature* **304:** 35–39.

Wheeler, E.F., D. Askew, S. May, J.N. Ihle, and C.J. Sherr. 1987. The v-*fms* oncogene induces factor-independent growth and transformation of the interleukin-3 dependent myeloid cell line FDC-P1. *Mol. Cell. Biol.* **7:** 1673–1680.

Woolford, J., A. McAuliffe, and L.R. Rohrschneider. 1988. Activation of the feline c-*fms* proto-oncogene: Multiple alterations are required to generate a fully transformed phenotype. *Cell* **55:** 965–977.

Yoshida, T., K. Miyagawa,, H. Odagiri, H. Sakamoto, P.F.R. Little, M. Terada, and T. Sugimura. 1987. Genomic sequence of *hst*, a transforming gene encoding a protein homologous to fibroblast growth factors and the *int*-2 encoded protein. *Proc. Natl. Acad. Sci.* **84:** 7305–7309.

Zhan, X., B. Bates, X. Hu, and M. Goldfarb. 1988. The human FGF-5 oncogene encodes a novel protein related to fibroblast growth factors. *Mol. Cell. Biol.* **8:** 3487–3495.

Zhan, X., A. Culpepper, M. Reddy, J. Loveless, and M. Goldfarb. 1987. Human oncogenes detected by a defined medium culture assay. *Oncogene* **1:** 369–376.

3

Growth Factors and Their Receptors

Gordon N. Gill
Department of Medicine, Division of Endocrinology and Metabolism
and Center for Molecular Genetics
School of Medicine, University of California, San Diego
La Jolla, California 92093

I. INTRODUCTION

During development, in regenerative and in reparative processes, growth is highly regulated to coincide with the overall needs of the organism for survival and reproduction. As with homeostatic metabolic adaptations to the environment, complex communication systems must function to integrate organ and cellular responses to the overall needs of the organism. In higher organisms, the nervous and endocrine systems serve this communicator function. Cells receive information via hormones and neurotransmitters that bind to allosteric proteins. These proteins (receptors) have both specific recognition and specialized activity functions. Interaction with these receptor molecules initiates biochemical processes that result in altered biological responses of the cell. The initial interaction of the signaling molecule with its receptor is a bimolecular reaction dependent on the concentration of each reactant as well as on intrinsic affinities dictated by their structures.

$$[\text{Ligand}] + \underset{\text{inactive}}{[\text{Receptor}]} \underset{k_{-1}}{\overset{k_1}{\rightleftharpoons}} \underset{\text{active}}{[\text{Ligand} \cdot \text{Receptor}]}$$

Oncogenes and the Molecular Origins of Cancer.

Extensive control systems determine the concentration of each of the reactants so that appropriate adaptive responses are initiated, modulated, and terminated.

Growth factors and their receptors were recognized initially by their effects on cell proliferation. Like other hormones, they regulate diverse cellular processes in addition to growth and, although the emphasis here is on cell proliferation, signaling information for specialized cell functions may prove equally important. During both development and regeneration, growth must be appropriately initiated and appropriately terminated. Regulation of the synthesis and metabolism of both growth factors and their cognate receptors provides one central mechanism for accomplishing this balance. Failure to do so would result in unrestrained proliferative responses inappropriate to nutrient availability and, ultimately, to survival of the organism.

Oncogenes have been increasingly recognized as mutations that bypass these normal, exquisite mechanisms that control cell growth. Mutations involving the ligand growth factor, the growth factor receptor, or one of the steps in the ordered cellular responses to the activated growth factor receptor result in either of two major types of change: qualitative or quantitative. Qualitative changes remove regulatory constraints so that proteins remain constitutively and inappropriately active. Quantitative changes result in overexpression of the protein with a similar result because constitutive overexpression of either ligand or receptor favors, by mass action, formation of the active ligand·receptor complex (see equation). Examples of each of these general mechanisms have been delineated for both retroviral oncogenes and for oncogenes isolated from human and animal tumors. Deletion of regulatory restraining genes or inactivation of their products may also tip the balance to unrestrained growth, resulting in tumor formation as delineated for the retinoblastoma gene (Friend et al. 1986; Huang et al. 1988).

Although it was recognized for some time that growth of cells in vitro required serum, and, therefore, serum must contain growth-promoting substances, the first growth factor was isolated from tissues. This peptide, nerve growth factor, was trophic for a specialized cell type, sympathetic neurons (Levi-Montalcini and Angeletti 1968). During purification of nerve growth factor, Stanley Cohen detected a second activity that promoted eyelid opening and incisor eruption in newborn mice and rats (Cohen 1962). Recognizing the importance of epithelial development for these processes, the factor was named epidermal growth factor (EGF). Purification of this growth factor allowed its radiolabeling and use to detect specific cell-surface receptors (Carpenter et al. 1975). The ability to identify the receptor by binding radiolabeled ligand permitted studies of the receptor resulting in purification, characterization as a ligand-stimulated protein tyrosine kinase (Ushiro and Cohen 1980), and structural analysis that identified it as the cellular progenitor of a retroviral oncogene, v-*erbB* (Downward et al. 1984b).

The EGF receptor is a 170-kD single-chain transmembrane glycoprotein with intrinsic protein tyrosine kinase activity (Gill et al. 1987; Carpenter 1987). The nucleotide sequence of the EGF receptor predicts an 1186-amino acid protein consisting of extra- and intracellular domains separated by a single hydrophobic transmembrane region (Ullrich et al. 1984) (Fig. 1). The N′ terminal cell-surface domain of 621 amino acids is glycosylated at 11–12 asparagine residues (Mayes and Waterfield 1984; Weber et al. 1984), a process essential for proper maturation and expression of the EGF receptor on the cell surface (Soderquist and Carpenter 1984; Feige and Scheffler 1987). The extracellular domain is replete with cysteines that are clustered in two regions (Fig. 1), each region being composed of an apparent gene duplication (Lax et al. 1988). The 1:1 stoichiometry of EGF binding predicts a single binding site in the extracellular domain of the EGF receptor (Weber et al. 1984). The K_d for binding of 10^{-10} M (Wiley and Cunningham 1981) indicates a high-affinity interaction with a calculated ΔG of -14 kcal mole^{-1}. Although there is a single EGF receptor gene and only one characterized EGF receptor protein, binding studies in vivo often reveal two affinity classes of binding sites (Carpenter 1987). Modifications of critical residues in the cytoplasmic domain appear to regulate the affinity of the extracellular domain for its ligand.

The EGF binding/recognition domain is separated from the intracellular domain by a region of 23 hydrophobic amino acids. The cytoplasmic boundary of this region is marked by multiple dibasic amino acids predicted to partition outside the membrane as a stop transfer sequence (Engelman et al. 1986). The cytoplasmic 542 C′ terminal amino acids consist of a proximal domain that is strongly homologous to the protein

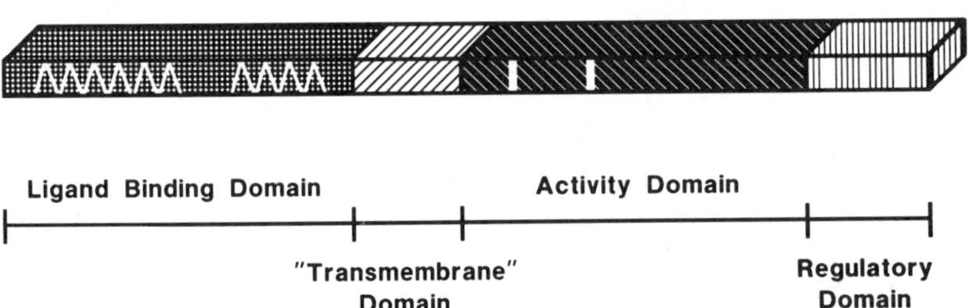

Figure 1 Schematic representation of the EGF receptor. Zigzag lines indicate cysteine-rich regions, and clear bars represent sites studied by in vitro mutagenesis. (Reprinted, with permission, from Gill et al. 1988.)

tyrosine kinase gene family (Lin et al. 1984; Ullrich et al. 1984; Xu et al. 1984; Hunter and Cooper 1985; see Chapter 6) and a C′ terminal region that is divergent from other members of this gene family (Fig. 1).

Binding sites for ATP and phosphate acceptor substrate proteins are located within the kinase core domain. The essential role of protein tyrosine kinase in mediating the biological effects of EGF was deduced from analysis of point mutations predicted to disrupt the ATP-binding site (Chen et al. 1987). The ATP-binding site is highly conserved among protein kinases and consists of a nucleotide-binding fold with a downstream lysine predicted to form a salt bridge to the β phosphate of ATP (Sternberg and Taylor 1984; Vogel et al. 1986). This site is located 50 amino acids from the inner membrane surface in all the growth factor receptors that possess intrinsic protein tyrosine kinase activity. Creation of mutants in which the essential lysine is replaced by a noncharged amino acid abolishes ligand-stimulated protein tyrosine kinase activity in the EGF receptor (Chen et al. 1987; Honegger et al. 1987a) and in the insulin receptor (Chou et al. 1987; Ebina et al. 1987; Russell et al. 1987), and abolishes the intrinsic protein tyrosine kinase activity of several retroviral oncogenes (Hannink and Donoghue 1985; Snyder et al. 1985; Weinmaster et al. 1986). The mutant kinase-inactive EGF receptor is synthesized as a cell-surface glycoprotein that binds EGF with expected affinity, but EGF fails to induce the biological responses seen in cells containing kinase-active EGF receptors.

The nonconserved C′ terminal region contains the major tyrosine sites of enzyme self-phosphorylation (Downward et al. 1984a). Self-phosphorylation, which occurs via an intramolecular mechanism (Weber et al. 1984), appears to remove an alternate substrate/competitive inhibitor providing a mechanism for achieving maximal enzyme activity (Bertics and Gill 1985). The C′ terminal region serves to control two processes: protein tyrosine kinase activity and ligand-induced receptor endocytosis (Gill et al. 1988).

The *Drosophila* homolog of the EGF receptor contains both the EGF-binding and tyrosine kinase domains, indicating that both activities have resided in the same molecule for over 800 million years (Livneh et al. 1985). These activities are dissociated in the protein encoded by the *erbB* oncogene of avian erythroblastosis virus, which lacks the extracellular ligand-binding domain (Yamamoto et al. 1983; Privalsky et al. 1984). The discovery that a retroviral oncogene was derived from a cellular growth factor receptor implied that deregulation of a normal growth-controlling pathway led to neoplastic transformation. Subsequent studies of the EGF receptor have shown that it can act as an oncogene-encoded protein (oncoprotein) not only when restraining structural features are deleted, but also when there is excessive expression of structurally normal receptors.

II. GROWTH FACTOR RECEPTORS WITH INTRINSIC PROTEIN TYROSINE KINASE ACTIVITY: MECHANISMS FOR CONVERSION TO ONCOPROTEINS

Because growth factor-activated protein tyrosine kinase is the essential biochemical mechanism through which one class of receptors act, understanding the control and effects of this activity is important to understanding cell growth control and the deregulation of this process that occurs with transformation. Covalent modification of proteins by the transfer of the γ phosphate of ATP to serine and threonine residues is an ancient and widely used signaling mechanism. Up to 10% of cell proteins are so modified, and there are many kinases that catalyze this reaction (Hunter 1987). Phosphotyrosine is much less abundant, accounting for about 0.03% of total cell protein phosphoamino acids (Hunter and Sefton 1980). Protein phosphotyrosine was initially discovered as a covalent modification of the middle T antigen of polyoma DNA tumor virus (Eckhart et al. 1979); this reaction was catalyzed by c-*src*, which was coprecipitated by anti-middle-T-antigen antibodies (Courtneidge and Smith 1984). Although rare, many of the enzymes catalyzing the phosphorylation of proteins on tyrosine residues have been discovered as retroviral oncogenes or as cell-surface growth factor receptors, implying a special role for this class of enzymes in regulating cell proliferation. Several cell-surface receptors possess intrinsic protein tyrosine kinase activity (Fig. 2).

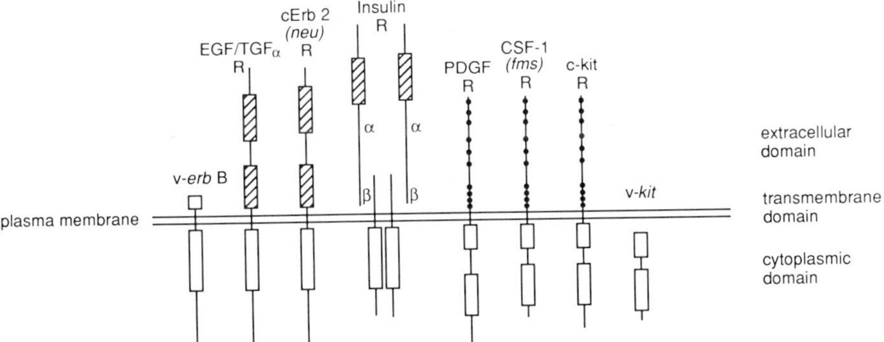

Figure 2 Schematic structures of some representative growth factor receptors with intrinsic protein tyrosine kinase activity. Hatched areas or closed circles in extracellular domains indicate locations of cysteine residues. Open boxed areas in cytoplasmic domains represent conserved protein tyrosine kinase core sequences. Note insertion in this area in PDGF, CSF-1, and c-*kit* receptors. The C′ terminus of v-*erbB* from AEV-H is truncated by 32 amino acids compared to the EGF receptor, the C′ terminus of the v-*fms* oncogene is truncated by 40 amino acids compared to the CSF-1 receptor, and the C′ terminus of v-*kit* is truncated by 49 amino acids compared to c-*kit*. (Derived from Yarden and Ullrich 1988.)

A. Qualitative: Activation by Deletion of Inhibitory Constraints

1. The Epidermal Growth Factor Receptor and erbB

v-*erbB* was identified in a retrovirus causing avian erythroblastosis (AEV) and erythroleukemia. This avian retrovirus contained two cell-derived genes: *erbA* and *erbB* (Vennstrom and Bishop 1982). Genetic analysis indicated that transforming activity resided in *erbB* (Frykberg et al. 1983). The v-*erbB* transforming protein is homologous to the transmembrane and cytoplasmic domains of the EGF receptor (Lin et al. 1984; Ullrich et al. 1984; Xu et al. 1984). It arose by insertion of viral DNA into the EGF receptor gene; this resulted in expression of a protein that lacked the amino-terminal ligand-binding domain (Fung et al. 1983; Nilsen et al. 1985). In the avian erythroblastosis virus strain H, 34 amino acids were also deleted from the C′ terminus (Yamamoto et al. 1983); other strains of virus contain progressive C′ terminal truncations in *erbB*, a change that extends their host range and enhances their transforming activity (Gamett et al. 1986). The finding that *erbB* retains the central protein tyrosine kinase domain of the EGF receptor implied that constitutive expression of this activity was the basis for its activity as a transforming oncoprotein. Although it was difficult to detect protein tyrosine kinase activity in *erbB*-transformed cells, recently such activity was clearly shown to be increased relative to untransformed cells (Gilmore et al. 1985; Kris et al. 1985).

Because viral isolates containing *erbB* consistently lack the amino-terminal ligand-binding domain, it appears that this region inhibits activity of the intrinsic protein tyrosine kinase domain. Genetic deletion of the ligand-binding domain from the EGF receptor is sufficient to create a transforming oncogene (Wells and Bishop 1988). Moreover, mutations within the protein tyrosine kinase domain of *erbB* abolish its transforming activity, whereas mutations in the C′ terminus do not (Ng and Privalsky 1986). *erbB* is thus transforming due to constitutively active protein tyrosine kinase resulting from deletion of the regulatory ligand-binding domain. Additional removal of carboxy-terminal regulatory sequences may enhance its transforming activity, but are not essential.

In in vitro cell transformation assays, *erbB* is less potent than several other retroviral and tumor-derived oncogenes (Di Fiore et al. 1987b). There are several possible explanations for this observation, including cell type expression and the active conformation of the transforming protein. Although EGF receptors are widely distributed, hematopoietic cells normally do not express the gene product. *erbB* may act more strongly on erythroid precursors both because of its constitutive activity and because expression is inappropriate for this cell type. *erbB* causes the outgrowth of erythroid progenitors that no longer require the growth factor erythropoietin (Beug et al. 1982). Although subsequent isolates of other independently arising avian viral strains contain only *erbB*, the AEV-H virus expressed two cellular genes: *erbA* and *erbB*. Although not transforming, *erbA*, which represents a mutated thyroid hormone receptor (Sap et al. 1986; Weinberger et al. 1986), strongly enhances transformation by *erbB* (Gandrillon et al. 1987), analogous to well-described synergism between peptide and steroid hormones.

Placement of the intact human EGF receptor in avian erythroid precursors caused ligand-dependent transformation (Khazaie et al. 1988). Short (32-amino-acid) C′ terminal deletions enhance transformation, but more extensive C′ terminal truncations both in *erbB* and in the human EGF receptor abolish their ability to transform erythroblasts, but not their ability to transform fibroblasts, suggesting that the structure of the C′ terminus provides an essential recognition feature in erythroblasts (Yamamoto et al. 1983; Khazaie et al. 1988). This resembles the requirement for an intact C′ terminus of the insulin receptor for insulin to stimulate glucose transport, although this region is not required for other insulin-stimulated events (Maegawa et al. 1988). The enhanced fibroblast-transforming activity of truncated *erbB* is consistent with the C′ terminus reversibly inhibiting the protein tyrosine kinase activity of the EGF receptor (Bertics and Gill 1985).

Constitutive expression of *erbB* is sufficient for transformation, but it remains possible that the ligand-activated EGF receptor has a different conformation from *erbB*, i.e., ligand binding not only may relieve inhibitory constraints, but also may induce the fully active conformation of the protein (Wedegaertner and Gill 1989).

*2. c-*erbB2 *and t-*neu

Creation of an oncoprotein by removal of the extracellular ligand-binding domain of the EGF receptor indicates this domain functions as a negative regulator. EGF binding to the holoreceptor must relieve this inhibitory constraint and allosterically activate the intracellular protein tyrosine kinase domain. The question of how signals are transduced across the plasma membrane by EGF binding to its receptor is important but unanswered. This issue is highlighted and made even more complex by study of an EGF receptor-related protein encoded by a gene known as c-*erbB2* or *neu*. This protein is potently activated to an oncoprotein by a distinct kind of structural change.

The c-*erbB2*/*neu* oncogene is encoded by a gene distinct from that which encodes the EGF receptor (Bargmann et al. 1986a). *neu*, initially isolated from mutagen-induced mouse neuroblastomas, contains a single point mutation in its transmembrane domain that renders the protein transforming (Bargmann et al. 1986b). Although the ligand for c-*erbB2* is still being sought, the single base change that alters the codon from valine to glutamic acid results in increased protein tyrosine kinase activity of the expressed protein (Bargmann and Weinberg 1988a). This qualitative change, which is far more limited than the large change that occurs in *erbB*, converts a normal cell-surface receptor into a transforming protein, presumably by inducing a conformational change that mimics the change induced by ligand binding. The mutation is specific for glutamic acid or glutamine; moreover, it exerts its transforming effect even with extensive N′ and C′ deletions (Bargmann and Weinberg 1988b).

*3. The Macrophage Colony Stimulating Factor-1 Receptor and v-*fms

v-*fms*, the oncogene of feline sarcoma virus, is derived from the proto-oncogene for the macrophage colony stimulating factor-1 (CSF-1) receptor (Sherr et al. 1985). Comparison of the primary sequences of the human CSF-1 receptor (c-*fms*) with feline v-*fms* reveals 84% amino acid homology (Coussens et al. 1986). At least two mutations appear to be required for conversion to a transforming protein. Like v-*src* and c-*src* (Cartwright et al. 1987; Kmiecik and Shalloway 1987; Piwnica-Worms et al. 1987), v-*fms* and c-*fms* differ in their C′ termini, with v-*fms* containing a deleted and altered C′ terminus. Placing the C′ terminus of c-*fms* onto v-*fms* reduces, but does not abolish its transforming activity (Roussel et al. 1987). Mutation of a tyrosine in this region to phenylalanine restores full transforming activity to the v-*fms*/c-*fms* chimera, suggesting that this residue, like the C′ terminal tyrosine in c-*src*, is inhibitory and its removal enhances activity. Although v-*fms* has transforming activity independent of ligand, c-*fms* is not transforming, even when the C′ terminal tyrosine is replaced with phenylalanine. Recent studies have identified the cell-surface ligand-binding domain as the site of the second transforming mutation, which confers ligand-independent, constitutively active protein tyrosine kinase activity (Roussel et al. 1988a). The major mutation responsible for transformation is conversion of leucine to serine at residue 301 with a second enhancing mutation at residue 374 (Roussel et al. 1988a; Woolford et al. 1988). Mutant c-*fms* binds CSF-1 with high affinity but does not require the ligand to transform cells, i.e., the change induces an active conformation without affecting the ligand-binding site.

Cotransfection of cells with a cDNA that directs production of the CSF-1 ligand and with the nontransforming c-*fms* results in cell transformation (Roussel et al. 1987). Mutations in the amino and carboxyl termini of the CSF-1 receptor thus convert a ligand-dependent growth factor receptor into a constitutively active, ligand-independent oncoprotein, v-*fms*. Mutations cause a state that mimics continuous activation of the growth factor receptor induced by binding its ligand. Ligand-dependent transformation is greater in the c-*fms* construction containing phenylalanine in its C′ terminal region than in the wild type containing tyrosine. Like the EGF receptor, the ligand-binding domain of the CSF-1 receptor appears to be the dominant regulator of activity, with the C′ terminus also serving a regulatory role.

Mutations in diverse regions of growth factor receptors thus abrogate restraints and convert ligand-dependent protein tyrosine kinases into constitutively active enzymes that are transforming. The fact that such diverse constraints exist in normal receptors emphasizes the strong evolutionary pressure to restrict growth to environmentally appropriate conditions. Mutations involving the ligand-binding domain (EGF and CSF-1 receptors), transmembrane domain (*neu*), and carboxyl terminus (EGF and CSF-1 receptors and c-*src*) all convert normal regulatory proteins into constitutively active oncoproteins. Additional cell-surface receptors with intrinsic protein tyrosine kinase activity have been identified as retroviral oncogenes, although the ligands for the proto-oncogene receptors have not been identified. Among these are the oncogenes v-*kit* (Yarden et al. 1987), *met* (Park et al. 1987), *ros* (Neckameyer et al. 1986), and *trk*, identified as a fusion gene in which the tyrosine kinase domain is fused to tropomyosin (Martin-Zanca et al. 1986; Oskam et al. 1988).

B. Quantitative: Activation by Increased Expression

Quantitative increases in either ligand or receptor are sufficient to perturb the mass action equilibrium and result in transformation. v-*sis*, the oncogene of the simian sarcoma virus, represents the B chain of platelet-derived growth factor (PDGF) (Doolittle et al. 1983; Waterfield et al. 1983). This structural identity provided the first evidence clearly linking growth factors to oncogenes. Constitutive overexpression of c-*sis* to form B-chain homodimers of PDGF results in activation of the PDGF receptor, a member of the growth factor receptor protein tyrosine kinase gene family (Fig. 2) (Yarden et al. 1986). Constitutive overproduction of tumor growth factor α (TGF-α), of EGF, and of CSF-1 encoded by cDNA constructs (Rosenthal et al. 1986; Roussel et al. 1987; Stern et al. 1987) similarly results in transformation, acting, as does v-*sis*, through structurally normal growth factor receptors (see Chapter 2). These examples provide strong support for the concept that tumorigenesis results from excessive activity of normal growth-controlling pathways.

There is controversy as to whether v-*sis* must be secreted to act via binding to PDGF receptors located on the cell surface or whether v-*sis*, during its synthesis and processing in the endoplasmic reticulum, activates nascent PDGF receptors within the cell during their synthesis and transit to the surface. Evidence for secretion and action at the cell surface derives from experiments in which removal of the signal peptide abolished the transforming activity of v-*sis* (Hannink and Donoghue 1984) and from experiments in which v-*sis* was placed under control of a heat-shock promoter (Hannink and Donoghue 1988). Heat-shock induction of v-*sis* expression resulted in PDGF receptor autophosphorylation and c-*fos* induction. Because these responses were blocked by monensin and suramin, it was argued that only secreted v-*sis* is active. Evidence for action within the cell derives from the inability to quantitatively block transforming activity with addition of anti-PDGF antibodies to the exterior of the cell (Huang et al. 1984), from detection of ligand-stimulated self-phosphorylation of immature PDGF receptors (Keating and Williams 1988), and from continued transforming activity of v-*sis* constructed to contain the endoplasmic reticulum retention sequence (T. Deuel, pers. comm.). Resolution of this question is conceptually important to the question of whether altered cellular distribution of kinases would bring them into contact with normally prohibited substrates. In the case of v-*src* and v-*erbB*, mutational analysis indicates these must localize to the normal expected position of their proto-oncogenes at the cell membrane to act as transforming proteins (Beug and Hayman 1984; Kamps et al. 1985; Pellman et al. 1985). Resolution of this problem may also clarify the importance of ligand-induced endocytosis and down-regulation of cell-surface receptors. This process, which decreases the concentration of cell-surface receptors, will only affect information provided by cell-surface receptors; nascent intracellular receptors will escape this form of inhibitory regulation.

Cells produce growth factors that may act on other cells or on the producer cell itself. Self-stimulation, termed autocrine to distinguish it from classic endocrine control via circulating hormones, was initially recognized as a property of many transformed cells (Todaro et al. 1979). Several growth factors, including agonists for the EGF receptor (TGF-α, PDGF, melanoma growth factor [Richmond et al. 1988] and insulin-like growth factors) have been identified. Autonomous production of growth factors by transformed cells provides a growth advantage via such autocrine loops. However, growth factor production is not limited to transformed cells; normal cells also produce growth factors. In fact, induction of genes encoding growth factors is one mechanism through which activated growth factor receptors work to integrate multicellular responses characteristic of developmental and reparative processes.

Insulin and insulin-like growth factor-I (IGF-I), which are structurally homologous (Blundell et al. 1978), are also produced in response to hormones to integrate responses. Synthesis of IGF-I depends on growth hormone (Salmon and Daughaday 1957); its synthesis is also regulated by thyroid hormone and nutritional status. The receptors for insulin and IGF-I are, like their ligands, structurally homologous (Fig. 2) (Ebina et al. 1985; Ullrich et al. 1985; Yarden and Ullrich 1988). The cloned cDNA for the insulin receptor predicts a precursor protein containing a signal peptide followed by the α chain and then the β chain in which the single transmembrane and protein tyrosine kinase domains are located. Cross-linking studies suggest the insulin receptor exists as a tetramer composed of two α and two β subunits (Massague et al. 1980); the α and β subunits are separable, indicating cleavage during maturation of the receptor. The close structural homology between insulin and IGF-I and their two receptors allows each ligand to bind and activate the opposite receptor, although with approximately one order of magnitude change in affinity (Rosen 1987). Oncogenes derived from these ligands and receptors have not yet been identified; however, production of IGFs by transformed cells is common and may contribute to autocrine-stimulated growth of the producer tumor cells (Todaro et al. 1979).

Provided even minute concentrations of ligand are available, formation of the active ligand · receptor complex will be favored by increasing the concentration of receptor. In human tumors, gene amplification is the most commonly occurring mechanism through which increased expression of growth factor receptors occurs. Other possible, but undocumented, mechanisms to increase receptor concentration are increased gene transcription due to mutations in regulatory elements and increased gene transcription due to stabilization of synthesized mRNA or protein. Increased receptor expression can be obtained experimentally by placing the receptor-encoding cDNA under control of strong viral promoters.

Human epidermoid carcinoma A-431 cells that express large numbers of EGF receptors were first shown to have amplified EGF receptor genes (Lin et al. 1984; Ullrich et al. 1984; Xu et al. 1984). Direct analysis of brain tumor specimens indicated that the EGF receptor gene is amplified in ~40% of human glioblastoma multiforme tumors (Libermann et al. 1985). Gene amplification occurs in epidermoid carcinomas, in breast cancer cells, and in other tumor types, although the frequency with which this occurs is uncertain and likely less than in glioblastoma multiforme. When clonal A-431 cells, selected for varying degrees of EGF receptor gene amplification, were implanted into athymic mice, the rate of tumor growth was directly proportional to the extent of gene amplification, consistent with increased receptors imparting a distinct growth advantage (Santon et al. 1986).

Analysis of breast cancer specimens from a well-characterized patient population revealed amplification of the *erbB2/neu* gene in the subset of patients whose tumors had the most aggressive behavior and whose survival was worst (Slamon et al. 1987). The clear implication is that amplification of this growth factor receptor gene imparts a growth advantage for involved breast cancer cells. Other studies have linked *erbB2/neu* amplification to a specific breast cancer cell type without identification of clear prognostic implications (van de Vijver et al. 1988). Because gene amplification is relatively easy to detect and because not all activating mutations have been defined, it is not yet possible to assess the relative contributions of qualitative versus quantitative alterations in growth factor receptors to human oncogenesis. Both likely result from mutations and both may have specific genetic backgrounds in which they occur.

Compared to the oncogenic allele of *erbB2/neu* with its glutamic acid substitution, the normal allele is not transforming (Hung et al. 1986). However, if *erbB2/neu* cDNA is placed under control of a strong viral transcription promoter, it behaves as a transforming protein in focus-forming, soft agar colony-forming, and athymic mice tumor-forming assay systems (Di Fiore et al. 1987a). Similarly, the EGF and CSF-1 receptors are transforming when transcription of their respective genes is enhanced by strong viral promoters. The latter two receptors are clearly ligand-dependent for their transforming activity. Thus, quantitative increases in the normal receptor as well as in the normal ligand can, by mass action, result in cell transformation.

III. GROWTH FACTOR RECEPTORS THAT OPERATE THROUGH OTHER SIGNALING MECHANISMS

Although less is known about the mechanisms through which growth factor receptors that lack intrinsic protein tyrosine kinase activity operate, elucidation of their structures is providing insight into this important question. Two general structures have been identified: those that span the membrane seven times, the "seven-membrane-spanning motif" initially identified in bacteriorhodopsin, eukaryotic photon receptor rhodopsins, and the acetylcholine receptor (Nathans and Hogness 1983; Kubo et al. 1986); and those that are predicted to contain a single membrane-spanning segment (described above). Among growth factor receptors, the angiotensin receptor is paradigmatic for the first class and the growth hormone receptor for the second.

Reasoning that focus-forming assays using NIH-3T3 cells might not detect certain classes of oncogenes, Wigler and colleagues (Fasano et al. 1984) developed an alternative assay. Tumor DNA was cotransfected along with plasmid DNA containing a selectable antibiotic-resistance marker. Successfully transfected cells were selected by antibiotic resistance and assayed for tumorigenicity by injection into athymic mice. Although the method is "leaky" in that rearrangements may occur revealing oncogenes irrelevant to the initial tumor, it can nonetheless reveal proto-oncogenes that are candidates for conversion to oncogenes by either qualitative or quantitative mechanisms. Through use of such an approach, a gene encoding a seven-membrane-spanning protein was isolated from a human epidermoid carcinoma and given the cognomen *mas* (Young et al. 1986) (Fig. 3). Like the adrenergic receptors that exhibit this structure (Dixon et al. 1986), the *mas* cDNA was produced from a gene that lacked introns. The isolated *mas* gene was rearranged in its 5′ end outside the coding region, an event which likely occurred, not in the original tumor,

A. Receptors With 7 Membrane Spanning Motif

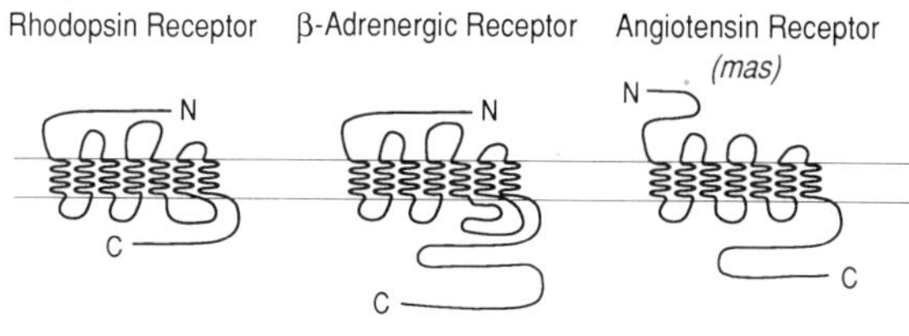

B. Receptors With a Single Membrane Spanning Domain

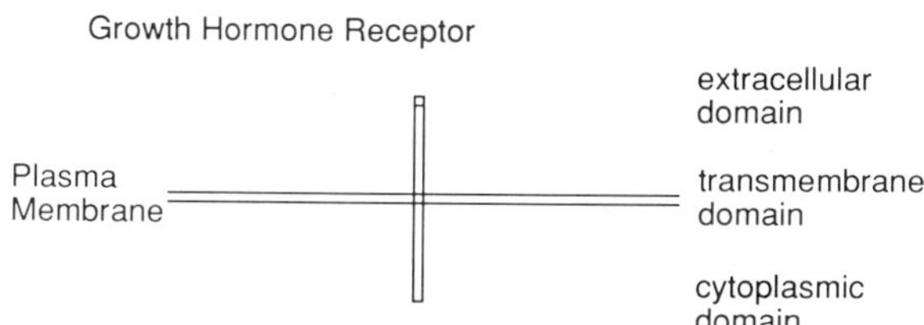

Figure 3 Schematic representation of receptors lacking intrinsic protein tyrosine kinase activity. (*A*) Receptors with seven predicted membrane-spanning domains. Sites of phosphorylation are located in the C′ terminus of the rhodopsin receptor and in the C′ terminus and cytoplasmic domain located between the fifth and sixth membrane-spanning domains of the β-adrenergic receptor. (Derived from Sibley et al. 1981 and Young et al. 1986.) (*B*) Receptor with a predicted single membrane-spanning domain. Structure of the growth hormone receptor is based on data of Leung et al. 1987.

but during transfection of the original human tumor DNA. The normal *mas* gene from placenta was transforming when placed in context of the rearranged 5′ end of oncogenic *mas* or behind the SV40 promoter. This indicated tumorigenicity likely resulted from quantitative alterations, rather than from a change in structure of the receptor itself.

The *mas* gene was subsequently identified as a receptor for angiotensin (Jackson et al. 1988). *Xenopus* oocytes injected with *mas* mRNA exhibited a dose-dependent inward current in response to angiotensins. Transfection of *mas* cDNA into a neural cell line and selection by antibiotic resistance yielded angiotensin-responsive clones. These clones increased cytosolic Ca^{++} in response to graded doses of angiotensin and, when serum starved, increased DNA synthesis in response to angiotensin. The *mas* gene thus behaved as a ligand-dependent growth factor. More than a decade previously, angiotensin had been shown to be mitogenic for cultured bovine adrenocortical cells, a physiological target for angiotensin (Gill et al. 1977).

A large body of pharmacological data indicates that angiotensin operates via stimulation of the phosphatidylinositol cycle to generate the two second messengers produced by this system: Ca^{++} and diacylglycerol (Kojima et al. 1984) (see below and Chapter 4). It is possible there is an angiotensin receptor subfamily analogous to the α and β adrenergic receptor and serotonin receptor subfamilies. Interestingly, overexpression of the serotonin receptor (Julius et al. 1988) results in transformation (Julius et al. 1989). Receptors with the seven-membrane-spanning motif may function as growth regulators during development in addition to their well-described roles in signal transduction.

An example of a non-tyrosine-kinase receptor having a single membrane-spanning domain is provided by the growth hormone receptor. Growth hormone, produced in the anterior pituitary gland, is essential for normal somatic growth with long-recognized syndromes of ateliotic dwarfism and gigantism resulting from prepubertal deficiences and excesses, respectively. Growth hormone is structurally closely related to prolactin, which regulates breast growth and milk production in mammals, and to chorionic somatomammotropin, the peptide hormone produced in greatest quantities by the placenta. Growth hormone stimulates production of IGF-I, a major mediator of many of the somatic growth-promoting properties of growth hormone. The cDNA clone for the growth hormone receptor predicts a 620-amino-acid protein with a single membrane-spanning domain (Leung et al. 1987) (Fig. 3). There are an 18-amino-acid signal sequence (precursor = 630 amino acids) and five potential N-linked glycosylation sites in the extracellular ligand-binding domain. The cysteine repeats evident in the extracellular domain of protein tyrosine kinase growth factor receptors are not present, nor are there recognizable protein kinase homologies in the cytoplasmic domain. The plasma growth-hormone-binding protein corresponds to the extracellular ligand portion of the receptor and is likely derived from the holoreceptor. Lorain dwarfs lack plasma human growth-hormone-binding activity and growth-hormone-stimulated IGF-I, although they have growth hormone itself (Daughaday et al. 1969). The genetic defect in this inherited form of dwarfism is thus likely due to a mutation involving the growth hormone receptor. Assuming that homologies between ligand structures extend to their receptors, those for prolactin and chorionic somatomammotropin can be predicted to have a structure similar to that of the growth hormone receptor.

IV. REGULATION OF RECEPTOR EXPRESSION AND ACTIVITY

Because the concentration of both ligand and receptor determines the concentration of the active ligand · receptor complex (see equation), extensive control mechanisms have evolved to regulate the concentration of each. The concentration of ligand is determined by a variety of mechanisms that operate not only at synthesis, but also at delivery in processes such as breakdown of platelets in wound healing (PDGF), recruitment of producer cells such as macrophages (fibroblast growth factor [FGF]) (Ross et al. 1986), binding protein delivery to receptors (IGF-I) (Clemmons et al. 1986), and perhaps cell-to-cell communication as in the sevenless · bride of sevenless system involved in development of the compound eye of *Drosophila*.

Receptor concentration is regulated both by cognate ligands and by other receptor-induced signals that serve to coordinate pathways in complex systems. Ligand binding serves to initiate signal (information) transduction and also to signal metabolic regulation of the receptor. On ligand binding, EGF receptors, which are diffusely distributed on the cell surface, undergo rapid lateral mobility, clustering in coated pits, endocytosis, and receptor degradation (Carpenter 1987). In contrast to receptors for low-density lipoproteins, asialoglycoproteins, transferrin, and α_2 macroglobulin, which recycle to the cell surface after delivery of their ligands to the cell interior (Brown et al. 1983), the receptor for EGF is extensively degraded after internalization, resulting in loss of 80–90% of cell-surface receptors (Stoscheck and Carpenter 1984). Although there is debate as to whether ligand-induced endocytosis is intimately involved in signaling per se, it clearly desensitizes the cell to ligand action, necessitating sustained high concentrations of ligand to elicit growth responses. Removal of a C′ terminal regulatory region from the EGF receptor (the CaIn domain) creates a kinase-active receptor that fails to undergo ligand-induced endocytosis and down-regulation (Chen et al. 1989). Failure to attenuate receptor signaling results in cell transformation. Conversely, anti-*neu* receptor antibodies that induce down-regulation revert cells transformed by the *erbB2*/*neu* oncogene (Drebin et al. 1985). For both EGF and insulin receptors, ligand-induced endocytosis and degradation depend on the intrinsic protein tyrosine kinase activity of the receptor. Whether this reflects self-phosphorylation-induced allosteric changes in the receptor itself, allowing interaction with the endocytic and routing mechanisms of the cell, or whether this represents phosphorylation of cellular proteins dictating these processes is not known (Glenney et al. 1988; Honegger et al. 1987b). Ligand-induced down-regulation of the PDGF receptor appears to occur independent of its intrinsic protein tyrosine kinase activity (Escobedo et al. 1988).

Although not defined for the angiotensin/*mas* receptor, rhodopsin and adrenergic receptors down-regulate via a phosphorylation process. On ligand binding, phosphorylation of these seven-membrane-spanning receptors by a cellular kinase occurs (Sibley et al. 1987); phosphorylation facilitates interaction with "arrestin," a cellular protein that sequesters the receptor, and may prevent activation of GTP-binding proteins and catalytic cGMP phosphodiesterase (rhodopsin) or cyclase (adrenergic) (Wilden et al. 1986; Bennett and Sitaramayya 1988). On dissociation of ligand, the sequestered receptors rapidly recycle to the cell surface (Levitzki 1988).

There is control of receptor synthesis as well as control of receptor metabolism. Both EGF and the tumor promoter TPA increase EGF receptor mRNA and protein (Clark et al. 1985; Earp et al. 1986; Bjorge et al. 1987). EGF-binding sites are reported to increase with administration of retinoic acid, thyroid hormone, and estrogen. Although the mechanism for this increased ligand binding is not defined, the 5′ promoter region of the EGF receptor contains DNA sequences that dictate inductive responses to EGF, cAMP, TPA, retinoic acid, and dexamethasone (Hudson et al. 1989). The 5′ promoter regions of both the EGF and insulin receptors are GC-rich, lacking classic TATA and CAAT sequences (Ishii et al. 1985). Analyses of control sequences within the 5′ end of the EGF receptor gene indicate a binding sequence for an EGF receptor transcription factor (Kageyama et al. 1988b), a TC-rich region that binds another protein factor (Johnson et al. 1988), sites for the transcription factor SP1 (Kageyama et al. 1988a), and a proximal 134-bp region sufficient to direct transcriptional induction by the five stimulators listed above (Hudson et al. 1989). Expression of the EGF receptor gene is, not surprisingly, extensively and exquisitely regulated by a variety of environmental factors, a paradigm likely necessary for growth factor receptors during development and postnatal life.

Because heterologous regulation of receptors serves a coordinating function, it may be either inhibitory or augmentatory. On addition of the tumor promoter TPA, which directly activates protein kinase C (Nishizuka 1988), or addition of stimulators of the phosphatidylinositol cycle to increase diacylglycerol, the endogenous activator of protein kinase C, high-affinity EGF receptor binding is diminished concomitant with decreased EGF-stimulated protein tyrosine kinase activity (Shoyab et al. 1979; Cochet et al. 1984). TPA in vivo and protein kinase C in vitro catalyze phosphorylation of the EGF receptor at threonine 654, an amino acid residue located between the inner membrane surface and the ATP-binding site (Hunter et al. 1984). Mutational removal of this phosphorylation site is reported to have variable effects: either abolition of the effects of TPA on high-affinity EGF binding (Lin et al. 1986) or abolition of the effects of TPA to decrease EGF-stimulated protein tyrosine kinase activity and biological consequences (Livneh et al. 1988). These mechanistic conclusions are not mutually exclusive, and varying results may depend on the particular EGF receptor clone used. Direct phosphorylation of the EGF receptor by protein kinase C and by other unidentified kinases (Davis and Czech 1987; Heisermann and Gill 1988) clearly occurs with significant effects on activity of the EGF receptor.

In addition to heterologous regulation of growth factor receptors by cellular kinases, phosphorylation of one receptor by another may occur. The EGF receptor catalyzes phosphorylation of c-*neu* (Stern and Kamps 1988); analysis of immunoprecipitated c-*neu* suggests its intrinsic protein tyrosine kinase activity is enhanced by this phosphorylation.

V. SIGNALING PATHWAYS

Signaling, initiated by activation of growth factor receptors, must be propagated and diffused throughout the cell to elicit complex cellular responses such as transit of the cell division cycle. A plethora of changes have been described; many of these likely represent supportive biochemical processes required for growth; others represent regulatory changes essential for a cell to progress through the cell cycle. Changes in response to stimuli must be considered in a temporal framework of events that precede them and of events that will occur as a consequence of their action.

A first question has been: What are the essential early substrates phosphorylated by activated protein tyrosine kinase growth factor receptors? Several cellular substrates have been identified either by their size and charge characteristics or as known cellular proteins (Hunter and Cooper 1985). A change in activity of one of the substrates that is due to tyrosine phosphorylation and in turn affects the process of transformation has not, however, been convincingly demonstrated. This difficulty is highlighted by studies of mutants of $p60^{v\text{-}src}$ that fail to localize to the cell membrane. Extensive cell tyrosine protein phosphorylation occurs in cells infected by virus-containing mutant enzyme, but transformation is limited to cells infected by wild-type virus containing membrane-associated $p60^{v\text{-}src}$ (Kamps et al. 1985; Pellman et al. 1985). This finding suggests that essential growth regulatory substrates may be localized at the inner surface of the plasma membrane. Identification of the substrates that are essential (and whose activity changes in response to phosphorylation) will require genetic and functional approaches in addition to biochemical approaches. The human cognate of a yeast serine/threonine protein kinase, cdc2 protein kinase, is phosphorylated on tyrosine in a cell-cycle-dependent manner (Draetta et al. 1988). Because this kinase is essential for yeast to progress through the cell division cycle, it is possible that information is transferred via a protein kinase cascade initiated by a protein tyrosine kinase, but changes in activity of a serine/threonine kinase in response to tyrosine phosphorylation have not yet been demonstrated. A similar question exists for other kinases stimulated in response to activated cell-surface receptors. Growth-controlling substrates for protein kinase C and Ca^{++} · calmodulin-dependent protein kinase enzymes activated in response to second messengers generated by the phosphatidylinositol cycle (angiotensin and the *mas* oncogene receptor activation) are yet to be convincingly demonstrated.

A second question has been: Which of the early responses are essential to initiation of growth and which are peripheral? An essential response can be considered one that, if lacking, abrogates cell growth. In response to growth factors such as EGF and PDGF, several rapid responses occur, including increased intracellular [Ca^{++}] concentrations (Moolenaar et al. 1984), activation of the Na^+/H^+ antiporter with a rise in intracellular pH (Pouyssegur et al. 1985), activation of the phosphatidylinositol cycle with generation of the two intracellular messengers diacylglycerol and inositol trisphosphate (Berridge 1987), and rapid induction of expression of a set of genes even in the absence of protein synthesis (Cochran et al. 1983). Although growth control mechanisms studied in diverse cell types may differ in detail, the basic pathways regulating growth and division are likely shared in common between all cells. The key questions concern how these central pathways are switched on following growth factor receptor activation.

Studies of protein regulators of transcription have suggested several mechanisms by which protein phosphorylation could stimulate entry into the cell growth cycle. Protein regulators of transcription are prominent members of the class of genes that are rapidly activated on growth factor addition to resting cells (Muller et al. 1984). *fos*, *myc*, and *jun* (AP-1) are especially interesting members of this class because each is the precursor of a strong retroviral oncogene (Kelly et al. 1983; Greenberg and Ziff 1984; Lamph et al. 1988). Additionally, expression of *myc* can largely, but not completely, abolish the requirement for growth factor addition (Armelin et al. 1984). Three mechanistic models for which there is experimental evidence are: (1) Phosphorylation of a transcription factor to enhance binding to its DNA recognition sequences and presumably its activity via dimer formation; evidence for this mechanism derives from studies of the protein that interacts with the DNA sequences specifying cAMP responses (cAMP response element binding, [CREB]) (Yamamoto et al. 1988). (2) Phosphorylation of an inhibitor that is complexed to a transcription factor to cause release of the transcription factor in an active form; evidence for this mechanism derives from studies of NF-κB, a transcriptional enhancer of immunoglobulin κ light-chain genes and a cytoplasmic protein that reversibly sequesters and inactivates it (Baeuerle and Baltimore 1988). (3) Phosphorylation of transcription factors outside their DNA-binding domain to enhance interaction with other components of the transcriptional apparatus; detailed studies of the yeast transcription factor GAL4 indicate that negative charge, positioned to the surface of an amphipathic helix, enhances transcription (Ptashne 1988). Covalent modification via phosphorylation could serve to reversibly add such negative charges to other transcription factors.

These models are neither inclusive nor exclusive; moreover, they are not meant to limit considerations of signal transduction to covalent modification of proteins via phosphorylation. They are presented as testable hypotheses that have important implications as biochemical mechanisms of cell growth control.

VI. GROWTH AND DEVELOPMENTAL PROGRAMS

Growth factors and their receptors, which play such well-documented roles in homeostasis and oncogenesis, are also centrally involved in regulating tissue development. Among the earliest developmental processes is formation of the mesoderm. Fertilized amphibian eggs exhibited polarity with the vegetal pole as precursor of endodermal structures and the animal pole as precursor of ectodermal structures. Microdissection indicated that mesoderm developed from animal pole cells in response to signals arising within the vegetal pole (Sudarwati and Nieuwkoop 1971). These signals include homologs of FGF and TFG-β, two well-characterized growth regulatory proteins. FGF and TGF-β act synergistically to induce mesodermal differentiation from animal pole cells (Kimelman and Kirschner 1987). Cloning of cDNAs from the developing blastula identified endogenous FGF- and TGF-β-like mRNAs, which formed a concentration gradient extending from vegetal to animal pole (Weeks and Melton 1987). Information directing amphibian mesoderm development from primitive ectoderm thus includes two growth factors initially characterized as mammalian growth regulators. FGF, a potent stimulator of mesodermal cell proliferation and of angiogenesis (Gospodarowicz et al. 1986), has been isolated as an oncogene from Kaposi's sarcoma (Deli Bovi et al. 1987). Mutations involving a structural homolog of FGF result in abnormal development in *Drosophila* (*int-2*) (Dickson et al. 1984). TGF-β, a member of a family of regulatory molecules, has profound and diverse effects on cell growth and function (Sporn and Roberts 1988).

Analysis of mutations that alter development supports the concept of reutilization of informational motifs. *notch*, a *Drosophila* mutation giving notched wings when heterozygous, results in abnormal neuroectodermal development when homozygous. Full expression of the *notch* mutation results in excessive development of precursor cells into neural derivatives with failure to adequately develop ectodermal progeny cells (Lehmann et al. 1983). Cloning of the *notch* locus reveals a predicted transmembrane precursor containing numerous EGF-like repeats (Wharton et al. 1985). Mutations in *notch* alter the EGF-like sequences (Kelley et al. 1987). *Lin 12*, a mutation affecting homeotic development in the nematode, *Caenorhabditis elegans*, involves a gene encoding 40 EGF-like repeat structures (Greenwald 1985). Both the *notch* and *Lin 12* mutations result in failure to provide proper developmental information via a sequence analogous to EGF, a growth factor originally identified in mouse submaxillary glands.

Development of the compound eye of *Drosophila* includes acquisition of the ability of the seventh cell of the ommatidia to sense UV light. The *sevenless* mutation affects a gene encoding a transmembrane protein with intrinsic tyrosine kinase activity analogous to other members of the growth factor protein tyrosine kinase gene family (Hafen et al. 1987). A second mutation, *bride of sevenless* (*boss*), also results in failure to develop the UV light sensing cell (R7) of the *Drosophila* eye (Reinke and Zipursky 1988). Genetic analysis of mosaic eyes indicates that the expression of this gene by the neighboring eighth cell of the retina is responsible for failure of development of R7, the UV sensing cell. These studies of developmental mutants indicate that the expression of *boss* by the photoreceptor cell R8 is required for R7 cell development. Environmental and positional information is provided by R8 expression of the probable ligand (*boss*) for the receptor expressed on R7 (*sevenless*). Mutants lacking either ligand or receptor fail to develop the ability to sense UV light due to failure of R7 development.

VII. SUMMARY

Many molecules have been identified that regulate cell proliferation occurring during development, growth, and repair. Among these, growth factors and their receptors play pleiotropic roles in providing cells with environmental information early during differentiation and development and later during regenerative and reparative growth. These molecules communicate information concerning both proliferation and expression of differentiated function. These regulators are themselves extensively regulated to provide multiple informational inputs to guide appropriate cell growth and development.

Information received at the cell surface must be processed by activated receptors through intermediates to stimulate a progressive series of gene activations that move a cell through the growth and division cycle. Mutations, acting via qualitative or quantitative changes in these regulators, can remove inhibitory constraints and result in uncontrolled cell proliferation. Oncogenes, originally identified in RNA tumor viruses and subsequently in human tumors, represent such mutated regulators. The biochemical mechanisms through which growth factors and receptors (both normal and mutated) operate are multiple, but covalent modification of proteins by phosphorylation is among the most common.

Oncogenes derived from growth factors and their receptors are largely dominant in action, i.e., enhanced activity as represented by the protein tyrosine kinase gene family. Growth inhibitors and tumor suppressors operate normally as part of the system of checks and balances on growth.

Deletion or inactivation of inhibitors has the effect of removing restraints to stimulators and results in unchecked cell proliferation, i.e., tumorigenesis. Inherited malignancies and the transforming activity of DNA tumor viruses, which do not themselves carry cellular oncogenes, may both result from loss or inactivation of these growth-restraining molecules.

Despite many advances, there are more unanswered than answered questions concerning growth control and oncogenesis. A framework is being provided by studies of normal growth control and of aberrations that occur in cancer. Two current lines of inquiry that build on this framework should provide deeper insights into central questions of growth control: (1) Mechanistic studies that define how signal transduction occurs, how information is processed within the cell via intermediates and interactive pathways, how gene transcription is regulated, and how the enzymology of DNA synthesis and cell division works; and (2) integrative studies that define temporal developmental programs, tumor suppressor genes and growth restraining processes, interactions between growth stimulatory and inhibitory gene products and pathways, and the influence of the genetic background on the occurrence of cancer.

ACKNOWLEDGMENTS

Studies from the author's laboratory were supported by grants from the National Institutes of Health, the American Cancer Society, the Council for Tobacco Research—U.S.A., Inc., and the Lucille P. Markey Charitable Trust.

REFERENCES

Armelin, H.A., M.C.S. Armelin, K. Kelly, T. Stewart, P. Leder, B.H. Cochran, and C.D. Stiles. 1984. Functional role for c-*myc* in mitogenic response to platelet-derived growth factor. *Nature* **310:** 655–660.

Baeuerle, P.A. and D. Baltimore. 1988. IKβ: A specific inhibitor of the NF-Kβ transcription factor. *Science* **242:** 540–546.

Bargmann, C.I. and R.A. Weinberg. 1988a. Increased tyrosine kinase activity associated with the protein encoded by the activated *neu* oncogene. *Proc. Natl. Acad. Sci.* **85:** 5394–5398.

———. 1988b. Oncogenic activation of the *neu*-encoded receptor protein by point mutation and deletion. *EMBO J.* **7:** 2043–2052.

Bargmann, C.I., M.-C. Hung, and R.A. Weinberg. 1986a. The *neu* oncogene encodes an epidermal growth factor receptor-related protein. *Nature* **319:** 226–230.

———. 1986b. Multiple independent activations of the *neu* oncogene by a point mutation altering the transmembrane domain of p185. *Cell* **45:** 649–657.

Bennett, N. and A. Sitaramayya. 1988. Inactivation of photoexcited rhodopsin in retinal rods: The roles of rhodopsin kinase and 48-kDa protein (arrestin). *Biochemistry* **27:** 1710–1715.

Berridge, M.J. 1987. Inositol trisphosphate and diacylglycerol: Two interacting second messengers. *Annu. Rev. Biochem.* **56:** 159–193.

Bertics, P.J. and G.N. Gill. 1985. Self-phosphorylation enhances the protein-tyrosine kinase activity of the epidermal growth factor receptor. *J. Biol. Chem.* **260:** 14642–14647.

Beug, H. and M.J. Hayman. 1984. Temperature-sensitive mutants of avian erythroblastosis virus: Surface expression of the *erbB* product correlates with transformation. *Cell* **36:** 963–972.

Beug, H., S. Palmieri, C. Freudenstein, H. Zentgraf, and T. Graf. 1982. Hormone-dependent terminal differentiation in vitro of chicken erythroleukemia cells transformed by ts mutants of avian erythroblastosis virus. *Cell* **28:** 907–919.

Bjorge, J.D. and J.E. Kudlow. 1987. Epidermal growth factor receptor synthesis is stimulated by phorbol ester and epidermal growth factor: Evidence for a common mechanism. *J. Biol. Chem.* **262:** 6615–6622.

Blundell, T.L., S. Bedarkar, E. Rinderknecht, and R.E. Humbel. 1978. Insulin-like growth factor: A model for tertiary structure accounting for immunoreactivity and receptor binding. *Proc. Natl. Acad. Sci.* **75:** 180–184.

Brown, M.S., R.G.W. Anderson, and J.L. Goldstein. 1983. Recycling receptors: The round-trip itinerary of migrant membrane proteins. *Cell* **32:** 663–667.

Carpenter, G.K., J. Lembach, M.M. Morrison, and S. Cohen. 1975. Characterization of the binding of ^{125}I-labeled epidermal growth factor to human fibroblasts. *J. Biol. Chem.* **250:** 4297–4304.

Carpenter, G. 1987. Receptors for epidermal growth factor and other polypeptide mitogens. *Annu. Rev. Biochem.* **56:** 881–914.

Cartwright, C.A., W. Eckhart, S. Simon, and P.L. Kaplan. 1987. Cell transformation by pp60$^{c\text{-}src}$ mutated in the carboxy-terminal regulatory domain. *Cell* **49:** 83–91.

Chen, W.S., C.S. Lazar, M. Poenie, R.Y. Tsien, G.N. Gill, and M.G. Rosenfeld. 1987. Requirement for intrinsic protein tyrosine kinase in the immediate and late actions of the EGF receptor. *Nature* **328:** 820–823.

Chen, W.S., C.S. Lazar, K.A. Lund, J.B. Walsh, C.-P. Chang, G.M. Walton, C.J. Dur, H.S. Wiley, G.N. Gill, and M.G. Rosenfeld. 1989. Functional independence of the epidermal growth factor receptor from a domain required for ligand-induced internalization and calcium regulation. *Cell* **59:** (in press).

Chou, C.K., T.J. Dull, D.S. Russell, R. Gherzi, D. Lebwohl, A. Ullrich, and O.M. Rosen. 1987. Human insulin receptors mutated at the ATP-binding site lack protein tyrosine kinase activity and fail to mediate postreceptor effects of insulin. *J. Biol. Chem.* **262:** 1842–1847.

Clark, A.J.L., S.Ishii, N. Richert, G.T. Merlino, and I. Pastan. 1985. Epidermal growth factor regulates the expression of its own receptor. *Proc. Natl. Acad. Sci.* **82:** 8374–8378.

Clemmons, D.R., R.G. Elgin, V.K. Han, S.J. Casella, A.J. D'Ercole, and J.J. Van Wyk. 1986. Cultured fibroblast monolayers secrete a protein that alters the cellular binding of somatomedin-C/insulin-like growth factor I. *J. Clin. Invest.* **77:** 1548–1556.

Cochet, C., G.N. Gill, J. Meisenhelder, J.A. Cooper, and T. Hunter. 1984. C-kinase phosphorylates the epidermal growth factor receptor and reduces its epidermal growth factor-stimulated tyrosine protein kinase activity. *J. Biol. Chem.* **259:** 2553–2558.

Cochran, B.H., A.C. Reffel, and C.D. Stiles. 1983. Molecular cloning of gene sequences regulated by platelet-derived growth factor. *Cell* **33:** 939–947.

Cohen, S. 1962. Isolation of a mouse submaxillary gland protein accelerating incisor eruption and eyelid opening in the new-born animal. *J. Biol. Chem.* **237:** 1555–1562.

Courtneidge, S.A. and A.E. Smith. 1984. The complex of polyoma virus middle-T antigen and pp60$^{c\text{-}src}$. *EMBO J.* **3:** 585–591.

Coussens, L., C. Van Beveren, D. Smith, E. Chen, R.A.L. Mitchell, C.M. Isacke, I.M. Verma, and A. Ullrich. 1986. Structural alteration of viral homologue of receptor proto-oncogene *fsm* at carboxyl terminus. *Nature* **320:** 277–280.

Daughaday, W.H., Z. Laron, A. Pertzelan, and J.N. Heins. 1969. Defective sulfation factor generation: A possible etiological link in dwarfism. *Trans. Assoc. Am. Physicians* **82:** 129–140.

Davis, R.J. and M.P. Czech. 1987. Stimulation of epidermal growth factor receptor threonine 654 phosphorylation by platelet-derived growth factor in protein kinase C-deficient human fibroblasts. *J. Biol. Chem.* **262:** 6832–6841.

Delli-Bovi, P., A.M. Curatola, F.G. Kern, A.Greco, M. Ittmann, and C. Basilico. 1987. An oncogene isolated by transfection of Kaposi's sarcoma DNA encodes a growth factor that is a member of the FGF family. *Cell* **50:** 729–737.

Dickson, C., R. Smith, S. Brookes, and G. Peters. 1984. Tumorigenesis by mouse mammary tumor virus: Proviral activation of a cellular gene in the common integration region *int*-2. *Cell* **37:** 529–536.

Di Fiore, P.P., J.H. Pierce, M.H. Kraus, O. Segatto, C.R. King, and S.A. Aaronson. 1987a. *erb*B-2 is a potent oncogene when overexpressed in NIH/3T3 cells. *Science* **237:** 178–182.

Di Fiore, P.P., J.H. Pierce, T.P. Fleming, R. Hazan, A. Ullrich, C.R. King, J. Schlessinger, and S.A. Aaronson. 1987b. Overexpression of the human EGF receptor confers an EGF-dependent transformed phenotype to NIH 3T3 cells. *Cell* **51:** 1063–1070.

Dixon, R.A.F., B.K. Kobilka, D.J. Strader, J.L. Benovic, H.G. Dohlman, T. Frielle, M.A. Bolanowski, C.D. Bennett, E. Rands, R.E. Diehl, R.A. Mumford, E.E. Slater, I.S. Sigal, M.G. Caron, R.J. Lefkowitz, and C.D. Strader. 1986. Cloning of the gene and cDNA for mammalian β-adrenergic receptor and homology with rhodopsin. *Nature* **321:** 75–79.

Doolittle, R.F., M.W. Hunkapiller, L.E. Hood, S.G. Devare, K.C. Robbins, S.A. Aaronson, and H.N. Antoniades. 1983. Simian sarcoma virus *onc* gene, v-*sis*, is derived from the gene (or genes) encoding a platelet-derived growth factor. *Science* **221:** 275–277.

Downward, J., P. Parker, and M.D. Waterfield. 1984a. Autophosphorylation sites on the epidermal growth factor receptor. *Nature* **311:** 483–485.

Downward, J., Y. Yarden, E. Mayes, G. Scrace, N. Totty, P. Stockwell, A. Ullrich, J. Schlessinger, and M.D. Waterfield. 1984b. Close similarity of epidermal growth factor receptor and v-*erb*-B oncogene protein sequences. *Nature* **307:** 521–527.

Draetta, G., H. Piwnica-Worms, D. Morrison, B. Druker, T. Roberts, and D. Beach. 1988. Human cdc2 protein kinase is a major cell-cycle regulated tyrosine kinase substrate. *Nature* **336:** 738–744.

Drebin, J.A., V.C. Link, D.F. Stern, R.A. Weinberg, and M.I. Greene. 1985. Down-modulation of an oncogene protein product and reversion of the transformed phenotype by monoclonal antibodies. *Cell* **41:** 695–706.

Earp, H.S., K.S. Austin, J. Blaisdell, R.A. Rubin, K.G. Nelson, L.W. Lee, and J.W. Grisham. 1986. Epidermal growth factor (EGF) stimulates EGF receptor synthesis. *J. Biol. Chem.* **261:** 4777–4780.

Ebina, Y., E. Araki, M. Taira, F. Shimada, M. Mori, C.S. Craik, K. Siddle, S.B. Pierce, R.A. Roth, and W.J. Rutter. 1987. Replacement of lysine residue 1030 in the putative ATP-binding region of the insulin receptor abolishes insulin- and antibody-stimulated glucose uptake and receptor kinase activity. *Proc. Natl. Acad. Sci.* **84:** 704–708.

Ebina, Y., L. Ellis, K. Jarnagin, M. Edery, L. Graf, E. Clauser, J.-H. Ou, F. Masiarz, Y.W. Kan, I.D. Goldfine, R.A. Roth, and W.J. Rutter. 1985. The human insulin receptor cDNA: The structural basis for hormone-activated transmembrane signalling. *Cell* **40:** 747–758.

Eckhart, W., M.A. Hutchinson, and T. Hunter. 1979. An activity phosphorylating tyrosine in polyoma T antigen immunoprecipitates. *Cell* **18:** 925–933.

Engelman, D.M., T.A. Steitz, and A. Goldman. 1986. Identifying nonpolar transbilayer helices in amino acid sequences of membrane proteins. *Annu. Rev. Biophys. Biophys. Chem.* **15:** 321–353.

Escobedo, J.A., P.J. Barr, and L.T. Williams. 1988. Role of tyrosine kinase and membrane-spanning domains in signal transduction by the platelet-derived growth factor receptor. *Mol. Cell. Biol.* **8:** 5126–5131.

Fasano, O., D. Birnbaum, L. Edlund, J. Fogh, and M. Wigler. 1984. New human transforming genes detected by a tumorigenicity assay. *Mol. Cell. Biol.* **4:** 1695–1705.

Feige, J.-J. and I.E. Scheffler. 1987. Analysis of the protein glycosylation defect of a temperature-sensitive cell cycle mutant by the use of mutant cells overexpressing the human EGF receptor after transfection of the gene. *J. Cell Physiol.* **133:** 461–470.

Friend, S.H., R. Bernards, S. Rogelj, R.A. Weinberg, J.M. Rapaport, D.M. Albert, and T.P. Dryja. 1986. A human DNA segment with properties of the gene that predisposes to retinoblastoma and osteosarcoma. *Nature* **323:** 643–646.

Frykberg, L., S. Palmieri, H. Beug, T. Graf, M.-J. Hayman, and B. Vennstrom. 1983. Transforming capacities of avian erythroblastosis virus mutants deleted in the *erbA* or *erbB* oncogenes. *Cell* **32:** 227–238.

Fung, Y.-K.T., W.G. Lewis, L.B. Crittenden, and H.-J. Kung. 1983. Activation of the cellular oncogene c-*erbB* by LTR insertion: Molecular basis for induction of erythroblastosis by avian leukosis virus. *Cell* **33:** 357–368.

Gamett, D.C., S.E. Tracy, and H.L. Robinson. 1986. Differences in sequences encoding the carboxyl-terminal domain of the epidermal growth factor receptor correlate with differences in the disease potential of viral *erbB* genes. *Proc. Natl. Acad. Sci.* **83:** 6053–6057.

Gandrillon, O., P. Jurdic, M. Benchaibi, J.-H. Xiao, J. Ghysdael, and J. Samarut. 1987. Expression of the v-*erb*A oncogene in chicken embryo fibroblasts stimulates their proliferation in vitro and enhances tumor growth in vivo. *Cell* **49:** 687–697.

Gill, G.N., P.J. Bertics, and J.B. Santon. 1987. Epidermal growth factor and its receptors. *Mol. Cell. Endocrinol.* **51:** 169–186.

Gill, G.N., C.R. Ill, and M.H. Simonian. 1977. Angiotensin stimulation of bovine adrenocortical cell growth. *Proc. Natl. Acad. Sci.* **74:** 5569–5573.

Gill, G.N., W.S. Chen, C.S. Lazar, J.R. Glenney, Jr., H.S. Wiley, H.A. Ingraham, and M.G. Rosenfeld. 1988. Role of intrinsic protein tyrosine kinase in function and metabolism of the epidermal growth factor receptor. *Cold Spring Harbor Symp. Quant. Biol.* **53:** 467–476.

Gilmore, T., J.E. McClue, and G.S. Martin. 1985. Protein phosphorylation at tyrosine is induced by the v-*erbB* gene product in vivo and in vitro. *Cell* **40:** 609–618.

Glenney, J.R., Jr., W.S. Chen, C.S. Lazar, G.M. Walton, L.M. Zokas, M.G. Rosenfeld, and G.N. Gill. 1988. Ligand-induced endocytosis of the EGF receptor is blocked by mutational inactivation and by microinjection of anti-phosphotyrosine antibodies. *Cell* **52:** 675–684.

Gospodarowicz, D., G. Neufeld, and L. Schweigerer. 1986. Fibroblast growth factor. *Mol. Cell. Endocrinol.* **46:** 187–204.

Greenberg, M.E. and E.B. Ziff. 1984. Stimulation of 3T3 cells induces transcription of the c-*fos* proto-oncogene. *Nature* **311:** 433–438.

Greenwald, I. 1985. *lin-12*, a nematode homeotic gene, is homologous to a set of mammalian proteins that includes epidermal growth factor. *Cell* **43:** 583–590.

Hafen, E., K. Basler, J.-E. Edstroem, and G.M. Rubin. 1987. *Sevenless*, a cell-specific homeotic gene of *Drosophila*, encodes a putative transmembrane receptor with a tyrosine kinase domain. *Science* **236:** 55–63.

Hannink, M. and D.J. Donoghue. 1984. Requirement for a signal sequence in biological expression of the v-*sis* oncogene. *Science* **226:** 1197–1199.

———. 1985. Lysine residue 121 in the proposed ATP-binding site of the v-mos protein is required for transformation. *Proc. Natl. Acad. Sci.* **82:** 7894–7898.

———. 1988. Autocrine stimulation by the v-*sis* gene product requires a ligand-receptor interaction at the cell surface. *J. Cell Biol.* **107:** 287–298.

Heisermann, G.-J. and G.-N. Gill. 1988. Epidermal growth factor receptor threonine and serine residues phosphorylated *in vivo*. *J. Biol. Chem.* **263:** 13152–13158.

Honegger, A.M., D. Szapary, A. Schmidt, R. Lyall, E. Van Obberghen, T.J. Dull, A. Ullrich, and J. Schlessinger. 1987a. A mutant epidermal growth factor receptor with defective protein tyrosine kinase is unable to stimulate proto-oncogene expression and DNA synthesis. *Mol. Cell. Biol.* **7:** 4568–4571.

Honegger, A.-M., T.J. Dull, S. Felder, E. Van Obberghen, F. Bellot, D. Szapary, A. Schmidt, A. Ullrich, and J. Schlessinger. 1987b. Point mutation at the ATP binding site of EGF receptor abolishes protein-tyrosine kinase activity and alters cellular routing. *Cell* **51:** 199–209.

Huang, H.-J.S., J.-K. Yee, J.-Y. Shew, P.-L. Chen, R. Bookstein, T. Friedmann, E.Y.-H. Lee, and W.-H. Lee. 1988. Suppression of the neoplastic phenotype by replacement of the RB gene in human cancer cells. *Science* **242:** 1563–1566.

Huang, J.S., S.S. Huang, and T.F. Deuel. 1984. Transforming protein of simian sarcoma virus stimulates autocrine growth of SSV-transformed cells through PDGF cell-surface receptors. *Cell* **39:** 79–87.

Hudson, L.G., J.B. Santon, and G.N. Gill. 1989. Regulation of epidermal growth factor receptor gene expression. *Mol. Endocrinol.* **3:** 400–408.

Hung, M.-C., A.L. Schechter, P.-Y.M. Chevray, D.F. Stern, and R.A. Weinberg. 1986. Molecular cloning of the *neu* gene: Absence of gross structural alteration in oncogenic alleles. *Proc. Natl. Acad. Sci.* **83:** 261–264.

Hunter, T. 1987. A thousand and one protein kinases. *Cell* **50:** 823–829.

Hunter, T. and J.A. Cooper. 1985. Protein-tyrosine kinases. *Annu. Rev. Biochem.* **54:** 897–930.

Hunter, T. and B.M. Sefton. 1980. Transforming gene product of Rous sarcoma virus. *Proc. Natl. Acad. Sci.* **77:** 1311–1315.

Hunter, T., N. Ling, and J.A. Cooper. 1984. Protein kinase C phosphorylation of the EGF receptor at a threonine residue close to the cytoplasmic face of the plasma membrane. *Nature* **311:** 480–483.

Ishii, S., Y.-H. Xu, R.H. Stratton, B.A. Roe, G.T. Merlino, and I. Pastan. 1985. Characterization and sequence of the promoter region of the human epidermal growth factor receptor gene. *Proc. Natl. Acad. Sci.* **82:** 4920–4924.

Jackson, T.R., L.A.C. Blair, J. Marshall, M. Goedert, and M.R. Hanley. 1988. The *mas* oncogene encodes an angiotensin receptor. *Nature* **335:** 437–440.

Johnson, A.C., Y. Jinno, and G.T. Merlino. 1988. Modulation of epidermal growth factor receptor proto-oncogene transcription by a promoter site sensitive to S1 nuclease. *Mol. Cell. Biol.* **8:** 4174–4184.

Julius, D., T.J. Livelli, T.M. Jessell, and R. Axel. 1989. Ectopic expression of the serotonin 1c receptor and the triggering of malignant transformation. *Science* **244:** 1057–1062.

Julius, D., A.B. MacDermott, R. Axel, and T.M. Jessell. 1988. Molecular characterization of a functional cDNA encoding the serotonin 1c receptor. *Science* **241:** 558–564.

Kageyama, R., G.T. Merlino, and I. Pastan. 1988a. Epidermal growth factor (EGF) receptor gene transcription. *J. Biol. Chem.* **263:** 6329–6336.

———. 1988b. A transcription factor active on the epidermal growth factor receptor gene. *Proc. Natl. Acad. Sci.* **85:** 5016–5020.

Kamps, M.P., J.E. Buss, and B.M. Sefton. 1985. Mutation of NH_2-terminal glycine of $p60^{src}$ prevents both myristoylation and morphological transformation. *Proc. Natl. Acad. Sci.* **82:** 4625–4628.

Keating, M.T. and L.T. Williams. 1988. Autocrine stimulation of intracellular PDGF receptors in v-*sis*-transformed cells. *Science* **239:** 914–916.

Kelley, M.T., S. Kidd, W.A. Deutsch, and M.W. Young. 1987. Mutations altering the structure of epidermal growth factor-like coding sequences at the *Drosophila notch* locus. *Cell* **51:** 539–548.

Kelly, K., B.H. Cochran, C.D. Stiles, and P. Leder. 1983. Cell-specific regulation of the c-*myc* gene by lymphocyte mitogens and platelet-derived growth factor. *Cell* **35:** 603–610.

Khazaie, K., T.J. Dull, T. Graf, J. Schlessinger, A. Ullrich, H. Beug, and B. Vennstrom. 1988. Truncations of the human EGF receptor leads to differential transforming potentials in primary avian fibroblasts and erythroblasts. *EMBO J.* **7:** 3061–3071.

Kimelman, D. and M. Kirschner. 1987. Synergistic induction of mesoderm by FGF and TGF-β and the identification of an mRNA coding for FGF in the early *Xenopus* embryo. *Cell* **51:** 869–877.

Kmiecik, T.E. and D. Shalloway. 1987. Activation and suppression of pp60$^{c\text{-}src}$ transforming ability by mutation of its primary sites of tyrosine phosphorylation. *Cell* **49:** 65–73.

Kojima, I., K. Kojima, D. Kreutter, and H. Rasmussen. 1984. The temporal integration of the aldosterone secretory response to angiotensin occurs via two intracellular pathways. *J. Biol. Chem.* **259:** 14448–14457.

Kris, R.M., I. Lax, W. Gullick, M.D. Waterfield, A. Ullrich, M. Fridkin, and J. Schlessinger. 1985. Antibodies against a synthetic peptide as a probe for the kinase activity of the avian EGF receptor and v-erbB protein. *Cell* **40:** 619–625.

Kubo, T., K. Fukuda, A. Mikami, A. Maeda, H. Takahashi, M. Mishina, T. Haga, K., Haga, A. Ichiyama, K. Kangawa, M. Kojima, H. Matsuo, T. Hirose, and S. Numa. 1986. Cloning, sequencing and expression of complementary DNA encoding the muscarinic acetylcholine receptor. *Nature* **323:** 411–416.

Lamph, W.W., P. Wansley, P. Sassone-Corsi, and I.M. Verma. 1988. Induction of proto-oncogene *JUN*/AP-1 by serum and TPA. *Nature* **334:** 629–631.

Lax, I., A. Johnson, T. Howk, J. Sap, F. Bellot, M. Winkler, A. Ullrich, B. Vennstrom, J. Schlessinger, and D. Givol. 1988. Chicken epidermal growth factor (EGF) receptor: cDNA cloning, expression in mouse cells, and differential binding of EGF and transforming growth factor alpha. *Mol. Cell. Biol.* **8:** 1970–1978.

Lehmann, R., F. Jimenez, U. Dietrich, and J.A. Campos-Ortega. 1983. On the phenotype and development of mutants of early neurogenesis in *Drosophila melanogaster* Roux's arch. *Dev. Biol.* **192:** 62–75.

Leung, D.W., S.A. Spencer, G. Cachianes, R.G. Hammonds, C. Collins, W.J. Henzel, R. Barnard, M.J. Waters, and W.I. Wood. 1987. Growth hormone receptor and serum binding protein: Purification, cloning and expression. *Nature* **330:** 537–543.

Levi-Montalcini, R. and P.U. Angeletti. 1968. Nerve growth factor. *Physiol. Rev.* **48:** 534–569.

Levitzki, A. 1988. From epinephrine to cyclic AMP. *Science* **241:** 800–806.

Libermann, T.A., H.R. Nusbaum, N. Razon, R. Kris, I. Lax, H. Soreq, N. Whittle, M.D. Waterfield, A. Ullrich, and J. Schlessinger. 1985. Amplification enhanced expression and possible rearrangement of EGF receptor gene in primary human brain tumours of glial origin. *Nature* **313:** 144–147.

Lin, C.R., W.S. Chen, C.S. Lazar, C.D. Carpenter, G.N. Gill, R.M. Evans, and M.R. Rosenfeld. 1986. Protein kinase C phosphorylation at Thr 654 of the unoccupied EGF receptor and EGF binding regulate functional receptor loss by independent mechanisms. *Cell* **44:** 839–848.

Lin, C.R., W.S. Chen, W. Kruijer, L.S. Stolarsky, W.Weber, R.M. Evans, I.M. Verma, G.N. Gill, and M.G. Rosenfeld. 1984. Expression cloning of human EGF receptor complementary DNA: Gene amplification and three related messenger RNA products in A431 cells. *Science* **224:** 843–848.

Livneh, E., L. Glazer, D. Segal, J. Schlessinger, and B.-Z. Shilo. 1985. The *Drosophila* EGF receptor gene homolog: Conservation of both hormone binding and kinase domains. *Cell* **40:** 599–607.

Livneh, E., T.J. Dull, E. Berent, R. Prywes, A. Ullrich, and J. Schlessinger. 1988. Release of a phorbol ester-induced mitogenic block by mutation at Thr-654 of the epidermal growth factor receptor. *Mol. Cell. Biol.* **8:** 2302–2308.

Maegawa, H., D.A. McClain, G. Freidenberg, J.M. Olefsky, T.J. Dull, J. Lee, and A. Ullrich. 1988. Properties of a human insulin receptor with a COOH-terminal truncation: II. Truncated receptors have normal kinase activity but are defective in signaling metabolic effects. *J. Biol. Chem.* **263:** 8912–8917.

Martin-Zanca, D., S.H. Hughes, and M. Barbacid. 1986. A human oncogene formed by the fusion of truncated tropomyosin and protein tyrosine kinase sequences. *Nature* **319:** 743–748.

Massague, J., P.F. Pilch, and M.-P. Czech. 1980. Electrophoretic resolution of three major insulin receptor structures with unique subunit stoichiometries. *Proc. Natl. Acad. Sci.* **77:** 7137–7141.

Mayes. E.L.V. and M.D. Waterfield. 1984. Biosynthesis of the epidermal growth factor receptor in A431 cells. *EMBO J.* **3:** 531–537.

Moolenaar, W.H., L.G.J. Tertoolen, and S.W. de Laat. 1984. Growth factors immediately raise cytoplasmic free Ca^{2+} in human fibroblasts. *J. Biol. Chem.* **259:** 8066–8069.

Muller, R., R. Bravo, and J. Burckhardt. 1984. Induction of c-*fos* gene and protein by growth factors precedes activation of c-*myc*. *Nature* **312:** 716–720.

Nathans, J. and D.S. Hogness. 1983. Isolation, sequence analysis, and intron-exon arrangement of the gene encoding bovine rhodopsin. *Cell* **34:** 807–814.

Neckameyer, W.S., M. Shibuya, M.-T. Hsu, and L.-H. Wang. 1986. Proto-oncogene c-ros codes for a molecule with structural features common to those of growth factor receptors and displays tissue-specific and developmentally regulated expression. *Mol. Cell. Biol.* **6:** 1478–1486.

Ng, M. and M.L. Privalsky. 1986. Structural domains of the avian erythroblastosis virus *erbB* protein required for fibroblast transformation: Dissection by in-frame insertional mutagenesis. *J. Virol.* **58:** 542–553.

Nilsen, T.W., P.A. Maroney, R.G. Goodwin, F.M. Rottman, L.B. Crittenden, M.A. Raines, and H.-J. Kung. 1985. c-*erbB* activation in ALV-induced erythroblastosis: Novel RNA processing and promoter insertion result in expression of an amino-truncated EGF receptor. *Cell* **41:** 719–726.

Nishizuka, Y. 1988. The molecular heterogeneity of protein kinase C and its implications for cellular regulation. *Nature* **334:** 661–665.

Oskam, R., F. Coulier, M. Ernst, D. Martin-Zanca, and M. Barbacid. 1988. Frequent generation of oncogenes by *in vitro* recombination of *TRK* protooncogene sequences. *Proc. Natl. Acad. Sci.* **85:** 2964–2968.

Park, M., M. Dean, K. Kaul, M.J. Braun, M.A. Gonda, and G.V. Woude. 1987. Sequence of *met* protooncogene cDNA has features characteristic of the tyrosine kinase family of growth-factor receptors. *Proc. Natl. Acad. Sci.* **84:** 6379–6383.

Pellman, D., E.A. Garber, F.R. Cross, and H. Hanafusa. 1985. Fine structural mapping of a critical NH_2-terminal region of $p60^{src}$. *Proc. Natl. Acad. Sci.* **81:** 1623–1627.

Piwnica-Worms, H., K.B. Saunders, T.M. Roberts, A.E. Smith, and S.H. Cheng. 1987. Tyrosine phosphorylation regulates the biochemical and biological properties of $pp60^{c\text{-}src}$. *Cell* **49:** 75–82.

Pouyssegur, J., J.-C. Chambard, A. Franchi, G. L'Allemain, S. Paris, and E. Van Obberghen-Schilling. 1985. Growth-factor activation of the Na^+/H^+ antiporter controls growth of fibroblasts by regulating intracellular pH. *Cancer Cells* **3:** 409–415.

Privalsky, M.L., R. Ralson, and J.M. Bishop. 1984. The membrane glycoprotein encoded by the retroviral oncogene v-*erb-B* is structurally related to tyrosine-specific protein kinases. *Proc. Natl. Acad. Sci.* **81:** 704–707.

Ptashne, M. 1988. How eukaryotic transcriptional activators work. *Nature* **335:** 683–689.

Reinke, R. and S.L. Zipursky. 1988. Cell-cell interaction in the *Drosophila* retina: The *bride of sevenless* gene is required in photoreceptor cell R8 for R7 cell development. *Cell* **55:** 321–330.

Richmond, A., E. Balentien, H.G. Thomas, G. Flaggs, D.E. Barton, J. Spiess, R. Bordoni, U. Francke, and R. Derynck. 1988. Molecular characterization and chromosomal mapping of melanoma growth stimulatory activity, a growth factor structurally related to β-thromboglobulin. *EMBO J.* **7:** 2025–2033.

Rosen, O.M. 1987. After insulin binds. *Science* **237:** 1452–1458.

Rosenthal, A., P.B. Lindquist, T.S. Bringman, D.V. Goeddel, and R. Derynck. 1986. Expression in rat fibroblasts of a human transforming growth factor-α cDNA results in transformation. *Cell* **46:** 301–309.

Ross, R., E.W. Raines, and D.F. Bowen-Pope. 1986. The biology of platelet-derived growth factor. *Cell* **46:** 155–169.

Roussel, M.F., J.R. Downing, C.W. Rettenmier, and C.J. Sherr. 1988a. A point mutation in the extracellular domain of the human CSF-1 receptor (c-*fms* proto-oncogene product) activates its transforming potential. *Cell* **55:** 979–988.

Roussel, M.F., J.R. Downing, R.A. Ashmun, C.W. Rettenmier, and C.J. Sherr. 1988b. Colony-stimulating factor 1-mediated regulation of a chimeric c-*fms*/v-*fms* receptor containing the v-*fms*-encoded tyrosine kinase domain. *Proc. Natl. Acad. Sci.* **85:** 5903–5907.

Roussel, M.F., T.J. Dull, C.W. Rettenmier, P. Ralph, A. Ullrich, and C.J. Sherr. 1987. Transforming potential of the c-*fms* proto-oncogene (CSF-1 receptor). *Nature* **325:** 549–552.

Russell, D.S., R. Gherzi, E.L. Johnson, C.-K. Chou, and O.M. Rosen. 1987. The protein-tyrosine kinase activity of the insulin receptor is necessary for insulin-mediated receptor down-regulation. *J. Biol. Chem.* **262:** 11833–11840.

Salmon, W.D., Jr. and W.H. Daughaday. 1957. A hormonally controlled serum factor which stimulates sulfate incorporation by cartilage in vitro. *J. Lab. Clin. Med.* **49:** 825–832.

Santon, J.B., M.T. Cronin, C.L. MacLeod, J. Mendelsohn, H. Masui, and G.N. Gill. 1986. Effects of EGF receptor concentration on tumorigenicity of A431 cells. *Cancer Res.* **46:** 4701–4705.

Sap, J., A. Munoz, K. Damm, Y. Goldberg, J. Ghysdael, A. Leutz, H. Beug, and B. Vennstrom. 1986. The c-*erb-A* protein is a high-affinity receptor for thyroid hormone. *Nature* **324:** 635–640.

Sherr, C.J., C.W. Rettenmier, R. Sacca, M.F. Roussel, A.T. Look, and E.R. Stanley. 1985. The c-*fms* proto-oncogene product is related to the receptor for the mononuclear phagocyte growth factor, CSF-1. *Cell* **41:** 665-676.

Shoyab, M., J.E. DeLarco, and G.J. Todaro. 1979. Biologically active phorbol esters specifically alter affinity of epidermal growth factor membrane receptors. *Nature* **279:** 387–391.

Sibley, D.R., J.L. Benovic, M.G. Caron, and R.J. Lefkowitz. 1987. Regulation of transmembrane signaling by receptor phosphorylation. *Cell* **48:** 913–922.

Slamon, D.J., G.M. Clark, S.G. Wong, W.J. Levin, A. Ullrich, and W.L. McGuire. 1987. Human breast cancer: Correlation of relapse and survival with amplification of the HER-2/*neu* oncogene. *Science* **235:** 177–182.

Snyder, M.A., J.M. Bishop, J.P. McGrath, and A.D. Levinson. 1985. A mutation at the ATP-binding site of pp60$^{v\text{-}src}$ abolishes kinase activity, transformation, and tumorigenicity. *Mol. Cell. Biol.* **5:** 1772–1779.

Soderquist, A.M. and G. Carpenter. 1984. Glycosylation of the epidermal growth factor receptor in A-431 cells. *J. Biol. Chem.* **259:** 12586–12594.

Sporn, M.B. and A.B. Roberts. 1988. Peptide growth factors are multifunctional. *Nature* **332:** 217–219.

Stern, D.F. and M.P. Kamps. 1988. EGF-stimulated tyrosine phosphorylation of p185^{neu}: A potential model for receptor interactions. *EMBO J.* **7:** 995–1001.

Stern, D.F., D.L. Hare, M.A. Cecchini, and R.A. Weinberg. 1987. Construction of a novel oncogene based on synthetic sequences encoding epidermal growth factor. *Science* **235:** 321–324.

Sternberg, M.J.E. and W.R. Taylor. 1984. Modelling the ATP-binding site of oncogene products, the epidermal growth factor receptor and related proteins. *FEBS Lett.* **175:** 387–392.

Stoscheck, C.M. and G. Carpenter. 1984. "Downregulation" of EGF receptors: Direct demonstration of receptor degradation in human fibroblasts. *J. Cell Biol.* **98:** 1048–1053.

Sudarwati, S. and P.D. Nieuwkoop. 1971. Mesoderm formation in the anuran *Xenopus laevis* (Daudin) Roux's arch. *Dev. Biol.* **166:** 189–204.

Todaro, G.J., J.E. De Larco, H. Marquardt, M.L. Bryant, S.A. Sherwin, and A.H. Sliski. 1979. Polypeptide growth factors produced by tumor cells and virus-transformed cells: A possible growth advantage for the producer cells. *Cold Spring Harbor Conf. Cell Proliferation* **6:** 113–127.

Ullrich, A., J.R. Bell, E.Y. Chen, R. Herrera, L.M. Petruzzelli, T.J. Dull, A. Gray, L. Coussens, Y.-C. Liao, M. Tsubokawa, A. Mason, P.H. Seeberg, C. Grunfeld, O.M. Rosen, and J. Ramachandran. 1985. Human insulin receptor and its relationship to the tyrosine kinase family of oncogenes. *Nature* **313:** 756–761.

Ullrich, A., L. Coussens, J.S. Hayflick, T.J. Dull, A. Gray, A.W. Tam, J. Lee, Y. Yarden, T.A. Libermann, J. Schlessinger, J. Downward, E.L.V. Mayes, N. Whittle, M.D. Waterfield, and P.H. Seeburg. 1984. Human epidermal growth factor receptor cDNA sequence and aberrant expression of the amplified gene in A431 epidermoid carcinoma cells. *Nature* **309:** 418–425.

Ushiro, H. and S. Cohen. 1980. Identification of phosphotyrosine as a product of epidermal growth factor-activated protein kinase in A-431 cell membranes. *J. Biol. Chem.* **255:** 8363–8365.

van de Vijver, M.J., J.L. Peterse, W.J. Mooi, P. Wisman, J. Lomans, O. Dalesio, and R. Nusse. 1988. *neu*-protein overexpression in breast cancer. *N. Eng. J. Med.* **319:** 1239–1245.

Vennstrom, B. and J.M. Bishop. 1982. Isolation and characterization of chicken DNA homologous to the two putative oncogenes of avian erythroblastosis virus. *Cell* **28:** 135–143.

Vogel, S., W. Freist, and J. Hoppe. 1986. Assignment of conserved amino acid residues to the ATP site in the protein kinase domain of the receptor for epidermal growth factor. *Eur. J. Biochem.* **154:** 529–532.

Waterfield, M.D., G.T. Scrace, N. Whittle, P. Stroobant, A. Johnsson, A. Wasteson, B. Westermark, C.-H. Heldin, J.S. Huang, and T.F. Deuel. 1983. Platelet-derived growth factor is structurally related to the putative transforming protein $p18^{sis}$ of simian sarcoma virus. *Nature* **304:** 35–39.

Weber, W., P.J. Bertics, and G.N. Gill. 1984. Immunoaffinity purification of the epidermal growth factor receptor: Stoichiometry of EGF binding and kinetics of self-phosphorylation. *J. Biol. Chem.* **259:** 14631–14636.

Weber, W., G.N. Gill, and J. Spiess. 1984. Production of an epidermal growth factor receptor-related protein. *Science* **224:** 294–297.

Wedegaertner, P.B. and G.N. Gill. 1989. Activation of the purified protein tyrosine kinase domain of the epidermal growth factor receptor. *J. Biol. Chem.* **264:** 11346–11353.

Weeks, D.L. and D.A. Melton. 1987. A maternal mRNA localized to the vegetal hemisphere in *Xenopus* eggs codes for a growth factor related to TGF-β. *Cell* **51:** 861–867.

Weinberger, C., C.C. Thompson, E.S. Ong, R. Lebo, D.J. Gruol, and R.M. Evans. 1986. The c-*erb-A* gene encodes a thyroid hormone receptor. *Nature* **324:** 641–646.

Weinmaster, G., M.J. Zoller, and T. Pawson. 1986. A lysine in the ATP-binding site of $P130^{gag\text{-}fps}$ is essential for protein-tyrosine kinase activity. *EMBO J.* **5:** 69–76.

Wells, A. and J.M. Bishop. 1988. Genetic determinants of neoplastic transformation by the retroviral oncogene v-*erbB*. *Proc. Natl. Acad. Sci.* **85:** 7597–7601.

Wharton, K.A., K.M. Johansen, T. Xu, and S. Artavanis-Tsakonas. 1985. Nucleotide sequence from the neurogenic locus notch implies a gene product that shares homology with proteins containing EGF-like repeats. *Cell* **43:** 567–581.

Wilden, U., S.W. Hall, and H. Kuhn. 1986. Phosphodiesterase activation by photoexcited rhodopsin is quenched when rhodopsin is phosphorylated and binds the intrinsic 48-kDa protein of rod outer segments. *Proc. Natl. Acad. Sci.* **83:** 1174–1178.

Wiley, H.S. and D.D. Cunningham. 1981. A steady state model for analyzing the cellular binding, internalization and degradation of polypeptide ligands. *Cell* **25:** 433–440.

Woolford, J., A. McAuliffe, and L.R. Rohrschneider. 1988. Activation of the feline c-*fms* proto-oncogene: Multiple alterations are required to generate a fully transformed phenotype. *Cell* **55:** 965–977.

Xu, Y.-H., S. Ishii, A.J.L. Clark, M. Sullivan, R.K. Wilson, D.P. Ma, B.A. Roe, G.T. Merlino, and I. Pastan. 1984. Human epidermal growth factor receptor cDNA is homologous to a variety of RNAs overproduced in A431 carcinoma cells. *Nature* **309:** 806–810.

Yamamoto, K.K., G.A. Gonzalez, W.H. Biggs III, and M.R. Montminy. 1988. Phosphorylation-induced binding and transcriptional efficacy of nuclear factor CREB. *Nature* **334:** 494–498.

Yamamoto, T., T. Nishida, N. Miyajima, S. Kawai, T. Ooi, and K. Toyoshima. 1983. The *erbB* gene of avian erythroblastosis virus is a member of the *src* gene family. *Cell* **35:** 71–78.

Yarden, T., J.A. Escobedo, W.-J. Kuang, T.L. Yang-Feng, T.O. Daniel, P.M. Tremble, E.Y. Chen, M.E. Ando, R.N. Harkins, U. Francke, V.A. Fried, A. Ullrich, and L.T. Williams. 1986. Structure of the receptor for platelet-derived growth factor helps define a family of closely related growth factor receptors. *Nature* **323:** 226–232.

Yarden, Y., W.-J. Kuang, T. Yang-Feng, L. Coussens, S. Munemitsu, T.J. Dull, E. Chen, J. Schlessinger, U. Francke, and A. Ullrich. 1987. Human proto-oncogene c-*kit*: A new cell surface receptor tyrosine kinase for an unidentified ligand. *EMBO J.* **6:** 3341–3351.

Yarden, Y. and A. Ullrich. 1988. Growth factor receptor tyrosine kinases. *Annu. Rev. Biochem.* **57:** 443–478.

Young, D., G. Waitches, C. Birchmeier, O. Fasano, and M. Wigler. 1986. Isolation and characterization of a new cellular oncogene encoding a protein with multiple potential transmembrane domains. *Cell* **45:** 711–719.

4

Signal Transduction and Intracellular Messengers

Henry R. Bourne* and Anthony L. DeFranco[†]
Departments of *Pharmacology, *Medicine, and
[†]Microbiology and Immunology
University of California, San Francisco, California 94143

I. OVERVIEW

Rapidly accumulating evidence indicates that many proto-oncogene proteins, especially those found in the cytoplasm and at the plasma membrane, act as detectors and generators of chemical signals in normal cells. These signals are called hormones or "second messengers," depending on whether they are found in the extracellular fluid or inside cells. This chapter describes several well-studied signaling pathways. Of these, some serve only to illustrate the organization and principles that underlie cellular regulation by chemical signals, whereas other pathways may, in addition, be directly affected by oncogene-encoded proteins.

Organisms have evolved a number of molecular strategies for transducing extracellular signals across the bilayer (Fig. 1). The simplest (S1 in the

Oncogenes and the Molecular Origins of Cancer.

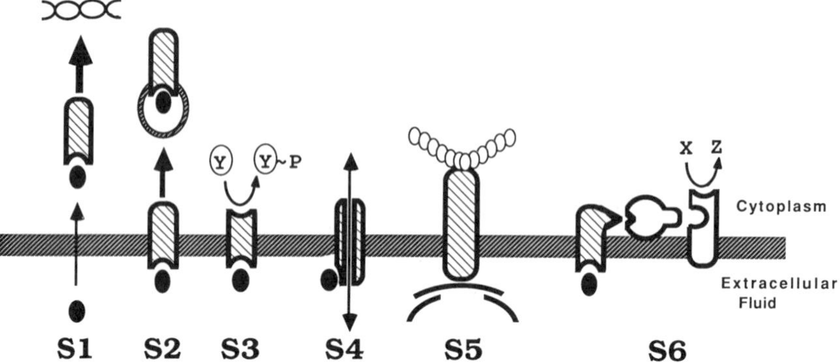

Figure 1 Known transmembrane signaling mechanisms include (1) lipid-soluble chemical signal crosses the plasma membrane and regulates transcription of specific genes; (2) the signal binds an extracellular receptor and is endocytosed; (3) the signal binds to the extracellular domain of a transmembrane protien, thereby activating an enzymatic activity of its cytoplasmic domain—in this case, phosphorylation of tyrosine residues (*Y*) in proteins; (4) the signal binds to and directly regulates the opening of an ion channel; (5) the signal, a component of the extracellular matrix, regulates cell shape and motility by binding to a transmembrane receptor system that interacts with actin microfilaments in the cytoplasm; (6) the signal binds to a cell-surface receptor linked via a G protein to an effector enzyme, which converts compound *X* to a second messenger, *Z*.

figure) uses a hormonal signal that is itself sufficiently lipid soluble to be able to cross the membrane and act on an intracellular receptor (e.g., cortisol, thyroid hormones). Alternatively, a receptor oriented toward the exterior of the cell can transport the extracellular ligand itself into the cell by endocytosis of membrane vesicles (S2, e.g., cholesterol carried by the low-density lipoprotein receptor). Some signal transducers are transmembrane receptor proteins, in which binding of the ligand (S3) to a site on the extracellular portion of the receptor triggers an enzymatic activity located in an intracellular domain of the same polypeptide; examples in the family of receptors with protein tyrosine kinase activity include receptors for insulin, epidermal growth factor (EGF), and platelet-derived growth factor (PDGF). At synapses and neuromuscular junctions, neurotransmitters (S4, including acetylcholine and γ-aminobutyric acid) act by binding to a transmembrane ion channel; rapid opening of the channel allows ions to cross the membrane, thereby changing the transmembrane electrical potential. A fifth class, receptors in the integrin family, are transmembrane proteins that link proteins of the extracellular matrix (S5) to microfilament components of the cytoskeleton and appear to regulate cell shape, attachment to extracellular matrix, motility, and growth. Finally, a large number of extracellular signals (S6) are detected by receptors that act through a family of GTP-binding proteins (G proteins) to regulate production of intracellular second messengers that then regulate activity of cytoplasmic proteins.

Once the signal has crossed the plasma membrane, the cell uses two basic strategies to coordinate an overall response that may involve tens or hundreds of different protein species within the cell. The first strategy is to alter the *activity* of preexisting proteins (enzymes, ion channels, cytoskeletal elements, etc.) either allosterically or by covalent modification (often by attaching or removing a phosphoryl group). The change in activity of an individual protein may also set in motion a response based on a second strategy—i.e., by regulating transcription of specific genes, the *number* of molecules of a specific protein may be altered. Regulatory effects of an extracellular signal within the cell may be propagated by either strategy, or both, regardless of the mechanism by which the signal crossed the plasma membrane.

Of the six mechanisms illustrated in Figure 1, this chapter focuses on three, chosen for their relevance to actions of proteins encoded by proto-oncogenes and oncogenes: The regulation of gene expression by lipid-soluble ligands (mechanism 1) and the cell-surface receptors with protein tyrosine kinase activity (mechanism 3) are briefly sketched because their structures and biochemical mechanisms have close parallels, respectively, in oncogene products that act in the nucleus (see Chapter 7) and in cytoplasmic oncogene products that are protein tyrosine kinases (see Chapters 3 and 6). In addition, this chapter places major emphasis on mechanism 6 for two related reasons. First, relative to the other mechanisms, the molecular basis of signaling by cell-surface receptors linked to G proteins and generation of intracellular second messengers is much better understood. Second, these signaling pathways exemplify key features of normal signaling systems that are often utilized (and sometimes deranged) by the actions of oncogene proteins.

II. SIGNALING BY G PROTEINS

The idea that hormones can regulate cells by causing the generation of intracellular second messengers began with the discovery of cyclic adenosine-3′,5′-monophosphate (cAMP) 30 years ago. Now cAMP has been joined by a number of other intracellular messenger molecules, including cyclic guanosine-3′,5′-monophosphate (cGMP), Ca^{++}, and products of phosphoinositide metabolism. Like an intracellular hormone, each of these messengers acts on multiple target proteins in the cell to mediate and coordinate the cell's response to an extracellular (first) messenger. In most cases, extracellular ligands stimulate production of second messengers through a G protein. In all these systems, the ligand is specifically detected by a transmembrane receptor. The receptor in turn triggers activation of an appropriate G protein, which is located on the cytoplasmic face of the plasma membrane. The activated G protein then changes the activity of an effector element, usually an enzyme or ion channel; the effector proteins are responsible for changing concentrations of intracellular second messengers. Each species of receptor for an extracellular ligand interacts with a specific member of the G-protein family. In turn, each G protein interacts with a specific class of effector molecules. For example, binding of certain hormones and neurotransmitters to specific receptors causes activation of G_s, a G protein that stimulates adenylyl cyclase; this effector enzyme in turn converts intracellular ATP to cAMP, the second messenger.

A. The G-protein Machine

A combination of biochemistry and molecular cloning has led to the discovery of at least six G proteins in addition to G_s (Table 1). Each member of the expanding G-protein family utilizes a common molecular mechanism for transducing signals and shares a common design (Stryer and Bourne 1986; Gilman 1987).

The molecular mechanism involves the following sequence of events (Fig. 2): (1) Interaction with a receptor that has been activated by ligand binding causes the G protein to release GDP, allowing GTP to enter the guanine-nucleotide-binding site; (2) in its GTP-bound conformation, the

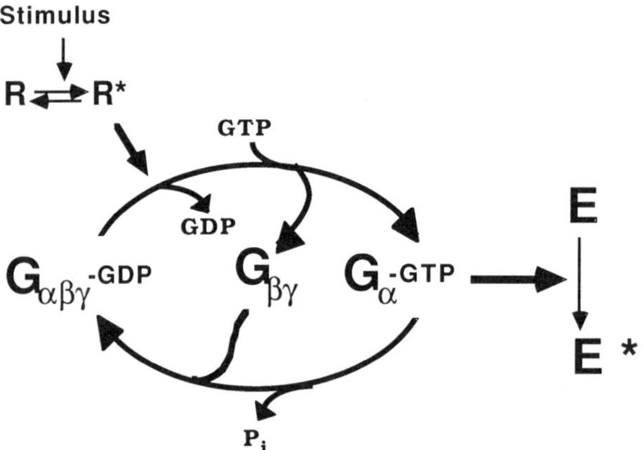

Figure 2 Guanine nucleotide-dependent activation/inactivation cycle of G proteins. The stimulus (hormone ligand, photon, etc.) activates the receptor (*R*), which promotes release of GDP from the α chain of the G protein (G_α), allowing GTP to bind and G_α to dissociate from the $\beta\gamma$ subunit ($G_{\beta\gamma}$). In its GTP-bound state (G_α-GTP), the α chain regulates activity of an effector enzyme or ion channel (*E*). Hydrolysis of GTP returns the α chain to the inactive, GDP-bound state, allowing reassociation with $G_{\beta\gamma}$. Further signaling requires that the $\alpha\beta\gamma$ complex interact once again with the activated receptor.

Table 1 Signal transduction by G proteins

Receptors for:	G Protein	ADP-ribosylated by:	Effector
β-Adrenergic catecholamines, glucagon, etc.	G_s	cholera toxin	↑ adenylyl cyclase
α_2-Adrenergic amines, somatostatin, acetylcholine, etc.	G_i (3 distinct α chains)	pertussis toxin	↓ adenylyl cyclase ↑ phospholipase C open K^+ channels
Unknown	G_0	pertussis toxin	unknown
α_1-Adrenergic catecholamines, vasopressin, etc.	G_x (or G_p)	none	↑ phospholipase C
Photons	rod and cone transducins	cholera and pertussis toxins	↑ cGMP-PDE

G protein regulates the effector molecule; (3) hydrolysis of bound GTP to GDP, mediated by an intrinsic GTPase activity of the G protein, terminates interaction of the G protein with the effector and sets the stage for reinitiation of the cycle by the receptor.

A key feature of the G-protein machine is that it allows amplification and regulation of the transduced signal by separating excitation of the receptor by its hormone ligand from activation of the effector. Thus, the encounter of a neurotransmitter such as norepinephrine with its membrane receptor may be quite short-lived, a matter of a few milliseconds. When the encounter generates a GTP-bound G_s molecule, however, the lifetime of the enzymatically active G_s-adenylyl cyclase complex depends on the longevity of GTP bound to G_s rather than on the tenacity with which the receptor binds norepinephrine. Indeed, like other G proteins, GTP-bound G_s characteristically remains active for tens of seconds; the result is an enormous amplification of the original signal.

In addition to G_s, the G-protein family includes two transducins, which mediate photoreception in rod and cone cells of the vertebrate retina; three G_i proteins, expressed in most mammalian cells; and G_o, which is highly abundant in brain membranes (Table 1). The three G_i proteins are named for the ability of one or more of them to mediate hormonal inhibition of adenylyl cyclase. This inhibition is one of several different cellular responses to hormones that bind to receptors distinct from those that stimulate adenylyl cyclase. The GTP-dependent inhibition of adenylyl cyclase by hormones was discovered before it was appreciated that G_i includes at least three distinct proteins, subsequently identified by molecular cloning. Although this group is now known to include proteins that mediate hormonal regulation of ion channels and production of second messengers derived from phospholipids (see below), it is not yet possible to assign any one of these signaling functions specifically to an individual member of the G_i family. Similarly, the function of G_o (the "other" type) has not yet been identified.

Despite their diverse functions, the G proteins are built on the same general plan, comprising three dissimilar polypeptide chains, α, β, and γ. The α chains bind and hydrolyze GTP; each member of the α-chain family confers on the corresponding G protein its specificities for interacting with receptors and effectors. The β and γ polypeptides, usually associated in a tight complex, serve to anchor the G protein to the membrane and to present the α chain to the receptor element. Activation of a G protein, triggered by binding of GTP to the α subunit, is accompanied by dissociation of α from the $\beta\gamma$ subunit (see Fig. 2). The α-GTP complex is responsible for stimulating the effector, at least in the case of G_s and transducin. Subsequent hydrolysis of the bound GTP terminates activity of the α chain. The inactive GDP-bound α chain rapidly reassociates with $\beta\gamma$, and is then ready to be activated by another hormone-receptor complex.

The different G proteins are distinguished by their α chains, because the β and γ chains are quite similar. These α chains are identified with subscripts corresponding to the G protein (α_s for G_s, α_o for G_o, α_t for transducin, etc.). Pairwise comparisons of primary sequences among six known α chains show various degrees of similarity (40–93% identical residues). Compared to the α chains, the β chains exhibit much less variety. (Two known β chains are 90% identical in amino acid sequence.) Indeed, the $\beta\gamma$ complexes associated with different G proteins appear to be functionally interchangeable. Although only one cDNA encoding a γ chain (that of retinal transducin) has been cloned and sequenced (Hurley et al. 1984), immunologic and other biochemical studies suggest that nonretinal tissues will contain more than one additional type of γ chain.

The highly conserved GTP-binding sites of the α chains closely resemble similar sites in the elongation and initiation factors of ribosomal protein synthesis, GTP-driven proteins whose structures are closely conserved from bacteria to man. The guanine-nucleotide-binding sites of both these protein families also resemble sites in a third family of GTP-binding proteins, the 21,000-dalton membrane-bound products (p21) of the *ras* oncogenes and proto-oncogenes (for review, see Masters et al. 1986). Structural and functional similarities between G proteins and $p21^{ras}$ strongly suggest that the latter proteins mediate transduction of signals that control cell proliferation. The ability of $p21^{ras}$ to substitute for a homologous protein as a regulator of yeast adenylyl cyclase makes this idea even more likely (see Chapter 5). Thus, the duplication and divergence of genes in evolution have adapted a single molecular machine for mediation of sensory transduction, control of cell proliferation, ribosomal protein synthesis, and cellular regulation by many hormones and neurotransmitters.

Despite important similarities, the G proteins differ from those of the $p21^{ras}$ family in three important ways: (1) Neither receptor nor effector components of the $p21^{ras}$ system so far have been identified. (2) The α and $\beta\gamma$ subunits of G proteins separate upon activation (i.e., upon binding of GTP); no cognate of the $\beta\gamma$ complex has been found for $p21^{ras}$. (3) GTP hydrolysis by $p21^{ras}$ is directly stimulated by a cytoplasmic protein (Trahey and McCormick 1987); in contrast, although GTPase activity of G-protein α chains is indirectly stimulated by hormone receptors (which promote replacement of GDP by GTP), the hydrolysis of a bound GTP molecule is thought to occur independently of whether the α chain binds effector, $\beta\gamma$, or any known protein.

Much of our knowledge of the G proteins derives from the fact that they serve as the primary targets of the bacterial exotoxins produced by *Vibrio cholerae* and *Bordetella pertussis*. Both toxins act by catalyzing transfer of ADP-ribose from NAD^+ to different amino acid residues on G-protein α chains (Stryer and Bourne 1986; Gilman 1987; see Table 1). Modification of α_s by cholera toxin stabilizes its GTP-bound active conformation and enhances stimulation of adenylyl cyclase; this effect is responsible for the elevated cAMP content in cells of the intestinal mucosa that causes the potentially lethal diarrhea of cholera. In contrast, G proteins modified by pertussis toxin cannot interact normally with receptors. Consequently, pertussis toxin blocks hormone effects mediated by G_i-like proteins, including inhibition of adenylyl cyclase, opening of K^+ channels, and stimulation of phosphoinositide metabolism (see Section II.C).

B. Receptors That Talk to G Proteins

In view of the remarkable conservation of structure and function among examples of the G-protein family, it is not surprising that the receptors coupled to G proteins comprise a related family of proteins. Recent investigations in a number of laboratories have led to molecular cloning of cDNAs encoding G-protein-coupled receptors for adrenergic catecholamines, muscarinic cholinergic agents, and photons (detected by virtue of conformational changes in a covalently attached lipid chromophore). For each of these receptor classes, more than one subtype has been cloned—three adrenoceptors, four muscarinic receptors, and four visual opsins (rhodopsin in rods and three color opsins in cones) (for review, see Dohlman et al. 1987).

These receptors show distinct family resemblances in amino acid sequence and in predicted membrane topology (Fig. 3). Each receptor polypeptide chain appears to cross the plasma membrane seven times, with the amino terminus lying in the extracellular space and the carboxyl terminus in the cytoplasm. The chromophore "ligand" of the opsins, 11-*cis*-retinal, lies parallel to the plane of the plasma membrane in a pocket created by transmembrane regions of the protein. It is likely that many of the hormonal ligands for this family of receptors bind similarly to intramembranous pockets in their receptors. The conservation of amino acid sequence in presumptive transmembrane regions of these receptors probably reflects a common mechanism of conformational change triggered by the binding of activating ligand.

Although sites for receptor interactions with the G proteins have not yet been identified, the carboxy-terminal tails of rhodopsin and the β-adrenergic receptors (adrenoceptors) do appear to regulate the ability of both receptors to interact with appropriate G proteins (for review, see Sibley et al. 1987). Upon activation, each of these receptor proteins becomes an excellent substrate for phosphorylation by rhodoposin kinase and β-adrenoceptor kinase, respectively. Attachment of phosphoryl groups to serine and threonine residues in their carboxy-terminal tails indirectly turns off (or desensitizes) the receptors by increasing their affinity for binding cytoplasmic "turnoff" proteins, such as retinal arrestin, that compete with and prevent activation of the G proteins. This desensitization

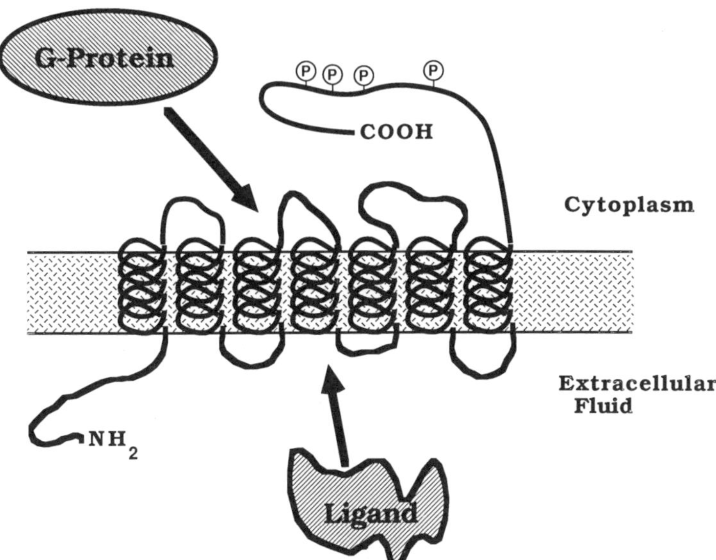

Figure 3 Schematic diagram of transmembrane receptors that talk to G proteins. These receptors comprise seven transmembrane regions (presumably α- helices). Amino and carboxyl termini are located on the extracellular and cytoplasmic faces of the membrane, respectively. The stimulatory ligand interacts with transmembrane helices and extracellular loops, whereas the G protein is thought to interact with intracellular loops. The receptor's carboxy-terminal tail contains multiple serine and threonine residues whose phosphorylation (*P*) by specific receptor kinases mediates receptor desensitization.

mechanism serves as an inhibitory feedback that limits the duration and intensity of receptor activation.

The number of receptors coupled to members of the G-protein family is quite large. More than 20 different hormones and neurotransmitters—amines, peptides, and lipids—stimulate adenylyl cyclase, whereas a slightly smaller number are known to interact with receptors coupled to the G_i-like proteins that inhibit adenylyl cyclase or activate other second-messenger pathways. It is not certain that all members of this large receptor family will share the same structural motif (i.e., seven transmembrane regions) and mechanism of action in stimulating G proteins. Conversely, however, any receptor molecule that shares the structural motif is strongly suspected of being linked to a G protein. For example, the receptor for a neuropeptide, substance K, has seven transmembrane domains and significant amino acid sequence similarities to β-adrenoceptors and the opsins (Masu et al. 1987); these features make it likely that substance K alters membrane potential via a G protein, even though the G protein itself has not been identified. Another apparent member of the family is the product of an oncogene: The *mas* oncogene, isolated from a human tumor by virtue of its ability to promote malignant transformation of NIH-3T3 cells, encodes a protein whose deduced primary structure places it within this class of receptors (Young et al. 1986). It is reasonable to speculate that the as yet unidentified ligand that is detected by the *mas* protein will turn out to be a growth-promoting hormone and that its signal will be transduced by a G protein.

C. Effector Targets of G Proteins

Although the previous discussion has emphasized the role of adenylyl cyclase as a target of G proteins, a variety of other effector molecules are regulated by G proteins (see Table 1). One of the best-characterized of these effectors is the cGMP phosphodiesterase (PDE) in the outer segments of retinal rod cells, which is stimulated by rod transducin. As in the case of adenylyl cyclase, the cGMP PDE is activated by binding the GTP-bound α subunit of the G protein (Stryer and Bourne 1986; Gilman 1987).

Details of G-protein–effector interactions in other signaling systems are less well understood. G_i was originally defined by its ability to mediate hormonal inhibition of adenylyl cyclase, but the biochemical mechanism(s) responsible for this effect are not clear. One view is based on the observations that G proteins activated by binding GTP dissociate into α-GTP and $\beta\gamma$ complexes (Fig. 2) and that addition of excess $\beta\gamma$ can reverse or inhibit the activation of α_s in vitro. According to this view, hormonal activation of G_i inhibits adenylyl cyclase by releasing $\beta\gamma$, which inhibits α_s (for review, see Gilman 1987). Alternatively, the α subunit of G_i could bind to adenylyl cyclase and inhibit it directly. The latter possibility is supported by the observation (Katada et al. 1984b) that G_i can inhibit adenylyl cyclase in a mutant cell line that totally lacks α_s.

In addition to inhibiting adenylyl cyclase, G_i-like proteins also mediate neurotransmitter opening of K^+ channels (Logothetis et al. 1987; Yatani et al. 1987a) and regulation of Ca^{++} channels. Interestingly, the countervailing effects of G_s and G_i on adenylyl cyclase reappear in regulation of Ca^{++} channels: A G_i-like protein sensitive to pertussis toxin mediates neurotransmitter closure of Ca^{++} channels in a pituitary cell line (Lewis et al. 1986), wherease G_s appears to open cardiac Ca^{++} channels (Yatani et al. 1987b).

Yet another target enzyme of G proteins is the phospholipase C involved in receptor-regulated hydrolysis of phosphatidylinositol-4,5-bisphosphate, a reaction that generates multiple intracellular messengers (see Section III.B). At least two different G proteins can regulate this phospholipase C. In neutrophils, pertussis toxin blocks hormonal stimulation of this enzyme; the G protein involved belongs to the G_i family (Table 1). In many other cells, including hepatocytes, astrocytoma cells, GH_3 pituitary cells, and B lymphocytes, pertussis toxin does not block receptor-stimulated phospholipase C activity. Receptor stimulation of phospholipase C in this latter group of cells requires GTP and is therefore thought to be mediated by a G protein. This postulated G protein is not classified as a G_i protein because it is insensitive to pertussis toxin; instead, it is called G_x or G_p (see Table 1). It is not certain that the protein that mediates pertussis-toxin-insensitive signals is a G protein at all; it is possible that the protein belongs to the p21^{ras} family, as suggested by observations that cells transfected with oncogenic or overexpressed *ras* genes exhibit increased metabolism of phosphoinositides (see Chapter 5).

GTP-binding signal transducers are beginning to be implicated in hormonal regulation of the generation of other lipid messengers, including arachidonic acid (Murayama and Ui 1985; see Section IV.B) and metabolites of phosphatidylcholine and phosphatidylethanolamine (Irving and Exton 1987). Observations that fibroblasts transformed by oncogenic *ras* genes contain increased amounts of the latter metabolites suggest that p21^{ras} may play a regulatory role in their metabolism (Lacal et al. 1987).

In summary, G proteins have been demonstrated to bind to and regulate adenylyl cyclase and cGMP PDE. Less rigorous but nonetheless convincing evidence indicates that other G proteins regulate phospholipases and ion channels.

D. Experimental Strategies for Testing Signaling Roles of G Proteins

The involvement of a G protein in a signal transduction system can be established on the basis of several kinds of evidence (Stryer and Bourne 1986; Gilman 1987). (1) Effects of bacterial toxins: Demonstration that pertussis toxin blocks or that cholera toxin enhances a signaling pathway strongly suggests that the pathway is mediated by a G protein and provides a strong hint as to the identity of its α chain (α_i or α_o for pertussis toxin, α_s for cholera toxin). (2) Stimulation by the ligand of the GTPase activity of an α chain in a membrane preparation. (3) Effects of guanine nucleotides on signal transduction in isolated membranes or in permeabilized or microinjected cells: Signaling should require GTP; note that endogenous GTP may obscure this requirement. Hydrolysis-resistant GTP analogs (e.g., GppNHp or GTPγS) cause persistent activation of G proteins and should stimulate effectors whose activity depends on G proteins. In contrast, GDPβS, a GDP analog that cannot be converted to GTP, may block signaling through G proteins by competing with endogenous GTP. (4) Stimulation of the effector by AlF_4^-, which is thought to activate the G-GDP complex by simulating the γ-phosphoryl of GTP (for review, see Gilman 1987). (5) Demonstration that guanine nucleotides lower receptor affinity for binding the activating ligand: This indirect consequence of G-protein involvement reflects the fact that receptor-G-protein complexes exhibit high affinity for stimulatory ligands; guanine nucleotides promote dissociation of the G protein from the receptor, thereby lowering the receptor's affinity for ligand.

Complete understanding of a G-protein-mediated signaling pathway ultimately requires purification of the receptor, effector, and G-protein components, followed by their functional reconstitution in vitro. Because membrane proteins are often difficult to handle biochemically, this level of analysis has so far been achieved only with hormone-sensitive adenylyl cyclase and the phototransduction system of retinal rod cells. Short of purifying all of the components, it may sometimes be possible to demonstrate G-protein involvement by using a signaling system that functions only upon addition of a resolved (but not necessarily pure) G protein. Thus, addition of G_s-containing extracts to membranes of a mutant lymphoma cell genetically deficient in α_s leads to assembly of an adenylyl cyclase complex that can be stimulated by hormones and guanine nucleotides (Ross et al. 1978); this in vitro complementation assay led to the discovery of G_s and eventually allowed it to be purified. Similarly, inactivation of endogenous G_i-like molecules by treatment with pertussis toxin allowed investigators to assess the abilities of exogenous G_i to mediate inhibition of adenylyl cyclase in platelets (Katada et al. 1984a) or opening of K^+ channels in heart membranes (Logothetis et al. 1987; Yatani et al. 1987a).

III. CYTOPLASMIC SECOND MESSENGERS

A. cAMP

In mammalian cells, the cyclic AMP (cAMP) generated by adenylyl cyclase mediates a wide spectrum of hormonal actions, including mobilization of stored energy (breakdown of carbohydrates in liver or triglycerides in fat cells, stimulated by β-adrenergic catecholamines), vasopressin-mediated conservation of water by the kidney, Ca^{++} homeostasis (regulated by parathyroid hormone), increased rate and force of contraction of heart muscle (β-adrenergic catecholamines), production of adrenal and sex steroids (in response to corticotropin or follicle-stimulating hormone), and regulation of many other endocrine and neural processes. Recent observations indicate also that cAMP mediates the sense of smell: Odorant stimuli activate adenylyl cyclase in olfactory epithelium, and the consequent rise in cAMP promotes electrical excitation of olfactory neurons (Lancet and Pace 1987).

cAMP exerts most of its effects in eukaryotes by binding to and activating the catalytic activity of cAMP-dependent protein kinases. The activated kinases phosphorylate specific proteins (Fig. 4). Two well-characterized cAMP-dependent protein kinases (A-kinases) are present in most cell types (Edelman et al. 1987); although they differ from cell to cell in relative abundance and subcellular distribution, the biological reasons underlying these differences are unknown. Both A-kinases are tetrameric, composed of a cAMP-binding regulatory (R) dimer and two catalytic (C) chains. cAMP binds to the R dimer. This causes release of catalytically active C chains, which are free to diffuse through the cytoplasm and nucleus, where they transfer phosphate from ATP to appropriate specific serine or threonine residues on appropriate target proteins.

Given this rather simple mechanism of action, how does cAMP produce specific regulatory effects in different cell types? The specificity resides in the specific polypeptide substrates of the kinase that are expressed in different cells. For example, liver is rich in phosphorylase kinase and glycogen synthase, enzymes whose reciprocal regulation by cAMP-dependent phosphorylation governs storage and release of carbohydrate; adipocytes are rich in a lipase whose cAMP-dependent phosphorylation mediates release of free fatty acids from fat cells. Other cell-specific

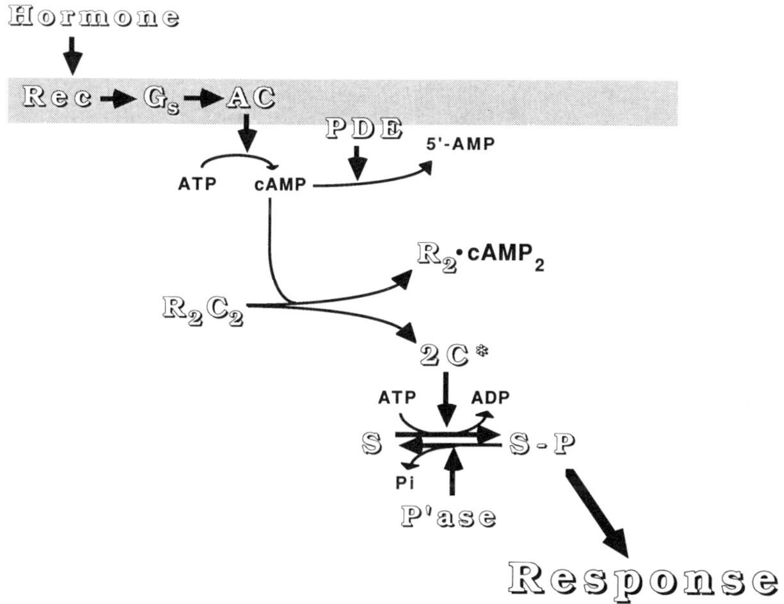

Figure 4 cAMP second-messenger pathway. Key proteins include hormone receptors (*Rec*), a stimulatory G protein (G_s), catalytic adenylyl cyclase (*AC*), phosphodiesterases (*PDE*) that hydrolyze cAMP, the A-kinase, with regulatory (*R*) and catalytic (*C*) subunits, protein substrates (*S*) of the kinase, and phosphatases (*P'ase*), which remove phosphate groups from the substrate proteins.

responses to cAMP as a second messenger similarly depend on the array of enzymes available for regulation by phosphorylation.

Only one regulatory effect of cAMP in eukaryotes is known *not* to be mediated by protein phosphorylation: The opening of sodium channels in olfactory neurons is induced by cAMP, which probably binds directly to the channel protein; no protein kinase activity is involved (Nakamura and Gold 1987). cAMP-mediated opening of these channels initiates action potentials in olfactory neurons that carry odorant information to the brain.

Upon cessation of the hormonal stimulus, the intracellular actions of cAMP are terminated by an elaborate series of enzymes. cAMP itself is degraded to 5′-AMP by a number of distinct cyclic nucleotide phosphodiesterases (PDEs) (Fig. 4), which differ in subcellular location, affinity for cAMP, and regulation by other intracellular molecules (such as Ca^{++}/calmodulin, as described below) (Beavo et al. 1982). Phosphorylation of A-kinase substrates is rapidly reversed by a diverse group of specific and nonspecific phosphatases (Cohen 1985), some of which are themselves regulated by cAMP-dependent phosphorylation. In addition, most cells express a protein, called protein kinase inhibitor (PKI) that specifically blocks the activity of C subunits of the A-kinase, but does not interact with R; PKI presumably also serves to damp responses to cAMP.

Upon discovery of a new hormone (or a new action of a known hormone), answers to a few simple questions allow one to determine whether the hormonal effect is mediated by cAMP. Positive answers to the following questions establish that cAMP does mediate the hormone response in question: (1) Does the hormone elevate cellular cAMP in parallel with other observed cellular responses? (2) Does the hormone stimulate adenylyl cyclase in broken cell preparations from the target organ or tissue? (3) Does forskolin, a drug that directly stimulates the catalytic unit of adenylyl cyclase, cause the cellular response observed with the hormone? (4) Does cholera toxin cause the response observed with hormone? (5) Do inhibitors of cAMP PDE, such as theophylline or methylisobutylxanthine, potentiate cellular responses to the hormone, including elevation of cAMP? (6) Do cAMP analogs (e.g., 8-bromo-cAMP, which is a poor PDE substrate but a quite satisfactory activator of A-kinase) elicit the same cellular response that is triggered by the hormone?

B. Phosphoinositides and Ca^{++}

Another well-studied second-messenger system involves hormonal stimulation of phosphoinositide hydrolysis (Abdel-Latif 1986; Berridge 1987) (Fig. 5). Receptors for hormones, neurotransmitters, and growth factors that act through this pathway stimulate—often via a G protein, but perhaps not always—the activity of a phospholipase C (PLC) that specifically hydrolyzes phosphatidylinositol-4,5-bisphosphate ($PtdInsP_2$), a phos-

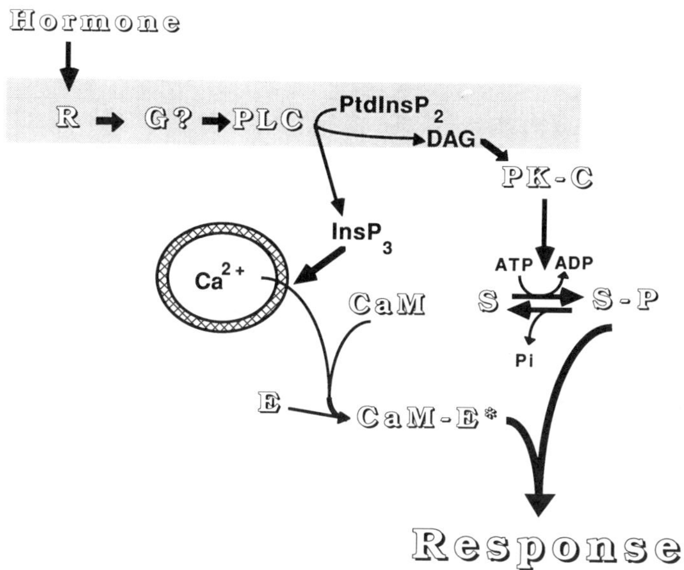

Figure 5 Ca^{++}/phosphoinositide signaling pathway. Key proteins include hormone receptors (*R*), a G protein (*G*), a phosphoinositide-specific phospholipase C (*PLC*), C-kinase (*PK-C*), substrates of the kinase (*S*), calmodulin (*CaM*), and calmodulin-binding enzymes (*E*), including kinases, PDEs, etc. *DAG* refers to diacylglycerol. See text for details.

pholipid component of the plasma membrane. $PtdInsP_2$ is split into two second messengers, diacylglycerol and inositol-1,4,5-trisphosphate ($InsP_3$). Diacylglycerol is confined to the membrane, where it activates protein kinase C (C-kinase). In contrast, the other messenger, $InsP_3$, is water-soluble and can diffuse through the cytoplasm, where it triggers release of Ca^{++} from storage vesicles inside the cell (Berridge and Irvine 1984). As a result, cytoplasmic Ca^{++} increases from approximately 0.1 μM to 0.5–1.0 μM. In turn, cytoplasmic Ca^{++} binds to the calcium-binding protein, calmodulin, which regulates activities of other enzymes, including Ca^{++}-dependent protein kinases. $InsP_3$ itself can be converted by phosphorylation into yet another potential second messenger, inositol-1,3,4,5-tetrakisphosphate ($InsP_4$). A second-messenger role for $InsP_4$ has not yet been firmly established.

In some systems, receptor stimulation of $PtdInsP_2$ breakdown is accompanied by phospholipase-C-catalyzed cleavage of phosphatidylinositol (PtdIns) and of phosphatidylinositol-4-phosphate (PtdInsP) (Imai and Gershengorn 1986). The products of head groups cleaved in these reactions (InsP and $InsP_2$ instead of $InsP_3$) do not release Ca^{++} from intracellular stores; if InsP and $InsP_2$ play roles in intracellular signaling, these roles have not been identified. As with cleavage of $PtdInsP_2$, hydrolysis of

PtdIns and PtdInsP by phospholipase C generates diacylglycerol; consequently, hydrolysis of PtdIns and PtdInsP, as well as $PtdInsP_2$, activates C-kinase.

The relative amounts of PtdIns, PtdInsP, and $PtdInsP_2$ are tightly regulated by kinases and phosphatases that act on the inositol head group. The kinases that interconvert these compounds are subject to regulation by oncogene proteins (e.g., $pp60^{v\text{-}src}$) and by receptor tyrosine kinases (see Chapters 3 and 6). Consequent changes in the amount of substrate ($PtdInsP_2$) available for cleavage by receptor-regulated phospholipase C may affect the $InsP_3$ and Ca^{++} responses to stimulation of these receptors.

Interestingly, tumor promoters such as phorbol esters (see Chapter 12), appear to act by stimulating C-kinase. It remains to be seen whether any of the multiple genes that encode C-kinase isozymes can be altered to produce an oncogene.

In broad outline, the C-kinase limb of the signaling system triggered by phospholipase C resembles the cAMP/A-kinase pathway. Although the C-kinase, unlike the A-kinase, lacks a separate regulatory subunit, both protein kinases catalyze phosphorylation of serine and threonine residues on multiple target proteins, and both are allosterically activated by second messengers.

The phosphoinositide signaling pathway is much more complex than the cAMP/A-kinase pathway, however. Indeed, the system is considerably more complex than shown in Figure 5 (Berridge 1987; Edelman et al. 1987). For example, different cell types may contain one or more quite specialized Ca^{++}/calmodulin-dependent kinases with limited substrate specificity (e.g., the enzyme that phosphorylates myosin light chains) in addition to a "general" Ca^{++}/calmodulin-dependent kinase capable of phosphorylating a wide variety of protein substrates. Also, at least four structurally distinct C-kinases have been identified (Edelman 1987; Ono and Kikkawa 1987); these enzymes differ in tissue distribution and may differ in regulatory or catalytic properties or in substrate specificity. Furthermore, the relative importance of the second messengers and kinases in this pathway may vary depending on the cell and the biological response.

Much of our understanding of the biological roles of phosphoinositide second messengers comes from the use of pharmacological agents that activate either the Ca^{++} or the C-kinase pathways. Cytosolic Ca^{++} can be elevated by calcium ionophores, compounds that facilitate transfer of Ca^{++} across the plasma membrane; ionophores raise intracellular Ca^{++} by allowing influx of the ion from outside the cell, where its concentration is usually 1000-fold greater than in the cytoplasm. C-kinase is directly stimulated by binding phorbol esters or synthetic diacylglycerols. One or both of these classes of agents may reproduce the biological response triggered by a physiological signal that utilizes the phosphoinositide pathway. For example, addition of Ca^{++} ionophores or microinjection of $InsP_3$ reproduces the cortical reaction of sea urchin oocytes that is physiologically triggered by fertilization which stimulates hydrolysis of $PtdInsP_2$.

In many phosphoinositide signaling systems, Ca^{++} and C-kinase exhibit a striking synergy in evoking the physiological response. In secretory systems, phorbol esters or synthetic diacylglycerols often produce a limited response, which is greatly augmented upon addition of a calcium ionophore (e.g., in platelets, neutrophils, parotid cells, T lymphocytes, and exocrine pancreatic cells) (Abdel-Latif 1986). In hepatocytes, vasopressin triggers $PtdInsP_2$ breakdown and enhanced degradation of glycogen: The Ca^{++} limb of the pathway acts via activation of phosphorylase kinase and stimulation of glycogen breakdown, whereas the C-kinase limb acts to turn off glycogen synthase.

The possibility should be noted that water-soluble products of $PtdInsP_2$ hydrolysis, including $InsP_3$ and $InsP_4$, may elicit intracellular messages distinct from elevation of cytoplasmic Ca^{++}. This could account for observations in some systems that effects of ligand-induced breakdown of phosphoinositides are not completely reproduced by elevation of cytoplasmic Ca^{++} activation of C-kinase. The possible roles of water-soluble $PtdInsP_2$ metabolites are difficult to test; because active analogs of $InsP_3$ and $InsP_4$ that can cross the plasma membrane are not available, direct effects of these agents can only be observed in permeabilized cells or by microinjection.

As in the cAMP system, multiple mechanisms are available to damp or terminate signaling by this pathway. $InsP_3$ and $InsP_4$ are rapidly dephosphorylated to inactive compounds; diacylglycerol can be phosphorylated to yield phosphatidic acid, which then is converted back into phospholipids, or it can be deacylated to yield arachidonic acid; Ca^{++} is actively removed from the cytoplasm by Ca^{++} pumps. Removal of second messengers does not always end the signaling process, however; in the case of the general calmodulin-dependent protein kinase, autophosphorylation produces an enzyme that is active in the absence of Ca^{++}—an example of molecular memory (Miller and Kennedy 1986).

Breakdown of $PtdInsP_2$ is not the only way stimulated cells can generate Ca^{++} or diacylglycerol as second messengers. Cytoplasmic Ca^{++} can be elevated by membrane depolarization and opening of voltage-gated Ca^{++} channels in the plasma membrane. Diacylglycerol can be generated by phospholipases C that act on lipids other than $PtdInsP_2$. For example, insulin has been reported to stimulate phospholipase C breakdown of a complex derivative of phosphatidylinositol (Saltiel et al. 1986) to generate diacylglycerol and a novel second messenger that can activate cAMP PDE. Receptor- and GTPγS-stimulated hydrolysis of phosphatidylcholine has also been reported (Irving and Exton 1987). Finally, cells transformed with a Ha-*ras* oncogene exhibit elevated amounts of diacylglycerol and phosphorylcholine, two metabolites of phosphatidylcholine produced by phospholipase C (Lacal et al. 1987).

C. Interplay between cAMP and Ca^{++} Pathways

As knowledge of the Ca^{++} phosphoinositide pathway has accumulated, investigators have discovered numerous examples of "cross talk" between this signaling pathway and the cAMP pathway. The two pathways oppose one another in some cells, whereas their actions are parallel in others (Berridge 1987; Edelman et al. 1987). For example, vasopressor agents that stimulate contraction of smooth muscle do so by $InsP_3$-mediated mobilization of Ca^{++}, whereas agents that relax smooth muscle often act by elevating cAMP. Part of the biochemical mechanism that underlies these opposing actions is known: Phosphorylation of the light chains of myosin, catalyzed by myosin light-chain kinase (MLCK), increases contractility of smooth muscle. The activity of MLCK increases when the enzyme binds Ca^{++}/calmodulin complexes, but decreases when the enzyme is phosphorylated by A-kinase (Edelman et al. 1987).

In contrast, cAMP and phosphoinositide second messengers act in concert to stimulate glucose release from the liver (Edelman et al. 1987). Epinephrine, for example, stimulates hepatic adenylyl cyclase through β-adrenoceptors and activates PLC via α_1-adrenoceptors. cAMP and Ca^{++} act in different ways to stimulate glycogen breakdown, the former by promoting cAMP-dependent phosphorylation (and activation) of phosphorylase kinase, the latter by calmodulin-mediated allosteric stimulation of the same enzyme. In turn, the activated phosphorylase kinase phosphorylates glycogen phosphorylase and thereby stimulates glycogen degradation. Similarly, by catalyzing phosphorylation of glycogen synthase, both C-kinase and the Ca^{++}/calmodulin-dependent protein kinase—like the A-kinase—can inhibit glycogen synthesis.

In addition to cross talk at the level of second-messenger *action*, the two signaling pathways talk to one another at the levels of *degradation* and *generation* of second messengers. For more information about these cross-talk mechanisms, see Beavo et al. (1982) on Ca^{++} regulation of cAMP PDEs; Salter et al. (1981) and Jakobs et al. (1985) on regulation of adenylyl cyclase by Ca^{++} or C-kinase; and Cohen (1985) on the complex regulatory loops that control dephosphorylation of proteins.

IV. OTHER CYTOPLASMIC SECOND MESSENGERS

Evolution has devised a number of second-messenger systems in addition to the well-characterized cAMP and Ca^{++}/phosphoinositide pathways. This section briefly sketches emerging knowledge of several of these "new" signaling systems.

A. cGMP

Unlike cAMP, the ubiquitous and versatile carrier of many and diverse messages, cGMP is a "specialist" messenger whose signaling roles have been established in only a few cell types. In intestinal mucosa and vascular smooth muscle, cGMP-based signal transduction closely parallels cAMP-mediated signaling: Ligands detected by cell-surface receptors stimulate membrane-bound guanylyl cyclase, and the resulting cGMP acts by stimulating a cGMP-dependent protein kinase (G-kinase). The actions of cGMP in these cells are terminated by enzymatic degradation of the cyclic nucleotide and by dephosphorylation of kinase substrates. Hydrolysis-resistant cGMP analogs reproduce the effects of ligands that stimulate guanylyl cyclase.

cGMP is thought to mediate the relaxation of smooth muscle triggered by atrial natriuretic factor and by a poorly characterized factor released from vascular endothelial cells in response to indirectly acting vasodilator molecules such as acetylcholine and histamine. In mucosal cells of the intestine, cGMP mediates the increased secretion of salt and water triggered by a heat-stable *Escherichia coli* exotoxin; it is likely that the same signaling pathway is utilized in normal regulation, although the relevant ligand is unknown (for review, see Murad 1986).

In sharp contrast to the conventional signaling mode, retinal rod cells use a *decrease* in cGMP to mediate visual phototransduction (Stryer 1986). Present at a high concentration in dark-adapted rods, cGMP occupies binding sites on Na^+ channels in the plasma membrane and keeps them open, thereby maintaining depolarization of the membrane. Photon activation of rhodopsin leads to activation of cGMP PDE in rod cells, a process mediated by a G protein, retinal transducin. Degradation of cGMP by the PDE causes a transient lowering of cGMP, which results in closure of cGMP-gated Na^+ channels and hyperpolarization of the membrane; this hyperpolarization decreases release of neurotransmitter from the cell, a change that is sensed by neural pathways that transmit the visual signal to the brain.

B. Arachidonic Acid Metabolites as Second Messengers

Arachidonic acid and many of its metabolites are released from a wide variety of cells in response to extracellular signals. Often these compounds act in a paracrine fashion to regulate the behavior of neighboring cells. In some cases, however, these mediators may also serve as intracellular second messengers. Although indirect evidence suggests that G proteins may be involved in mediating hormonal regulation of arachidonic acid release, the precise mechanisms of regulation are presently obscure. Arachidonic acid is released from phospholipids either by the direct action of phospholipase A_2 or by the sequential actions of phospholipase C and diacylglycerol lipase; in most cases, the former pathway is thought to be more important. Arachidonic acid is then converted by different enzyme pathways (cycloxygenase, lipoxygenase, and epoxygenase) into at least three distinct and well-characterized families of metabolites that are involved in inter- and intracellular signaling (Needleman et al. 1986). Metabolites of arachidonic acid participate in glucose stimulation of insulin release from pancreatic islet cells, hormonal release of luteinizing hormone from pituitary cells, and hormonal regulation of K^+ channels in sensory neurons of *Aplysia* (Piomelli et al. 1987).

The phospholipase A_2 that releases arachidonic acid is stimulated by hormone receptors that may act through G proteins. Such responses are stimulated by α_2-adrenoceptor responses in a rat thyroid cell line (Burch et al. 1986), by light in retinal rod cells (Jelsema 1987), and by microinjection of oncogenic *ras* proteins in fibroblasts (Bar-Sagi and Feramisco 1986).

C. Cytoplasmic pH

Cytoplasmic pH appears to act as a second messenger in several cell types. Stimulation of fibroblasts by growth factors or of sea urchin oocytes by fertilization leads to rapid alkalinization of the cytoplasm by about 0.2 pH units. The changes in pH are physiologically important in both systems: Blockade of the pH change in oocytes causes inhibition of oocyte activation, and artificial elevation of pH induces the increase in protein synthesis normally seen following fertilization (Whitaker and Steinhardt 1982). In fibroblasts, the Na^+/H^+ antiporter prevents acidification of the cytoplasm by exchanging intracellular proteins for extracellular Na^+. Mutations that inactivate this antiporter also produce a decreased mitogenic response to growth factors (Pouyssegur et al. 1984); the decrease can be relieved by manipulations that artificially induce elevation of intracellular pH.

The pH of the cytoplasm is regulated by two transport systems, the Na^+/H^+ antiporter and a bicarbonate antiporter. Of these two systems, the former plays a dominant role in mediating the pH response to extracellular stimuli, as shown by experimental manipulation of extracellular HCO_3^- and Na^+ and pharmacologic inhibition of the Na^+/H^+ antiporter by amiloride and its congeners.

The best-understood regulator of cytoplasmic pH is C-kinase. Phorbol esters, presumably acting through C-kinase, induce cytoplasmic alkalinization in fibroblasts and lymphocytes by a mechanism that requires the Na^+/H^+ antiporter. Whether the C-kinase directly phosphorylates the antiporter is not known, however. Some agents (e.g., EGF and insulin) can elevate fibroblast pH by a mechanism that does not require C-kinase (Vara and Rozengurt 1985). Thus, extracellular stimuli can regulate the Na^+/H^+ antiporter by at least two different mechanisms. Interestingly, microinjection of an oncogenic Ha-v-*ras*-encoded protein, which stimulates C-kinase and mitogenesis, also increases cytoplasmic pH by stimulating the Na^+/H^+ antiporter (Hagag et al. 1987).

V. PROTEIN TYROSINE KINASES

In the transmembrane signaling systems discussed so far, the receptor elements activate catalytic activities on separate, distinct proteins. Receptors with protein tyrosine kinase activity exemplify a quite different solution to the problem of signaling across a lipid bilayer—i.e., ligand bound to a receptor domain on one side of the bilayer activates an enzymatic domain of the *same receptor molecule* on the other side of the membrane. The enzymatic function used by many transmembrane receptors is a protein tyrosine kinase activity. The superfamily of tyrosine kinases includes a large (and apparently still increasing) number of receptors for hormones and growth factors, including those for insulin, insulin-like growth factor I (IGF-I), EGF, PDGF, and colony-stimulating factor 1 (CSF-1) (see Chapter 2); structure and function of these receptors are detailed in Chapter 3 (for reviews, see also Carpenter 1987; Deuel 1987). This superfamily also includes a series of structurally related protein tyrosine kinases (e.g., c-*src*); although these are not covalently associated with transmembrane receptors, they may interact with receptors and transmit signals from them. As described in Chapters 3 and 6, recent investigations in many laboratories have revealed common elements in the primary structures of these proteins and have established unequivocally that tyrosine phosphorylation plays an essential role in signaling by receptor tyrosine kinases. None of this work has succeeded in defining precisely what that role may be. It has, however, revealed postreceptor mechanisms that parallel or overlap those of the better-understood signaling processes mediated by cAMP, phosphoinositides, and Ca^{++}. This brief section highlights the similarities among these different signaling pathways.

A. Targets of Receptor Tyrosine Kinases

As soon as the receptor tyrosine kinases were discovered, investigators began to search for the elusive "next steps" in these signaling pathways. Site-directed mutations quickly proved that ablation of the tyrosine kinase activities of several receptors prevents signaling. Searches for physiologically relevant protein substrates have proved disappointing, however. Investigators have found several cellular proteins that are phosphorylated on tyrosine residues in response to insulin, EGF, PDGF, etc.; some of these proteins are also phosphorylated by oncogene protein tyrosine kinases (see chapters 3 and 6). The physiological importance of these phosphorylations remains unclear, however, because the physiological functions of the substrate proteins are obscure.

Several postreceptor processes have been studied in some detail. Not surprisingly, these differ from receptor to receptor. Growth factors that work through the EGF receptor and the PDGF receptor, for example, stimulate the Ca^{++}/phosphoinositide pathway and activation of C-kinase in many (but not all) cell types (Carpenter 1987; Deuel 1987). These growth factors also stimulate the Na^{+}/H^{+} antiporter and elevate cytoplasmic pH. In some cells, these extracellular signals even elevate cAMP, possibly by an indirect pathway involving arachidonic acid release and prostaglandin receptors that stimulate adenylyl cyclase. Responses to insulin include uptake of glucose and amino acids, as well as regulation of a number of enzymes and metabolic processes.

So far, however, signaling links between the receptor tyrosine kinases and any of these responses remain to be identified in molecular terms. It is quite possible, of course, that some effects of insulin or growth factor receptors may be mediated by signaling mechanisms that do not depend on their tyrosine kinase activities. For example, some postreceptor processes initiated by these receptors may also involve G proteins, as suggested by the ability of pertussis toxin to block part of the response to PDGF in fibroblasts (Murayama and Ui 1987). It is also possible that the c-*ras* proteins play a role in signal transduction by these receptors, although the evidence to date is not compelling (see Chapter 5).

Growth factors like EGF and PDGF induce expression of a number of genes, including those for c-*myc* and c-*fos* (see Chapter 7). The steps that intervene between activation of second-messenger systems by the growth factor receptors and the subsequent activation of gene expression are quite unclear. Enhancer elements in these genes appear to mediate responses to cAMP and to phorbol esters (see Section VI).

B. Signal Termination and Receptor Endocytosis

We have seen that the cAMP and Ca^{++}/phosphoinositide systems incorporate multiple mechanisms designed to terminate signal response pathways; these include receptor turnoff by phosphorylation, degradation of second messengers, and dephosphorylation of kinase substrates. Although less well understood, the mechanisms that turn off receptor tyrosine kinases include specific phosphatases, which can remove the phosphates from tyrosine residues on receptors such as the insulin receptor that activate themselves by self-phosphorylation (Rosen 1987); receptor endocytosis (Carpenter 1987; Deuel 1987); and receptor phosphorylation by C-kinase (for review, see Deuel 1987). Chapter 5 describes these mechanisms in greater detail.

VI. MESSAGE TRANSMISSION TO THE NUCLEUS

Until now, this chapter has focused on receptor-mediated changes in second-messenger concentrations and consequent changes in activities of cytosolic proteins. Frequently, however, stimulation of receptors results in altered transcription of specific genes, such as c-*fos* and c-*myc*, as mentioned above. How is the regulatory message conveyed from receptor to the nucleus?

Two classes of mechanisms for regulation of gene expression by external signals are coming into view (Maniatis et al. 1987). The first class utilizes hormonal ligands whose hydrophobicity relieves them of the chore of transmitting signals across the lipid bilayer of the plasma membrane. Instead, these ligands—including corticosteroids, mineralocorticoids, sex steroids, vitamin D, and thyroid hormone—cross the membrane by themselves and bind to intracellular receptors; in turn, these receptors stimulate transcription of genes in the nucleus by binding directly to specific enhancer DNA sequences near the gene whose expression is to be regulated. The second class of mechanisms involves cell-surface receptors that generate intracellular second messengers. Second messengers could travel to the nucleus and act directly there on proteins that regulate transcription (transcription factors). So far this has not been reported. As described below, however, several examples have been reported of proteins that are first altered by second messengers acting in the cytoplasm and then travel to the nucleus to regulate transcription.

Signal transduction by the first class of ligands is reasonably well understood: Many of the receptors have been purified, and their cDNAs have been cloned; the relevant enhancer sequences are well defined; structural domains of the receptors that participate in binding ligand and DNA have been identified (Gehring 1987). Removal of the steroid-binding domain of the glucocorticoid receptor yields a truncated protein that still binds to appropriate enhancer DNA sequences and stimulates transcription of genes in the absence of glucocorticoids. Thus the steroid-binding domain seems to inhibit transcription-stimulating activity of the intact receptor, and this inhibition is relieved by binding of the steroid ligand. Ligand binding to the glucocorticoid receptor also induces its translocation from the cytoplasm to the nucleus. Receptors for estrogen and thyroid hormone, however, seem to be located in the nucleus even in the absence of their ligands.

Many physiological ligands regulate gene transcription by causing generation of second messengers that in turn modulate the activity of transcription factors. cAMP, for example, induces the expression of a number of genes. Related DNA sequences comprising a "cAMP response element" have been shown to mediate induction by cAMP. These sequences have been used to isolate a specific DNA-binding protein that can be phosphorylated by A-kinase in vitro (Montminy and Bilezikjian 1987). Phosphorylation does not affect binding of this protein to DNA, and it is not yet known whether the phosphorylation affects its ability to regulate transcription. The protein is clearly distinct from the R subunit of the A-kinase. The variety of DNA sequences in different cAMP response elements suggests that cAMP-mediated regulation of gene expression involves more than one enhancer-binding protein.

Although in principle cAMP could activate transcription through either of the two classes of A-kinase subunits, the subunit involved is probably C, the catalytic subunit. This conclusion is supported by experiments that utilized a recombinant active fragment of the PKI protein (Section III.A), which specifically inhibits the kinase activity of C subunits but does not interact with R. Expression of the recombinant PKI fragment in COS cells blocks cAMP-induced transcription of a cAMP-responsive reporter gene (Grove et al. 1987). Although this experiment strongly suggests that cAMP regulates transcription by stimulating phosphorylation, it does not identify the relevant kinase substrate(s) or specify whether it is located in the cytoplasm or the nucleus.

Activation of C-kinase by phorbol esters (and presumably by the diacylglycerol produced upon receptor stimulation of phospholipase C) induces expression of many genes, including those that encode metallothionein IIA, c-*myc*, collagenase, and immunoglobulin κ light chain. The enhancer sequences responsible for this induction are targets for at least three proteins, activator protein-1 (AP-1), AP-2, and nuclear factor-κB (NF-κB). In B lymphocytes, NF-κB binds to the κ light-chain enhancer, where it stimulates expression of κ light chains (Sen and Baltimore 1986). In several other cell types, however, phorbol ester treatment is required to promote binding of this protein to enhancer sequences. It is not known whether C-kinase directly phosphorylates NF-κB or whether intermediate proteins are involved.

Regulatory sequences in many of the genes turned on by phorbol esters bind the transcription factors AP-1 or AP-2. Both AP-1 and AP-2 can stimulate transcription in vitro (Angel et al. 1987; Imagawa et al. 1987). Furthermore, DNA elements constructed from multiples of AP-1 or AP-2 binding sequences exhibit enhancer activity that is increased substantially by treatment with phorbol esters. Phorbol esters increase binding of AP-1 to its enhancer sequences. In contrast, AP-2 binds equally well to its DNA-binding sites whether or not the cells have been exposed to phorbol esters, suggesting that its ability to stimulate transcription may be altered. In none of these cases has it been established whether or not C-kinase acts directly to phosphorylate the identified DNA-binding protein.

Interestingly, AP-2-dependent transcription is stimulated not only by phorbol esters, but also by agents that mimic or elevate cAMP. AP-2 may represent an additional site for convergence of two different signaling systems, as in the case of c-*fos*, a gene whose transcription is turned on by both the cAMP and the Ca^{++}/phosphoinositide pathways.

Two oncogenes are known to be derived from normal genes for transcriptional activators involved in cellular responses to external stimuli. The v-*erbA* and v-*jun* oncogenes are derived from the genes for thyroid hormone receptors and AP-1, respectively (Sap et al. 1986; Weinberger et al.

1986; Bohmann et al. 1987). These genes are described in greater depth in the discussion of nuclear oncogenes (Chapter 7).

VII. CONCLUSIONS

In view of the importance of transmembrane signaling pathways for regulation of cell proliferation, it is not surprising that mutations that affect these pathways can produce dominantly acting genes that induce inappropriate proliferation. In a few cases, the actions of oncogenes can be straightforwardly interpreted in relation to receptor signal transduction pathways. For the most part, however, understanding the relation between oncogene action and signal transduction remains a challenge. Two additional comments seem justified:

1. Relations between oncogenes and signaling pathways that utilize cAMP and G proteins can be predicted, although some of the actual oncogenes remain to be discovered. For example, G proteins stimulate phospholipase C, and the results of this stimulation—elevated cytoplasmic Ca^{++} and activated C-kinase—are known to promote cell proliferation. Consequently, we can predict the existence of a class of yet to be discovered oncogenes that will encode amplified or constitutively activated G-protein subunits and other enzymes (e.g., phospholipase C) involved in signaling through phosphoinositides. As noted above, the *mas* oncogene (Young et al. 1986) may encode a receptor that normally stimulates a G protein whose activity somehow promotes cell proliferation. Similarly, it is safe to predict that G_s, the stimulatory regulator of adenylyl cyclase, will prove to be the target of an oncogene in cells whose proliferation normally depends on stimulation by hormones that utilize cAMP as a second messenger—e.g., pituitary somatotrophs and endocrine target cells of the thyroid, ovary, and adrenal (Bourne 1987).
2. Finally, the signaling mechanisms described in this chapter are certainly not the only ones employed by mammalian cells. The number of hormones and growth factors that do *not* act through these pathways is very large. For example, no signaling mechanism has yet been identified for transforming growth factor-β, the interferons, many of the interleukins, growth hormone, etc. It is reasonable to predict that elucidation of these as yet unexplored signaling pathways will be accelerated by discovery and characterization of new oncogenes, just as known oncogenes have already contributed to elucidation of signaling by receptor tyrosine kinases.

REFERENCES

Abdel-Latif, A.A. 1986. Calcium-mobilizing receptors, polyphosphoinositides, and the generation of second messengers. *Pharmacol. Rev.* **38:** 227–272.

Angel, P., M. Imagawa, R. Chiu, B. Stein, R.J. Imbra, H.J. Rahmsdorf, C. Jonat, P. Herrlich, and M. Karin. 1987. Phorbol ester-inducible genes contain a common *cis* element recognized by a TPA-modulated *trans*-acting factor. *Cell* **49:** 729–739.

Bar-Sagi, D. and J.R. Feramisco. 1986. Induction of membrane ruffling and fluid-phase pinocytosis in quiescent fibroblasts by *ras* proteins. *Science* **233:** 1061–1068.

Beavo, J.A., R.S. Hansen, S.A. Harrison, R.L. Hurwitz, T.J. Martins, and M.C. Mumby. 1982. Identification and properties of cyclic nucleotide phosphodiesterases. *Mol. Cell. Endocrinol.* **28:** 387–410.

Berridge, M.J. 1987. Inositol trisphosphate and diacylglycerol: Two interacting second messengers. *Annu. Rev. Biochem.* **56:** 159–193.

Berridge, M.J. and R.F. Irvine. 1984. Inositol trisphosphate, a novel second messenger in cellular signal transduction. *Nature* **312:** 315–321.

Bohmann, D., T.J. Bos, A. Admon, T. Nishimura, P.K. Vogt, and R. Tjian. 1987. Human proto-oncogene c-*jun* encodes a DNA binding protein with structural and functional properties of transcription factor AP-1. *Science* **238:** 1386–1392.

Bourne, H. 1987. G proteins and cAMP. Discovery of a new oncogene in pituitary tumors? *Nature* **330:** 517–518.

Burch, R.M., A. Luini, and J. Axelrod. 1986. Phospholipase A_2 and phospholipase C are activated by distinct GTP-binding proteins in response to a_1-adrenergic stimulation in FRTL5 thyroid cells. *Proc. Natl. Acad. Sci.* **83:** 7201–7205.

Carpenter, G. 1987. Receptors for epidermal growth factor and other polypeptide mitogens. *Annu. Rev. Biochem.* **56:** 881–914.

Cohen, P. 1985. The role of protein phosphorylation in the hormonal control of enzyme activity. *Eur. J. Biochem.* **151:** 439–448.

Deuel, T.F. 1987. Polypeptide growth factors: Roles in normal and abnormal cell growth. *Annu. Rev. Cell Biol.* **3:** 443–492.

Dohlman, H.G., M.G. Caron, and R.J. Lefkowitz. 1987. A family of receptors coupled to guanine nucleotide regulatory proteins. *Biochemistry* **26:** 2657–2664.

Edelman, A.M., D.K. Blumenthal, and E.G. Krebs. 1987. Protein serine/threonine kinases. *Annu. Rev. Biochem.* **56:** 567–613.

Gehring, U. 1987. Steroid hormone receptors: Biochemistry, genetics, and molecular biology. *Trends Biochem. Sci.* **12:** 399–402.

Gilman, A.G. 1987. G proteins: Transducers of receptor-generated signals. *Annu. Rev. Biochem.* **56:** 615–649.

Grove, J.R., D.J. Price, H.M. Goodman, and J. Avruch. 1987. Recombinant fragment of protein kinase inhibitor blocks cyclic AMP-dependent gene transcription. *Science* **238:** 530–533.

Hagag, N., J.C. Lacal, M. Graber, S. Aaronson, and M.V. Viola. 1987. Microinjection of *ras* p21 induces a rapid rise in intracellular pH. *Mol. Cell. Biol.* **7:** 1984–1988.

Hurley, J.B., H.K.W. Fong, D.B. Teplow, W.J. Dreyer, and M.I. Simon. 1984. Isolation and characterization of a cDNA clone for the γ subunit of bovine retinal transducin. *Proc. Natl. Acad. Sci.* **81:** 6948–6952.

Imagawa, M., R. Chiu, and M. Karin. 1987. Transcription factor AP-2 mediates induction by two different signal-transduction pathways: Protein kinase C and cAMP. *Cell* **51:** 251–260.

Imai, A. and M.C. Gershengorn. 1986. Phosphatidyl 4,5 bisphosphate turnover is transient while phosphatidylinositol turnover is persistent in thyrotropin-releasing hormone-stimulated rat pituitary cells. *Proc. Natl. Acad. Sci.* **83:** 8540–8544.

Irving, H.R. and J.H. Exton. 1987. Phosphatidylcholine breakdown in rat liver plasma membranes. Roles of guanine nucleotides and P_2-purinergic agonists. *J. Biol. Chem.* **262:** 3440–3443.

Jakobs, K.H., S. Bauer, and Y. Watanabe. 1985. Modulation of adenylate cyclase of human platelets by phorbol ester impairment of the hormone-sensitive inhibitory pathway. *Eur. J. Biochem.* **151:** 425–430.

Jelsema, C.L. 1987. Light activation of phospholipase A_2 in rod outer segments of bovine retina and its modulation by GTP-binding proteins. *J. Biol. Chem.* **262:** 163–168.

Katada, T., G.M. Bokoch, J.K. Northup, M. Ui, and A.G. Gilman. 1984a. The inhibitory guanine nucleotide-binding regulatory component of adenylate cyclase. *J. Biol. Chem.* **259:** 3568–3577.

Katada, T., G.M. Bokoch, M.D. Smigel, M. Ui, and A.G. Gilman. 1984b. The inhibitory guanine nucleotide-binding regulatory component of adenylate cyclase. Subunit dissociation and the inhibition of adenylate cyclase in S49 lymphoma *cyc*$^-$ and wild type membranes. *J. Biol. Chem.* **259:** 3586–3595.

Lacal, J.C., J. Moscat, and S.A. Aaronson. 1987. Novel source of 1,2-diacylglycerol elevated in cells transformed by Ha-*ras* oncogene. *Nature* **330:** 269–272.

Lancet, D. and U. Pace. 1987. The molecular basis of odor recognition. *Trends Biochem. Sci.* **12:** 63–66.

Lewis, D.H., F.F. Weight, and A. Luini. 1986. A guanine nucleotide-binding protein mediates the inhibition of voltage-dependent calcium current by somatostatin in a pituitary cell line. *Proc. Natl. Acad. Sci.* **83:** 9035–9039.

Logothetis, D.E., Y. Kurachi, J. Galper, E.J. Neer, and D.E. Clapham. 1987. The $\beta\gamma$ subunits of GTP-binding proteins activate the muscarinic K^+ channel. *Nature* **325:** 321–326.

Maniatis, T., S. Goodbourn, and J.A. Fischer. 1987. Regulation of inducible and tissue-specific gene expression. *Science* **236:** 1237–1245.

Masters, S.B., R.M. Stroud, and H.R. Bourne. 1986. Family of G protein α chains: Amphipathic analysis and predicted structure of functional domains. *Protein Engineering* **1:** 47–54.

Masu, Y., K. Nakayama, H. Tamaki, Y. Harada, M. Kuno, and S. Nakanishi. 1987. cDNA cloning of bovine substance-K receptor through oocyte expression system. *Nature* **329:** 836–838.

Miller, S.G. and M.B. Kennedy. 1986. Regulation of brain Type II Ca^{2+}/calmodulin-dependent protein kinase by autophosphorylation: A Ca^{2+}-triggered molecular switch. *Cell* **44:** 861–870.

Montminy, M.R. and L.M. Bilezikjian. 1987. Binding of a nuclear protein to the cyclic-AMP response element of the somatostatin gene. *Nature* **328:** 175–178.

Murad, F. 1986. Cyclic guanosine monophosphate as a mediator of vasodilation. *J. Clin. Invest.* **78:** 1–5.

Murayama, T. and M. Ui. 1985. Receptor-mediated inhibition of adenylate cyclase and stimulation of arachidonic acid release in 3T3 fibroblasts. *J. Biol. Chem.* **260:** 7226–7233.

———. 1987. Possible involvement of a GTP-binding protein, the substrate of islet-activating protein, in receptor-mediated signaling responsible for cell proliferation. *J. Biol. Chem.* **262:** 12463–12467.

Nakamura, T. and G.H. Gold. 1987. A cyclic nucleotide-gated conductance in olfactory receptor cilia. *Nature* **325:** 442–444.

Needleman, P., J. Turk, B.A. Jakschik, A.R. Morrison, and J.B. Lefkowith. 1986. Arachidonic acid metabolism. *Annu. Rev. Biochem.* **55:** 69–102.

Ono, Y. and U. Kikkawa. 1987. Do multiple species of protein kinase C transduce different signals? *Trends Biochem. Sci.* **12:** 421–423.

Piomelli, D., A. Volterra, N. Dale, S.A. Siegelbaum, E.R. Kandel, J.H. Schwartz, and F. Belardetti. 1987. Lipoxygenase metabolites of arachidonic acid as second messengers for presynaptic inhibiton of *Aplysia* sensory cells. *Nature* **328:** 38–43.

Pouyssegur, J., C. Sardet, A. Franchi, G. L'Allemain, and S. Paris. 1984. A specific mutation abolishing Na^+/H^+ antiport activity in hamster fibroblasts precludes growth at neutral and acidic pH. *Proc. Natl. Acad. Sci.* **81:** 4833–4837.

Rosen, O.M. 1987. After insulin binds. *Science* **237:** 1452–1458.

Ross, E.M., A.C. Howlett, K.M. Ferguson, and A.G. Gilman. 1978. Reconstitution of hormone-sensitive adenylate cyclase activity with resolved components of the enzyme. *J. Biol. Chem.* **253:** 6401–6412.

Salter, R.S., M.H. Krinks, C.B. Klee, and E.J. Neer. 1981. Calmodulin activates the isolated catalytic unit of brain adenylate cyclase. *J. Biol. Chem.* **256:** 9830–9833.

Saltiel, A.R., J.A. Fox, P. Sherline, and P. Cuatrecasas. 1986. Insulin-stimulated hydrolysis of a novel glycolipid generates modulators of cAMP phosphodiesterase. *Science* **233:** 967–972.

Sap, J., A. Monoz, K. Damm, Y. Goldberg, J. Ghysdael, A. Leutz, H. Beug, and B. Vennstrom. 1986. The c-*erb*-A protein is a high-affinity receptor for thyroid hormone. *Nature* **324:** 635–640.

Sen, R. and D. Baltimore. 1986. Inducibility of κ immunoglobulin enhancer-binding protein NF-κB by a posttranslational mechanism. *Cell* **47:** 921–928.

Sibley, D.R., J.L. Benovic, M.G. Caron, and R.J. Lefkowitz. 1987. Regulation of transmembrane signaling by receptor phosphorylation. *Cell* **48:** 913–922.

Stryer, L. 1986. Cyclic GMP cascade of vision. *Annu. Rev. Neurosci.* **9:** 87–119.

Stryer, L. and H.R. Bourne. 1986. G proteins: A family of signal transducers. *Annu. Rev. Cell Biol.* **2:** 391–419.

Trahey, M. and McCormick, F. 1987. A cytoplasmic protein stimulates normal N-*ras* p21 GTPase, but does not affect oncogenic mutants. *Science* **238:** 542–545.

Vara, F. and E. Rozengurt. 1985. Stimulation of Na^+/H^+ antiport activity by epidermal growth factor and insulin occurs without activation of protein kinase C. *Biochem. Biophys. Res. Commun.* **130:** 646–653.

Weinberger, C., C.C. Thompson, E.S. Ong, R. Lebo, D.J. Gruol, and R.M. Evans. 1986. The c-*erb*-A gene encodes a thyroid hormone receptor. *Nature* **324:** 641–646.

Whitaker, M.J. and R.A. Steinhardt. 1982. Ionic regulation of egg activation. *Q. Rev. Biophys.* **15:** 593–666.

Yatani, A., J. Codina, A.M. Brown, and L. Birnbaumer. 1987a. Direct activation of mammalian atrial muscarinic potassium channels by GTP regulatory protein G_k. *Science* **235:** 207–211.

Yatani, A., J. Codina, Y. Imoto, J.P. Reeves, L. Birnbaumer, and A.M. Brown. 1987b. A G protein directly regulates mammalian cardiac calcium channels. *Science* **238:** 1288–1292.

Young, D., G. Waitches, C. Birchmeier, O. Fasano, and M. Wigler. 1986. Isolation and characterization of a new cellular oncogene encoding a protein with multiple potential transmembrane domains. *Cell* **45:** 711–719.

5

ras Oncogenes

Frank McCormick
Cetus Corporation
Emeryville, California 94608

I. DISCOVERY OF *ras* GENES

ras oncogenes were first recognized as the transforming genes of Harvey and Kirsten murine sarcoma viruses (Ha-MSV, Ki-MSV). These highly oncogenic retroviruses were generated during passage of murine leukemia viruses through laboratory strains of rats (Harvey 1964; Kirsten and Mayer 1967). Subsequent molecular analysis showed that Ha-MSV and Ki-MSV contained sequences in their genomes that were not present in the genomes of the parental viruses; these newly acquired sequences appeared to be the result of viral transduction of cellular genes and were thus likely to be responsible for oncogenic transformation. This was directly confirmed when it was shown that subgenomic fragments of Ha-MSV containing only cell-derived sequences were able to transform cells (Chang et al. 1980; De Feo et al. 1981; Ellis et al. 1981).

The proteins produced by Ha-MSV and Ki-MSV were identified using antibodies from rats bearing tumors induced by these viruses; these antibodies reacted with a 21,000-dalton phosphoprotein (p21) produced by Ha-MSV transformed cells. The gene for Ha-MSV p21 was mapped to the region of viral DNA known to be of cellular origin. Furthermore, p21 proteins could be detected in normal, untransformed cells (Langbeheim et al. 1980). Therefore, it was concluded that the p21 gene was the oncogene of Ha-MSV and Ki-MSV (and other closely related viruses) and that this oncogene was derived from a proto-oncogenic form present in normal cells. The genes encoding p21 proteins are now referred to as *ras* genes (from *ra*t *s*arcoma genes).

Oncogenes and the Molecular Origins of Cancer.

Since these early studies, the cellular genes encoding *ras* proteins have been cloned and thoroughly characterized. Mammalian cells express three closely related *ras* genes. Two of these are the proto-oncogene homologs of Ha-MSV and Ki-MSV oncogenes and are referred to as Ha-*ras-1* and Ki-*ras-2*. In addition, the Ki-*ras-2* gene is able to generate two forms of p21 (Ki-*ras2A* and Ki-*ras2B*) by alternative splicing of its fourth exon. The third mammalian *ras* gene has no known retroviral homolog and was detected by transfecting DNA from neuroblastoma cells into NIH-3T3 cells. Molecular analysis of the transfected gene indicated homology with known *ras* genes, and it was designated N-*ras* (Hall et al. 1983; Shimizu et al. 1983). In addition to these expressed genes, two pseudogenes (Ha-*ras-2* and Ki-*ras-1*) have been identified in mammalian cells.

ras p21 proteins bind guanine nucleotides with high affinity (Scolnick et al. 1979) and are localized on the inner surface of the plasma membrane (Willingham et al. 1980). The four species of *ras* proteins produced by mammalian cells (Ha-*ras*, Ki-*ras2A*, Ki-*ras2B*, and N-*ras*) share many common properties. The first 85 amino acids are in fact identical, and the next 80 amino acids are 85% identical. These 165 amino acids make up the guanine-nucleotide-binding region, the crystal structure of which is now known (de Vos et al. 1988; Pai et al. 1989), as well as other regions essential for *ras* action. This high degree of conservation between mammalian *ras* proteins suggests a common function for these proteins. On the other hand, sequences between amino acids 165 and 185 differ greatly between different *ras* proteins, suggesting that each protein species also has a unique activity. Three amino acids from the carboxyl terminus of each p21 protein are a cysteine residue, to which a polyisoprenoid group is covalently attached (Hancock et al. 1989). This modification is essential for membrane localization and oncogenic activity (Willumsen et al. 1984). This has led to the notion that the site of action of the normal and oncogenic forms of p21 is the inner surface of the plasma membrane.

In addition to Ha-*ras*, Ki-*ras*, and N-*ras* genes, mammalian cells contain a family of *ras*-related genes. The closest relatives are *ral* and R-*ras* (50% and 35% identical to the *ras* genes, respectively); other members of the family include *rho*, *rab-1*, *rab-2*, *rab-3*, *rab-4*, *rap-1*, and *rap-2*, all of which encode guanine-nucleotide-binding proteins of 21,000–26,000 molecular weights with similar predicted structures including the cysteine residues close to the carboxyl terminus (Gallwitz et al. 1983; Madaule and Axel 1985; Chardin and Tavitian 1986; Lowe et al. 1987; Touchot et al. 1987; Pizon et al. 1988). Homologs of many of these genes have been identified in lower eukaryotic species, including yeast, *Drosophila*, and the mollusk *Aplysia*. Properties of some of these genes will be discussed below.

Much of the interest in mammalian *ras* genes is focused on the possibility that they play a causative role in human cancers. The series of experiments that led to this suggestion began in 1979, when it was demonstrated that high molecular weight genomic DNA from transformed cells induced morphological transformation of NIH-3T3 cells (Shih et al. 1979; Cooper et al. 1980; Perucho et al. 1981). These experiments suggested the existence of dominant acting transforming genes in these cells and provided an assay for their identification. A number of cell lines and tumor types were tested, and it was soon realized that, in many cases, the same genes were responsible for transformation (Krontiris and Cooper 1981; Perucho et al. 1981).

One of these genes, derived from the EJ/T24 bladder carcinoma cell line, was quickly identified as the human homolog of the Ha-MSV *ras* gene (Der et al. 1982; Parada et al. 1982; Santos et al. 1982). This startling discovery immediately raised the question as to how this gene differed from its normal proto-oncogene counterpart, which was apparently unable to transform NIH-3T3 cells in this assay. Again, this issue was resolved quickly when it was reported that a single base change accounted for the activation of the EJ/T24 bladder carcinoma Ha-*ras-1* gene. (Tabin et al. 1982; Reddy et al. 1982; Taparowsky et al. 1983). This change altered the twelfth codon of the *ras* p21 gene product from glycine to valine. Using DNA transfection, other activating mutations were later discovered in a variety of cell lines (e.g., Yuasa et al. 1983) and solid tumors (Pulciani et al. 1982). With simpler and more sensitive detection methods, several hundred human tumors have now been analyzed for the presence of activated *ras* genes. The incidence of these mutations varies greatly between different tumor types and raises many questions as to the exact role of activated *ras* oncogenes in these diseases (see Section V). However, it is clear that the detection of a specific genetic change in DNA from a human tumor represented a major milestone in understanding the molecular biology of tumorigenesis, especially since the transforming ability of this mutant gene had already been established from earlier studies on murine retroviruses.

II. MECHANISM OF ACTIVATION

Like the G proteins described in Chapter 4, which transduce signals from cell-surface receptors (e.g., the β-adrenergic receptor and rhodopsin) to internal second-messenger systems, the *ras* proteins were found to bind GDP and GTP. Because of this and their similar intracellular localization on the inner surface of the plasma membrane, Scolnick and co-workers (1979) suggested that *ras* proteins and G proteins may have functional similarities. G proteins possess intrinsic GTPase activity that converts bound GTP to GDP. However, such an activity could not be detected in p21 proteins purified from virus-transformed cells. Moreover, Ha-MLV and Ki-MLV-encoded p21 proteins had been shown to use GTP for autophosphorylation, and in this respect also appeared to differ from the classic

G proteins. When recombinant human Ha-*ras-1* p21 and its oncogenic homolog (the valine-12 mutant from EJ/T24 bladder carcinoma) were expressed in *Escherichia coli*, the reasons for these discrepancies became clear, and the analogy with G-protein function was strengthened once again.

It was found that normal Ha-*ras-1* p21 does indeed possess intrinsic GTPase activity, although this activity is slow compared with classic G proteins. The valine-12 mutant also possessed this activity but at tenfold lower levels. This was the first demonstration of a biochemical difference between oncogenic and proto-oncogenic p21 proteins and immediately led to the model shown in Figure 1 (Gibbs et al. 1984; McGrath et al. 1984; Sweet et al. 1984; Manne et al. 1985).

The model implies that p21 functions as an intermediate in a signal-transducing pathway, acquiring a signal from an upstream element and passing it on to a downstream target. According to this model, p21 bound to GDP (p21.GDP) is inactive and is converted to an active state by a signal that impinges on p21, causing release of GDP and its replacement by GTP. This is analogous to the exchange of GDP from GTP seen on G proteins following binding of ligand to a G-protein-coupled receptor. p21.GTP (the active state) then activates a downstream target that serves as its effector and subsequently returns to its resting state by hydrolyzing bound GTP to GDP. The valine 12 mutant, being defective in GTPase activity, would remain in the active state for a prolonged period, emitting

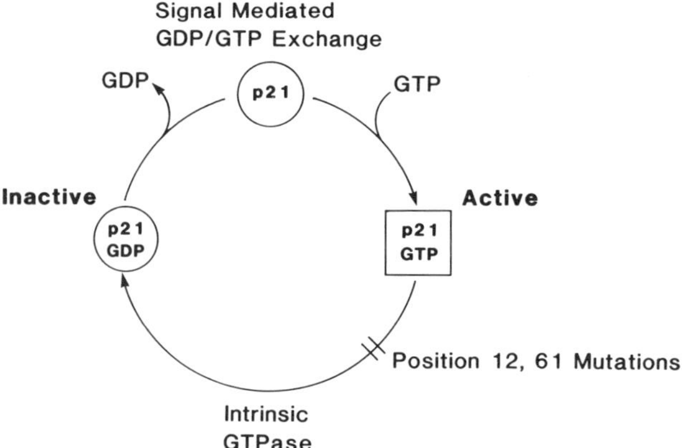

Figure 1 Control of p21 function by guanine nucleotides. In this scheme, inactive p21.GDP is converted to the active form (p21.GTP) by a signal that promotes exchange of bound GDP for GTP. The nature of this signal is not known. Conversion of p21.GTP to p21.GDP was thought to be mediated by intrinsic GTPase activity, as shown here, but is now known to be greatly accelerated by GAP, as shown in Fig. 4A. Positions 12 and 61 mutants reduce intrinsic GTPase activity, as discussed in the text.

signals to its effector. This deregulated excitation of the effector was thought to lead ultimately to uncontrolled proliferation.

This model sharply focused research into mechanisms of *ras* activation and inactivation. Many mutants were tested for GTPase activity as well as GDP- and GTP-binding properties and transforming potential. Mutations at codons 13 and 61 were discovered in DNA from transformed cells and were also shown to be able to convert the protein to an oncogenic form. Using site-directed mutagenesis, it was discovered that any mutation at position 12, except proline, and any mutation at position 61, except glycine, activated transforming potential (Seeburg et al. 1984; Der et al. 1986). Relatively large deletions around position 12 were also found to be activating, as were certain mutations at positions 59 and 63 (Fasano et al. 1984; Chipperfield et al. 1985). When such mutant proteins were examined, they were invariably found to have a reduced GTPase activity, in consonance with the model.

This work also shed light on why the biochemical properties of Ha-MSV and Ki-MSV *ras* proteins differed from the normal proto-oncogenic counterparts and from classic G proteins. These oncogenes carry point mutations in codon 12 (arginine for glycine in Ha-MSV and serine for glycine in Ki-MSV) and therefore have reduced GTPase. Furthermore, both proteins have mutations at position 59, resulting in replacement of alanine with threonine. This substitution further decreases intrinsic GTPase activity and decreases the affinity for GDP (Feig et al. 1986; Clanton et al. 1987), but also creates a site for autophosphorylation. Thus, the γ phosphate of bound GTP is transferred to the hydroxyl group of threonine instead of to water. Substitution of threonine for alanine is itself an activating mutation and, thus, contributes to the biological activity of the highly oncogenic phosphoprotein originally described as the *ras* oncogene product. As yet, such mutations affecting position 59 have not yet been identified in human tumors.

Analysis of more mutant p21 proteins created in vitro and expressed in *E. coli* revealed a second class of activating mutations. Proteins of this second class have greatly reduced affinity for guanine nucleotides rather than having an altered GTPase, and they become activated by rapidly exchanging bound GDP for GTP (Feig et al. 1986; Sigal et al. 1986b; Walter et al. 1986). This exchange occurs because cellular guanine nucleotide pools are mostly GTP (about 1 mM), with very little GDP. Thus, GDP lost through rapid dissociation from these mutant proteins is replaced by GTP, resulting in biological activation. Mutations of this type have been detected in animals exposed to carcinogens but have not yet been detected in human tumors. The reason for this discrepancy is not clear but may reflect the relatively low transforming potency of these mutant alleles.

All this would suggest that oncogenic mutations cause biochemical changes that either trap p21 in the active GTP-bound state by reducing

GTPase or destabilize the inactive GDP-bound form. However, as biochemical properties of mutant and normal p21 proteins were examined in more detail, it became clear that several oncogenic mutants retained substantial GTPase activity and that reductions in GTPase did not correlate invariably with biological activity. For example, the aspartate 12 mutant of N-*ras* p21 (which is particularly prevalent in human leukemias) only differs from normal N-*ras* p21 by a twofold drop in GTPase measured in vitro, and yet it is a fully active transforming protein (Trahey et al. 1987). Therefore, it was concluded that reduced intrinsic GTPase could not adequately account for oncogenic activation and that other biochemical differences may exist between normal and oncogenic proteins.

These conclusions led to the examination of biochemical properties of *ras* proteins in living cells, where the biochemical activities can be measured under physiological conditions. Using this approach, a protein was discovered in extracts of *Xenopus* oocytes that greatly stimulated normal p21 GTPase activity without affecting GTPase of oncogenic mutants. In the presence of this protein, referred to as GAP (GTPase-activating protein), normal p21 had about 500 times more GTPase activity than aspartate 12 or valine 12 mutants (Trahey and McCormick 1987). This suggested that these in vivo conditions (specifically the presence of the GAP) revealed the true difference between normal and oncogenic p21 proteins. Indeed, when tested in these in vivo assays, the differences in GTPase rates among various oncogenic mutants are small compared to the difference between these mutants and wild-type p21. Thus, the original model could be reformulated: In the presence of appropriate ancillary proteins (i.e., GAP), the oncogenic activity of a *ras* protein strongly correlates with its reduced GTPase activity. It was further proposed that GAP maintains normal p21 in its inactive, GDP-bound state and that oncogenic mutants escape this control and thus remain in their active GTP-bound states constitutively. This model is similar to that shown in Figure 1, except that GTP hydrolysis is mediated by a GAP-p21 complex rather than being intrinsic to p21 alone. The possible significance of GAP will be discussed in more detail below.

III. DETAILED STRUCTURE/FUNCTION OF p21

The biochemical properties of two other classes of GTP-binding proteins have been studied in detail for several years. One of these classes includes signal-transducing G proteins, as described above. The other includes proteins involved in polypeptide chain elongation, of which bacterial elongation factor EF-Tu is the best known.

The possibility that EF-Tu resembles p21 structurally as well as biochemically was proposed by Halliday (1985), who showed that the primary sequences of EF-Tu and p21 had a surprising degree of similarity and could be aligned throughout most of the p21 sequence. Shortly thereafter, the crystal structure of EF-Tu in its GDP-bound form was determined (Jurnak 1985; LaCour et al. 1985). Models could therefore be built for the structure of p21 bound to GDP (p21.GDP) based on the structure of EF-Tu (Jurnak 1985; McCormick et al. 1985). Recently, the three-dimensional structure of c-Ha-*ras* p21 in its GDP-bound form was solved (de Vos et al. 1988). The structure of the GTP-bound form has also been solved, in this case at high resolution (Pai et al. 1989). This structure confirmed that the nucleotide-binding site of p21 is very similar in most respects to that of EF-Tu; these similarities between these otherwise unrelated proteins suggest that a basic G-binding/hydrolytic domain is used for regulating a number of disparate switches in the cell's signaling apparatus. Furthermore, the structure revealed several important new insights relating to p21 structure and function, which provide a basis for future comparisons between inactive and active forms of p21 that should eventually lead to a clear understanding for the mechanism by which guanine nucleotides control p21 function.

A. The GTP-binding Site

Figure 2 is a schematic representation of the p21 protein in its active, GTP-bound form, as deduced by Pai and co-workers (1989). p21 amino acids that contact the purine group of GTP are Asp-119 and Ala-146. Asp-119 is part of the sequence Asn-Lys-X-Asp, which occurs in most GTP-binding proteins and is responsible for specificity of these proteins for guanine nucleotides. Asn-116 and lysine hydrogen bond to main-chain carbonyl groups of amino acids 13 and 14, respectively. Mutations in the 116-119 region reduce the affinity of p21 proteins and in some cases alter the specificity of nucleotide binding (Sigal et al. 1986b; McCormick et al. 1987). Phe-28 also contributes to nucleotide binding, in this case by providing part of a hydrophobic pocket for the purine ring. Furthermore, the main-chain carbonyl group of this amino acid hydrogen bonds to the sugar moiety of GTP.

The phosphate groups of GTP interact with p21 through hydrogen bonds to the γ phosphate from Lys-16, Gly-60, and Thr-35, and to the α phosphate through a hydrogen bond to the main-chain amido group of residue 18. Other contacts are to a magnesium ion, which itself interacts with Ser-16 and Thr-35. Each of these amino acids is highly conserved among GTP-binding proteins. The region of p21 around position 12 forms a rigid cage around the bound phosphates by virtue of these contacts. Currently, it is not clear how mutations at positions 12, 13, 61, and other sites cause oncogenic activation; nor is it clear how switching GDP for GTP alters the biological potency of the *ras* protein. Obviously, it will be of great interest to compare the structures of GTP- and GTP-bound forms as well as normal and mutant proteins at high resolution.

B. The Variable Region

This region is carboxy-terminal to the guanine-nucleotide-binding region, and in mammalian *ras* proteins, it corresponds to amino acids 165–185. This region is most divergent among all *ras* proteins and even differs in length between mammalian and *Saccharomyces cerevisiae* proteins. The variable regions of *ras* family members are highly conserved between mammalian species (human and mouse N-*ras* p21 proteins only differ by three amino acids, for example), suggesting that these sequences are more than simply nonfunctional spacer sequences and may perform conserved functions. In oncogenic forms of *ras* proteins, the variable region is dispensable for transforming activity. This has led to speculation that variable regions of each type of *ras* protein normally receive signals from a distinct upstream pathway and all *ras* proteins then transmit their signal to the same downstream pathway. Oncogenic mutants are always activated and thus do not require their variable regions to receive these signals. At the mechanistic level, it is tempting to speculate that incoming signals interact with specific variable regions to promote exchange of GDP for GTP on normal p21 proteins. This exchange will be unnecessary for oncogenic mutants that are always GTP-bound. Other interpretations are also possible: For example, the variable regions may direct different p21 proteins to specific sites in the cell such as different types of membrane. The mechanism of signal input and output may be identical for all types of mammalian *ras* proteins according to this particular model.

C. The Effector-binding Region

It is now well established that the biological activity of p21 proteins is controlled by guanine nucleotides: GTP-bound p21 is active; GDP-bound p21 is inactive. This relationship was inferred from genetic and biochemical analysis of a number of p21 mutants, as described above, and confirmed by microinjecting p21 proteins preloaded with one or the other guanine nucleotide into *Xenopus* oocytes (Trahey and McCormick 1987) or rat PC12 pheochromocytoma cells (Satoh et al. 1987). In both systems, it was shown that normal p21 is inactive when bound to GDP, but can be activated by binding of GppNHp (a nonhydrolyzable GTP analog) prior to injection.

p21-bound GTP is expected to have a different conformation than p21 bound to GDP. Presumably, the active conformation interacts specifically with a cellular target and in doing so transmits a signal. In *Xenopus* oocytes, this signal initiates meiosis; in PC12 cells, the signal initiates differentiation; in fibroblasts in culture, the signal causes transformation (see below). A region of p21 that appears to be necessary for signal transmission has been defined genetically and is referred to as the effector-binding region. This region was first identified by analysis of the transforming ability of a large number of v-Ha-*ras* p21 deletion mutants (Willumsen et al. 1986). This revealed a region corresponding to amino acids 32–40 that was necessary for transforming activity. Similarly, it was shown that certain point mutations in this region destroyed transforming ability (Sigal et al. 1986a). These deletion and point mutants did not affect nucleotide binding or membrane localization and appeared to define a region required for "effector" or target binding. This region is identical in all Ha-*ras*, Ki-*ras*, and N-*ras* proteins (and in *ras* proteins from other species), suggesting that they all send signals down the same pathway. R-*ras*, *rap-1*, and *rap-2* proteins have virtually identical effector-binding sequences. However, none of these proteins can transform cells. Other sequences must therefore participate in sending signals involved in transformation. In the three-dimensional structure of p21.GDP, the effector region is on an external surface (Fig. 2), supporting the notion that this region interacts with other cellular components. In EF-Tu, the equivalent region has been shown to interact with aminoacyl-tRNA in a GTP-dependent manner, suggesting that the conformation of this region is sensitive to the presence of bound GTP or GDP. Clearly, it will be of great interest to determine whether this region of p21 undergoes a conformational change when GDP is exchanged for GTP.

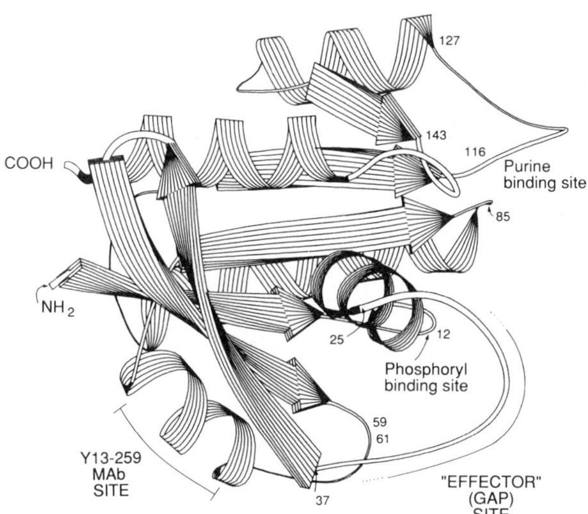

Figure 2 Tertiary structure of Ha-*ras* p21. (Figure printed, with permission, from E.F. Pai, Max-Planck-Institut, Heidelberg.)

IV. BIOCHEMICAL FUNCTIONS CONTROLLED BY *ras* PROTEINS

Despite the extensive structural, biological, and biochemical evidence that has been accumulated from the study of mammalian p21 proteins, the exact mechanisms of action of these proteins are not yet known. However, study of *ras* proteins in the yeast *S. cerevisiae* has been more successful in this respect, and it is now well established that a major function of the yeast *ras* proteins is regulation of adenylate cyclase activity. This discovery was the result of genetic analysis of *S. cerevisiae* strains containing defective or mutant *ras* genes (Tatchell et al. 1985; Toda et al. 1985).

S. cerevisiae contains two *ras* genes, referred to as *RAS1* and *RAS2*. Either one of these genes can be deleted without loss of viability, but deletion of both is lethal (Kataoka et al. 1985; Tatchell et al. 1985). *RAS1* and *RAS2* both encode proteins of about 40,000 daltons (*RAS1* encodes 309 amino acids; *RAS2* encodes 322 amino acids). The guanine-nucleotide-binding regions of these proteins are highly homologous to equivalent regions in mammalian *ras* genes, and their effector regions are identical. The majority of the sequence differences between *S. cerevisiae RAS* proteins and mammalian *ras* proteins, and between *RAS1* and *RAS2* themselves, lie in the variable regions. However, the carboxy-terminal four amino acids are similar to those of other *ras* family members and include the cysteine residue known to be involved in membrane localization.

Since the guanine-nucleotide-binding regions of *RAS1* and *RAS2* are very similar to those of mammalian proteins, it was possible to make mutants with biochemical properties similar to oncogenic p21 proteins. The best-characterized mutant of this type is *RAS2* valine 19: This is equivalent to the valine 12 mutant of mammalian p21 proteins (*RAS2* proteins have an additional seven amino-terminal residues). Introduction of *RAS2* valine 19 into wild-type *S. cerevisiae* generated a phenotype characterized by altered response to nutritional stress and low sporulation efficiency (Kataoka et al. 1985; Toda et al. 1985). The altered phenotype of *RAS2* valine 19 resembled that of a mutant known as bcy1 characterized previously by Matsumoto and co-workers (Matsumoto et al. 1982): This mutant suppresses the requirement for adenylate cyclase by inducing constitutive activation of a cAMP-dependent protein kinase. Furthermore, expression of bcy1 suppressed the requirement for *RAS1* and *RAS2* genes, indicating that bcy1 affects a function that operates downstream from *RAS* in a signal transduction pathway (Fig. 3).

Further genetic analysis has clearly shown that *RAS* gene products activate adenylate cyclase and that the valine 19 mutant causes uncontrolled production of high levels of cAMP. As a result, the cAMP-dependent kinase is constitutively activated, just as it is in bcy1 mutants. Consistent with results of genetic analyses, *RAS* proteins in their GTP-bound states are able to activate adenylate cyclase in *S. cerevisiae* membranes.

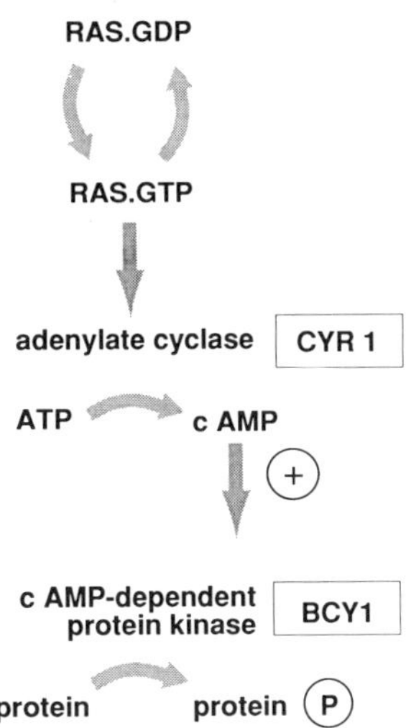

Figure 3 Control of adenylate cyclase by *RAS* proteins in *S. cerevisiae*. RAS.GTP activates adenylate cyclase (the CYR1 gene product), which catalyzes conversion of ATP to cAMP. cAMP activates cAMP-dependent protein kinase, the regulatory subunit of which is referred to as BCY1. Valine 19 mutants of *RAS* genes remain in their GTP-bound forms constitutively and thus cause elevated cAMP levels. Cells lacking *RAS* genes can be rescued by mutations in BCY1 that allow cAMP-independent protein kinase activity.

Mutants with alterations in their effector-binding domain (the region equivalent to amino acids 32–40 in mammalian *ras* proteins) fail to activate adenylate cyclase in vitro. The interaction of *S. cerevisiae* proteins with their target may therefore be similar, if not identical, to the interaction of mammalian p21 proteins. Indeed, mammalian *ras* proteins can substitute for *RAS1* or *RAS2* genes in yeast strains lacking these gene products. Similarly, *S. cerevisiae RAS2* genes can transform mammalian cells, although this requires removal of part of the RAS2 variable region and inclusion of an activating mutation such as valine 19.

These data imply that mammalian *ras* proteins also function by controlling adenylate cyclase activity; however, this does not appear to be the case. Adenylate cyclase levels are lower in *ras*-transformed cells than in normal cells, and purified p21 proteins do not activate adenylate cyclase membranes from mammalian cells. The resemblance between yeast *RAS* proteins and mammalian p21 proteins may therefore be restricted to the mechanical aspects of protein-protein signaling; presumably, the protein with which mammalian p21 proteins interact in a GTP-dependent manner shares structural but not functional similarities with *S. cerevisiae* adenylate cyclase. Another interpretation must also be considered: *S. cerevisiae* may use a second pathway that is controlled by *RAS* proteins and more closely resembles a *ras*-controlled pathway operating in mammalian cells. Evidence for such a second pathway comes from the observation that deletion of both *RAS* genes is lethal for the yeast cell, whereas deletion of adenylate cyclase is not. Thus, *RAS* genes perform functions in addition to regulation of adenylate cyclase activity that may yet shed light on the role of *ras* proteins in mammalian cell growth control.

The search for a biochemical pathway controlled by mammalian *ras* proteins has often involved introduction of *ras* genes or proteins into mammalian cells, followed by analysis of biochemical responses that are likely candidates for *ras*-controlled pathways. For example, it has been well established that cellular transformation frequently involves increased rates of phospholipid turnover (see Chapter 4). Therefore, it is important to determine whether activated *ras* proteins control these events. Several approaches have been taken to address this kind of question, including injection of oncogenic p21 proteins into mammalian cells (or *Xenopus* oocytes) and analysis of phospholipid metabolism in cells containing inducible levels of *ras* proteins. These studies point to an effect of *ras* proteins on diacylglycerol production (Lacal et al. 1987), arachidonic acid production (Bar-Sagi and Feramisco 1986), and inositol phosphate turnover (Yu et al. 1988). These approaches do not prove direct effects of *ras* proteins on these pathways; this will require in vitro biochemical analysis or genetic analysis. For example, variant cells resistant to *ras* transformation have been isolated (Noda et al. 1989), and these may well be mutant in steps downstream from *ras* p21 in a signaling pathway. The genes involved in these steps could in principle be identified by gene-transfer techniques.

Another approach has involved introduction of antibodies against *ras* proteins into cells with the aim of blocking *ras* function. These studies have shown that active *ras* proteins are required for serum-stimulated DNA synthesis and division, and for transformation of cells by tyrosine kinase oncogenes (Mulcahy et al. 1985; Smith et al. 1986). Likewise, insulin-dependent maturation of *Xenopus* oocytes is blocked by anti-p21 antibodies (Deshpande and Kung 1987; Korn et al. 1987). On the other hand, cellular transformation by cytosolic serine/threonine kinase oncogenes (such as *raf* and *mos*) does not require *ras* activity, indicating that their normal counterparts may be downstream from *ras* on a signal pathway or on a parallel, independent pathway.

One candidate for a mammalian *ras* effector protein has recently been identified by biochemical means (Trahey and McCormick 1987; Adari et al. 1988; Cales et al. 1988). This is the GTPase-activating protein (GAP) referred to above. This protein interacts with p21.GTP at the site defined as the effector-binding site. Thus, mutations that destroy the transforming ability of v-Ha-*ras* or prevent mammalian *ras* proteins from activating *S. cerevisiae* adenylate cyclase also fail to interact with GAP. Furthermore, GAP only binds to the GTP-bound form of p21 (Vogel et al. 1988), another criterion for a *ras* effector protein. It will be recalled that GAP was identified as a protein that regulated GTPase activity of wild-type p21 but failed to affect GTPase of oncogenic mutants (above) and was therefore shown to be a potential regulator of GAP action. Figure 4 shows a scheme in which GAP is an effector as well as a regulator of *ras* action.

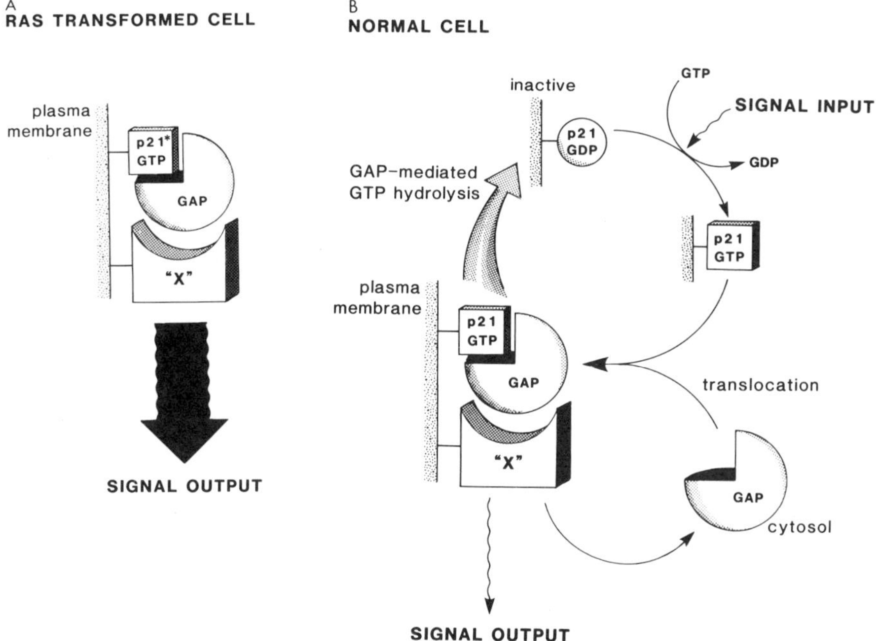

Figure 4 (*A*) Control of p21 activity in normal cells. This scheme is similar to Fig. 1, except that conversion of p21.GTP to p21.GDP is mediated by GAP rather than by intrinsic GTPase activity. p21.GTP bound to GAP may be the active state that sends a signal to the next component of the pathway, shown here as X. This is proposed to be a membrane component, since p21 must be membrane-bound to function. (*B*) Activity of mutant *ras* p21: Oncogenic mutants form complexes with GAP, but conversion to p21.GDP is not stimulated. Thus, p21.GTP remains in the active state constitutively.

In this scheme, p21.GDP in the plasma membrane is normally converted to p21.GTP by an unknown mechanism and can now interact with GAP. GAP appears to be a cytosol protein and can form a brief association with the membrane-associated *ras* p21. During this association, p21.GTP.GAP sends a mitogenic signal to the cell. The lifetime of the p21.GTP.GAP complex and the duration of the signal emission is limited by the ability of GAP to stimulate conversion of p21.GTP to p21.GDP by *ras* p21. Once GTP hydrolysis has occurred, the complex dissociates, GAP returns to a fully cytosolic state, and the signal ceases. In transformed cells, mutant p21 is not provoked by GAP to hydrolyze GTP, so the p21-GAP association and signal output can continue indefinitely.

The validity of this model is currently under investigation. If, indeed, GAP is an effector of *ras* action, it is clear that elucidation of the biochemical properties of GAP will help us understand *ras* action. The structure of GAP gives few clues as to its function: It is a 125,000-dalton protein with a hydrophobic amino terminus and weak homology with the regulatory region of *S. cerevisiae* adenylate cyclase (Trahey et al. 1988; Vogel et al. 1988). This homology is encouraging, for reasons discussed above, but its significance is unclear. More helpful, perhaps, GAP has significant homology with regulatory regions of nonreceptor tyrosine kinases, phospholipase C, and the *crk* oncogene. Identification of cellular factors that interact at common sites on all these proteins will help us understand more about the pathways they may control.

V. *ras* IN THE CONTEXT OF CELL BIOLOGY AND CANCER

The discovery of an activated Ha-*ras*-1 gene in the bladder carcinoma line EJ/T24, as discussed above, was a major breakthrough in the effort to understand the molecular basis of human cancer. This observation raised many urgent questions. The most obvious, perhaps, was the generality of the observation and whether it applied to primary tumors as well as to cell lines. Almost as obvious was the necessity to ask whether *ras* gene activation is a causative step in malignant transformation and, if so, whether this step is sufficient for conversion of normal cells to tumor cells. Many aspects of these questions have now been answered; the more central question of the mechanism by which *ras* oncogenes cause transformation has not.

The incidence of *ras* mutations in human cancers is summarized in Table 1. These data were acquired first by transfecting DNA from tumors onto NIH-3T3 cells to determine focus-forming activity and identity of the transforming gene and more recently by DNA-probe techniques that allow detection of single base mutations directly from genomic DNA. One of these techniques involves amplification of DNA sequences around position 12 or 61 (for example) using the polymerase chain reaction (PCR) (for review, see Bos 1988). The product of this reaction is typically a DNA fragment of about 100 bp, in which mutations can easily be detected by stringent hybridization to allele-specific oligonucleotide probes. Since PCR requires very little sample preparation and can be performed on archival material such as paraffin-embedded sections, it has been possible to analyze a large number of samples from clinically characterized specimens. The following generalizations can now be made: (1) The incidence of *ras* mutations varies substantially between different types of cancer. For example, most, if not all, carcinomas of the exocrine pancreas contain activated *ras* genes, whereas these mutations are very rare in mammary carcinomas. Similarly, about 30% of acute myeloid leukemias contain *ras* mutations (Farr et al. 1988), but analysis of more than 100 cases of chronic lymphocytic leukemia and non-Hodgkin's lymphoma failed to reveal any such mutations (Neri et al. 1988). (2) In a particular kind of cancer, a particular

Table 1 Incidence of *ras* gene mutations in human cancer

Tumor type	Incidence (%)	Predominant *ras* gene activated
Lung (adenocarcinoma)	30	Ki-*ras*
Colon (adenocarcinoma)	50	Ki-*ras*
Pancreatic carcinoma	90	Ki-*ras*
Seminoma	40	Ki-*ras*, N-*ras*
Melanoma	20	N-*ras*
Bladder carcinoma	6	Ha-*ras*
Thyroid	50	all types
Myeloid (myelodysplasia)	30	N-*ras*
Myeloid (acute myelogenous leukemia)	30	N-*ras*
Myeloid (chronic myelogenous leukemia)	10	N-*ras*
Lymphoid (acute lymphocytic leukemia)	10	

Cancers in which less than 5% of tumors contan *ras* mutations: breast, ovarian, cervical, esophageal, glioblastoma, neuroblastoma, stomach, lung (epidermoid, large cell), chronic lymphocytic leukemia, and non-Hodgkin's lymphoma.

ras oncogene often predominates. For example, activated Ki-*ras* oncogenes occur in many types of carcinoma, whereas N-*ras* oncogenes are prevalent in certain leukemias. The reasons for this bias are not yet understood. An obvious interpretation would be that the occurrence of activated *ras* genes simply reflects tissue-specific expression of proto-oncogenic forms in the normal cells that were precursors to the tumor. However, this does not appear to be the case. For example, it has been reported that cells from acute myeloid leukemias with activated N-*ras* oncogenes express both Ha-*ras* and Ki-*ras* p21 proto-oncogene proteins (Shen et al. 1987). However, the possibility of specific expression within the normal precursor cell from which the leukemia arose cannot yet be formally excluded. Another interpretation is that different *ras* genes perform different functions, even in their activated states; most available data argue against this possibility, but again this cannot be formally excluded. (3) In general, the presence of activated *ras* genes does not correlate with the stage of development of a particular tumor. In colorectal cancer, for example, in which adenomas are thought to progress to become malignant carcinomas, the incidence of *ras* mutations is the same in both stages. This indicates that in these tumors, *ras* activation occurs relatively early in the multistep process of tumor progression (see Chapter 12). Detection of *ras* mutations, therefore, does not yet have any clear diagnostic implication that could be useful in a clinical setting.

These extensive studies have established that *ras* gene activation is a frequent event in many, but not all, kinds of human cancer (see also Chapter 13). However, the biological role is still far from clear. For example, in certain leukemias such as AML and ALL, it has been possible to detect two different *ras* mutations in DNA from the same patient. It is likely, although not yet proven, that these mutations are responsible for clonal growth of two independent tumor cell lines, both derived from a common preleukemic population. If so, it would appear that *ras* activation is not the initiating event in this disease but contributes toward later progression.

On the other hand, experiments on carcinogen-induced tumors in rats and mice strongly argue that in these tumors, *ras* mutation is indeed an initiating event equivalent to the first step in tumor progression. For example, a single dose of nitrosomethylurea (NMU) during puberty causes the development of mammary carcinomas, most (if not all) of which contain activated Ha-*ras-1* oncogenes (Sumukar et al. 1984). NMU is known to induce mutations by methylating guanine residues, resulting in substitution of G for A at affected sites in DNA. In NMU-induced mammary carcinomas, *ras* genes are activated by G to A transitions at the second base of codon 12, resulting in replacement of glycine with glutamic acid in the Ha-*ras-1* p21 protein. When a different carcinogen was used (dimethylbenz[a]anthracene), activated *ras* oncogenes again appeared, and again the mutations reflected the mode of action of the carcinogen. These results strongly suggest that in this system at least, *ras* genes are the direct target of these carcinogen molecules. Similarly, treatment of mice with different carcinogens gave rise to skin papillomas and carcinomas containing activated Ha-*ras-1* oncogenes. Once more, the substitution observed in the Ha-*ras-1* gene corresponded to the known mechanism of mutation (Quintanilla et al. 1986). *ras* oncogenes can, therefore, initiate carcinogenesis in appropriate animal models; in humans, their exact role in this process has yet to be resolved.

One difficulty initially perceived with the concept that *ras* oncogenes cause tumors arose from estimates of spontaneous mutation rates in animal cells, which are sufficiently high to ensure that all animals contain thousands of activated *ras* oncogenes at any given moment. Obviously, very few of these oncogenes succeed in triggering tumor production. Therefore, it was apparent that a single point mutation in a *ras* gene would not be sufficient to convert a normal cell to a tumor cell, and, indeed, it was reported that the valine 12 Ha-*ras-1* oncogene is unable to transform primary cells in culture (Land et al. 1983; Newbold and Overell 1983; Ruley 1983). This difficulty was resolved by the demonstration that nuclear oncogenes such as c-*myc*, adenovirus E1A, or polyomavirus large T antigen cooperate with activated *ras* genes, enabling them to transform primary cells (Land et al. 1983; Ruley 1983). Established cell lines, such as NIH-3T3 cells, presumably contain functions equivalent to these nuclear oncogenes that facilitate transformation by *ras* oncogenes (see Chapter 12). *ras* activation was therefore seen as one of several interactive steps in the progression from a normal to a malignant phenotype. Another set of experiments may shed light on the molecular basis of cooperation between *ras* and nuclear oncogenes: It was reported that *ras* oncogenes can transform primary cells if transfected cells are maintained at low cell density (Spandidos 1986). This implies that at high density, inhibitory factors somehow suppress the ability of *ras* to transform cells; nuclear oncogenes may act by preventing these factors from exerting their effects. These possibilities are currently under active investigation.

VI. SUMMARY AND FUTURE PROSPECTS

In the 10 years since *ras* oncogenes were first identified, remarkable progress has been made toward understanding their mode of action and significance in human cancer; however, neither goal has yet been completely fulfilled. The structures of the genes encoding *ras* proteins have been thoroughly documented, and many new members of the *ras* gene family have been recently identified. The occurrence of *ras* oncogenes in human cancers has been a major focus of attention, and several hundred tumor specimens have been analyzed. This is no small technical feat when one considers that a single base change on one of three genes, at one of several possible positions, may be responsible for oncogenic activation. Animal models have provided many useful insights into the mechanism of oncogenic activation, and in vitro systems have revealed that *ras* oncogenes require cooperation with other types of oncogenes to bring about transformation. These fundamental insights will certainly be applicable to a full understanding of the role of *ras* oncogenes in human cancer.

At the biochemical level, the properties of more than 100 p21 mutants have been studied, and the three-dimensional structure of one p21 protein has been determined. Progress has been made in understanding how single amino changes can activate the transforming potential of p21 proteins, and one candidate for an effector protein is currently under scrutiny. In the future, biochemical pathways that *ras* controls will be identified, and the mechanism by which normal p21 proteins are converted from inactive to active states will also be revealed. These developments should lead to a full understanding of *ras* function and may lead to profound insights into the mechanisms by which cells control their growth and differentiation. Perhaps they will also lead to a better understanding of neoplastic transformation and eventually to new and rational ways of treating human cancer.

REFERENCES

Adari, H., D.G. Lowy, B. Willumsen, C.J. Der, and F. McCormick. 1988. Guanosine triphosphatase activating protein (GAP) interacts with the p21 *ras* effector binding domain. *Science* **240:** 518–521.

Bar-Sagi, D. and J.R. Feramisco. 1986. Induction of membrane ruffling and fluid-phase pinocytosis in quiescent fibroblasts by *ras* proteins. *Science* **233:** 1061–1068.

Bos, J.L. 1988. The *ras* gene family and human carcinogenesis. *Mutat. Res.* **195:** 255–271.

Cales, C., J.F. Hancock, C.J. Marshall, and A. Hall. 1988. The cytoplasmic protein GAP is implicated as the target for regulation by the *ras* gene product. *Nature* **332:** 548–551.

Chang, E.H., J.M. Maryak, C.M. Wei, T.Y. Shih, R. Shober, H.L. Cheung, R.W. Ellis, G.L. Hager, E.M. Scolnick, and D.R. Lowy. 1980. Functional organization of the Harvey murine sarcoma virus genome. *J. Virol.* **35:** 76–92.

Chardin, P. and A. Tavitian. 1986. The *ral* gene: A new *ras*-related gene isolated by the use of a synthetic probe. *EMBO J.* **5:** 2203–2209.

Chipperfield, R.G., S.S. Jones, K.-M. Lo, and R.A. Weinberg. 1985. Activation of Ha-*ras* p21 by substitution, deletion, and insertion mutations. *Mol. Cell. Biol.* **5:** 1809–1818.

Clanton, D.J., Y. Lu, D.G. Blair, and T.Y. Shih. 1987. Structural significances of the GTP binding domain of *ras* p21 studies by site-directed mutagenesis. *Mol. Cell. Biol.* **7:** 3092–3097.

Cooper, G.M., S. Okenquist, and L. Silverman. 1980. Transforming activity of DNA of chemically transformed and normal cells. *Nature* **284:** 418–421.

DeFeo, D., M.A. Gonda, H.A. Young, E.H. Chang, D.R. Lowy, E.M. Scolnick, and R.W. Ellis. 1981. Analysis of two divergent rat genomic clones homologous to the transforming gene of Harvey murine sarcoma virus. *Proc. Natl. Acad. Sci.* **78:** 3328–3332.

Der, C.J., T. Finkel, and G.M. Cooper. 1986. Biological and biochemical properties of human *ras*H genes mutated at codon 61. *Cell* **44:** 167–176.

Der, C.J., T.G. Krontiris, and G.M. Cooper. 1982. Transforming genes of human bladder and lung carcinoma cell lines are homologous to the *ras* gene of Harvey and Kirsten sarcoma viruses. *Proc. Natl. Acad. Sci.* **79:** 3637–3640.

Deshpande, A.K. and H.F. Kung. 1987. Insulin induction of *Xenopus laevis* oocyte maturation is inhibited by monoclonal antibody against p21 *ras* proteins. *Mol. Cell. Biol.* **7:** 1285–1288.

de Vos, A.M., L. Tong, M.V. Milburn, P.M. Matias, J. Jancarik, S. Noguchi, S. Nishimura, K. Miura, E. Ohtsuka, and S.-H. Kim. 1988. Three dimensional structure of an oncogene protein: Catalytic domain of human c-H-*ras* p21. *Science* **239:** 888–893.

Ellis, R.W., D. DeFeo, T.Y. Shih, M.A. Gonda, H.A. Young, N. Tsuchida, D.R. Lowy, and E.M. Scolnick. 1981. The p21 *src* genes of Harvey and Kirsten sarcoma virus originate from divergent members of a family of normal vertebrate genes. *Nature* **292:** 506–511.

Farr, C.J., R.K. Saiki, H.A. Erlich, F. McCormick, and C.J. Marshall. 1988. Analysis of *RAS* gene mutations in acute myeloid leukemia by polymerase chain reaction and oligonucleotide probes. *Proc. Natl. Acad. Sci.* **85:** 1629–1633.

Fasano, O., T. Aldrich, F. Tamanoi, E. Taparowsky, M. Furth, and M. Wigler. 1984. Analysis of the transforming potential of the human H-*ras* gene by random mutagenesis. *Proc. Natl. Acad. Sci.* **81:** 4008–4012.

Feig, L.A., B.-T. Pan, T.M. Roberts, and G.M. Cooper. 1986. Isolation of *ras* GTP-binding mutants using an *in situ* colony-binding assay. *Proc. Natl. Acad. Sci.* **83:** 4607–4611.

Gallwitz, D., C. Donath, and C. Sander. 1983. A yeast gene encoding a protein homologous to the human c-*ras*/*bas* proto-oncogene product. *Nature* **306:** 704–707.

Gibbs, J.B., I.S. Sigal, M. Poe, and E.M. Scolnick. 1984. Intrinsic GTPase activity distinguishes normal and oncogenic *ras* p21 molecules. *Proc. Natl. Acad. Sci.* **81:** 5704–5708.

Hall, A., C.J. Marshall, N.K. Spurr, and R.A. Weiss. 1983. Identification of transforming gene in two human sarcoma cell lines as a new member of the *ras* gene family located on chromosome 1. *Nature* **303:** 396–400.

Hancock, J.F., A.I. Magee, J.E. Childs, and C.J. Marshall. 1989. All *ras* proteins are polyisoprenylated but only some are palmitoylated. *Cell* **57:** 1167–1177.

Harvey, J.J. 1964. An unidentified virus which causes the rapid production of tumors in mice. *Nature* **204:** 1104–1105.

Jurnak, F. 1985. Structure of the GDP domain of EF-Tu and location of the amino acids homologous to *ras* oncogene proteins. *Science* **230:** 32–36.

Kataoka, T., S. Powers, S. Cameron, O. Fasano, M. Goldfarb, J. Broach, and M. Wigler. 1985. Functional homology of mammalian and yeast *RAS* genes. *Cell* **40:** 19–26.

Kirsten, W.H. and L.A. Mayer. 1967. Morphologic responses to a murine erythroblastosis virus. *J. Natl. Cancer Inst.* **39:** 311–335.

Korn, L.J., C.W. Siebel, F. McCormick, and R.A. Roth. 1987. *ras* p21 as a potential mediator of insulin action in *Xenopus* oocytes. *Science* **236:** 840–843.

Krontiris, T.G. and G.M. Cooper. 1981. Transforming activity of human tumor DNAs. *Proc. Natl. Acad. Sci.* **78:** 1181–1184.

Lacal, J.C., P. de la Pena, J. Moscat, P. Garcia-Barreno, P.S. Anderson, and S.A. Aaronson. 1987. Rapid stimulation of diacylglycerol production in *Xenopus* oocytes by microinjection of H-*ras* p21. *Science* **238:** 533–536.

la Cour, T.F.M., J. Nyborg, S. Thirup, and B.F.C. Clark. 1985. Structural details of the binding of guanosine diphosphate to elongation factor Tu from *E. coli* as studied by x-ray crystallography. *EMBO J.* **4:** 2385–2388.

Land, H., L.F. Parada, and R.A. Weinberg. 1983. Tumorigenic conversion of primary embryo fibroblasts requires at least two cooperating oncogenes. *Nature* **304:** 596–602.

Langbeheim, H., T.Y. Shih, and E.M. Scolnick. 1980. Identification of a normal vertebrate cell protein related to the p21 *src* of Harvey sarcoma virus. *Virology* **106:** 292–300.

Lowe, D.G., D.J. Capon, E. Delwart, A.Y. Sakaguchi, S. Naylor, and D.V. Goeddel. 1987. Structure of the human and murine R-*ras* genes, novel genes closely related to *ras* proto-oncogenes. *Cell* **48:** 137–146.

Madaule, P. and R. Axel. 1985. A novel *ras*-related gene family. *Cell* **41:** 31–40.

Manne, V., E. Bekesi, and H.F. Kung. 1985. Ha-*ras* proteins exhibit GTPase activity: Point mutations that activate Ha-*ras* gene products result in decreased GTPase activity. *Proc. Natl. Acad. Sci.* **82:** 376–380.

Matsumota, K., I. Uno, Y. Oshima, and T. Ishikawa. 1982. Isolation and characterization of yeast mutants deficient in adenylate cyclase and cAMP-dependent protein kinase. *Proc. Natl. Acad. Sci.* **79:** 2555–2559.

McCormick, F., C. Levenson, G. Cole, M. Innis, and R. Clark. 1987. Genetic and biochemical analysis of *ras* p21 structure. In *Critical determinants in carcinogenesis* (ed. F.F. Becker and T.J. Slaga), vol. 39, pp. 137–145. University of Texas Press, Austin.

McCormick, F., B.F. Clark, T.F. la Cour, M. Kjeldgaard, L. Norskov-Lauritsen, and J. Nyborg. 1985. A model for the tertiary structure of p21, the product of the *ras* oncogene. *Science* **230:** 78–82.

McGrath, J.P., D.J. Capon, D.V. Goeddel, and A.D. Levinson. 1984. Comparative biochemical properties of normal and activated human *ras* p21 protein. *Nature* **310:** 644–649.

Mulcahy, L.S., M.R. Smith, and D.W. Stacey. 1985. Requirement for *ras* proto-oncogene function during serum-stimulated growth of NIH 3T3 cells. *Nature* **313:** 241–243.

Neri, A., D.M. Knowles, A. Greco, F. McCormick, and R. Dalla-Favera. 1988. Analysis of *RAS* oncogene mutations in human lymphoid malignancies. *Proc. Natl. Acad. Sci.* **85:** 9268–9272.

Newbold, R.F. and R.W. Overell. 1983. Fibroblast immortality is a prerequisite for transformation by EJ c-Ha-*ras* oncogene. *Nature* **304:** 648–651.

Noda, M., T. Matsuzaki, M. Kitayama, Y. Sugimoto, H. Okayama, R.H. Bassin, and Y.

Ikawa. 1989. Detection of genes with a potential for suppressing the transformed phenotype associated with activated *ras* genes. *Proc. Natl. Acad. Sci.* **86:** 162–166.

Pai, E.F., W. Kabsch, K.C. Holmes, J. John, and A. Wittinghofer. 1989. Structure of the guanine nucleotide binding domain of the H-*ras* oncogene product p21 in the triphosphate conformation. *Nature* (in press).

Parada, L.F., C.J. Tabin, C. Shih, and R.A. Weinberg. 1982. Human EJ bladder carcinoma oncogene is homologue of Harvey sarcoma virus *ras* gene. *Nature* **297:** 474–478.

Perucho, M., M. Goldfarb, K. Shimizu, C. Lama, J. Fogh, and M. Wigler. 1981. Human-tumor-derived cell lines contain common and different transforming gene. *Cell* **27:** 467–476.

Pizon, V., P. Chardin, I. Lerosey, B. Olofsson, and A. Tavitian. 1988. Human cDNAs *rap*1 and *rap*2 homologous to the Drosophila gene D*ras*3 encode proteins closely related to *ras* in the effector region. *Oncogene* **3:** 201–204.

Pulciani, S., E. Santos, A.V. Lauver, L.K. Long, K.C. Robbins, and M. Barbacid. 1982. Oncogenes in human tumor cell lines: Molecular cloning of a transforming gene from human bladder carcinoma cells. *Proc. Natl. Acad. Sci.* **79:** 2845–2849.

Quintanilla, M., K. Brown, M. Ramsden, and A. Balmain. 1986. Carcinogen-specific mutation and amplification of Ha-*ras* during mouse skin carcinogenesis. *Nature* **322:** 78–80.

Reddy, E.P., R.K. Reynolds, E. Santos, and M. Barbacid. 1982. A point mutation is responsible for the acquisition of transforming properties of the T24 human bladder carcinoma oncogene. *Nature* **300:** 149–152.

Ruley, H.E. 1983. Adenovirus early region 1A enables viral and cellular transforming genes to transform primary cells in culture. *Nature* **304:** 602–605.

Santos, E., S.R. Tronick, S.A. Aaronson, S. Pulciani, and M. Barbacid. 1982. T24 human bladder carcinoma oncogene is an activated form of the normal human homologue of BALB- and Harvey-MSV transforming genes. *Nature* **298:** 343–347.

Satoh, T., S. Nakamura, and Y. Kaziro. 1987. Induction of neurite formation in PC12 cells by microinjection of proto-oncogenic Ha-*ras* protein preincubated with guanosine-5′-*O*-(3-thiotriphosphate). *Mol. Cell. Biol.* **7:** 4553–4556.

Scolnick, E.M., A.G. Papageorge, and T.Y. Shih. 1979. Guanine nucleotide-binding activity as an assay for *src* protein of rat-derived murine sarcoma viruses. *Proc. Natl. Acad. Sci.* **76:** 5355–5359.

Seeburg, P.H., W.W. Colby, D.J. Capon, D.V. Goeddel, and A.D. Levinson. 1984. Biological properties of human c-Ha-*ras*1 genes mutated at codon 12. *Nature* **312:** 71–75.

Shen, W.P.V., T.H. Aldrich, G. Venta-Perez, B.R. Franza, Jr., and M.E. Furth. 1987. Expression of normal and mutant *ras* proteins in human acute leukemia. *Oncogene* **1:** 157–165.

Shih, C., B.-Z. Shilo, M.P. Goldfarb, A. Dannenberg, and R.A. Weinberg. 1979. Passage of phenotypes of chemically transformed cells via transfection of DNA and chromatin. *Proc. Natl. Acad. Sci.* **76:** 5714–5718.

Shimizu, K., M. Goldfarb, Y. Suard, M. Perucho, Y. Li, T. Kamata, J. Feramisco, E. Stavnezer, J. Fogh, and M.H. Wigler. 1983. Three human transforming genes are related to the viral *ras* oncogenes. *Proc. Natl. Acad. Sci.* **80:** 2112–2116.

Sigal, I., J.B. Gibbs, J.S. D'Alonzo, and E.M. Scolnick. 1986a. Identification of effector residues and a neutralizing epitope of a-*ras*-encoded p21. *Proc. Natl. Acad. Sci.* **83:** 4725–4729.

Sigal, I.S., J.B. Gibbs, J.S. D'Alonzo, G.L. Temeles, B.S. Wolanski, S.H. Socher, and E.M. Scolnick. 1986b. Mutant *ras*-encoded proteins with altered nucleotide binding exert dominant biological effects. *Proc. Natl. Acad. Sci.* **83:** 951–956.

Smith, M.R., S.J. DeGudicibus, and D.W. Stacey. 1986. Requirement for c-*ras* proteins during viral oncogene transformation. *Nature* **320:** 540–543.

Spandidos, D.A. 1986. *Anticancer Res.* **6:** 259–262.

Sukumar, S., S. Pulciani, J. Doniger, J.A. DiPaolo, C.H. Evans, B. Zbar, and M. Barbacid. 1984. A transforming *ras* gene in tumorigenic guinea pig cell lines initiated by diverse chemical carcinogens. *Science* **223:** 1197–1199.

Sweet, R.W., S. Yokiyama, T. Kamata, J.R. Feramisco, M. Rosenberg, and M. Gross. 1984. The product of *ras* is a GTPase and the T24 oncogenic mutant is deficient in this activity. *Nature* **311:** 273–275.

Tabin, C.J., S.M. Bradley, C.I. Bergman, R.A. Weinberg, A.G. Papageorge, E.M. Scolnick, R. Dhar, D.R. Lowy, and E.H. Chang. 1982. Mechanism of activation of a human oncogene. *Nature* **300:** 143–149.

Taparowsky, E., K. Shimizu, M. Goldfarb, and M. Wigler. 1983. Structure and activation of the human N-*ras* gene. *Cell* **34:** 581–586.

Tatchell, K., L.C. Robinson, and M. Breitenbach. 1985. *RAS*2 of *Saccharomyces cerevisiae* is required for gluconeogenic growth and proper response to nutrient limitation. *Proc. Natl. Acad. Sci.* **82:** 3785–3789.

Toda, T., I. Uno, T. Ishikawa, S. Powers, T. Kataoka, D. Broek, S. Cameron, J. Broach, K. Matsumoto, and M. Wigler. 1985. In yeast, *RAS* proteins are controlling elements of adenylate cyclase. *Cell* **40:** 27–36.

Touchot, N., P. Chardin, and A. Tavitian. 1987. Four additional members of the *ras* super-family isolated by an oligonucleotide strategy: Molecular cloning of YPT-related cDNAs from a rat brain. *Proc. Natl. Acad. Sci.* **84:** 8210–8214.

Trahey, M. and F. McCormick. 1987. A cytoplasmic protein regulates GTPase of normal N-*ras* p21, but does not affect oncogenic mutants. *Science* **238:** 542–545.

Trahey, M., R.J. Milley, G.E. Cole, M. Innis, H. Paterson, C.J. Marshall, A. Hall, and F. McCormick. 1987. Biochemical and biological properties of the human N-*ras* p21 protein. *Mol. Cell. Biol.* **7:** 541–544.

Trahey, M., G. Wong, R. Halenbeck, B. Rubinfeld, G.A. Martin, M. Ladner, C.M. Long, W.J. Crosier, K. Watt, K. Koths, and F. McCormick. 1988. Molecular cloning of two types of GAP complementary DNA from human placenta. *Science* **242:** 1697–1700.

Vogel, U., R.A.F. Dixon, M.D. Schaber, R.E. Diehl, M.S. Marshall, E.M. Scolnick, I.S. Sigal, and J. Gibbs. 1988. Cloning of bovine GAP and its interaction with oncogenic *ras* p21. *Nature* **335:** 90–93.

Walter, M., S.G. Clark, and A.D. Levinson. 1986. The oncogenic activation of human p21 *ras* by a novel mechanism. *Science* **233:** 649–652.

Willingham, M.C., I. Pastan, T.Y. Shih, and E.M. Scolnick. 1980. Localization of the *src* gene product of the Harvey strain of MSV to plasma membrane of transformed cells by electron microscopic immunocytochemistry. *Cell* **19:** 1005–1014.

Willumsen, B.M., A. Christensen, N.L. Hubbert, A.G. Papageorge, and D.R. Lowy. 1984. The p21 *ras* C-terminus is required for transformation and membrane association. *Nature* **310:** 583–586.

Willumsen, B.M., A.G. Papageorge, H.-F. Kung, E. Bekesi, T. Robins, M. Johnsen, W.C. Vass, and D.R. Lowy. 1986. Mutational analysis of a *ras* catalytic domain. *Mol. Cell. Biol.* **6:** 2646–2654.

Yu, C.-L., M.-H. Tsai, and D.W. Stacey. 1988. Cellular *ras* activity and phospholipid metabolism. *Cell* **52:** 63–71.

Yuasa, Y., S.K. Srivastava, C.Y. Dunn, J.S. Rhim, E.P. Reddy, and S.A. Aaronson. 1983. Acquisition of transforming properties by alternative point mutations within c-*bas*/*ras* human proto-oncogene. *Nature* **303:** 775–779.

6

Oncogene Products in the Cytoplasm: The Protein Kinases

Tony Hunter
Molecular Biology and Virology Laboratory
The Salk Institute
San Diego, California 92138

I. INTRODUCTION

The dogma emerging from the study of prokaryotic regulatory systems in the 1960s led many investigators to suspect that the majority of mammalian oncoproteins would function in the nucleus where they would perturb gene expression and thus induce the transformed phenotype. When it was proved in the mid-1970s that the papovavirus nuclear T antigens were indeed the virally encoded transforming proteins, this surmise appeared to be borne out. The mold was soon broken, however, with the demonstration in 1978 that the transforming protein of Rous sarcoma virus, pp60$^{v\text{-}src}$, was a cytoplasmic protein. In the ensuing years, a surprisingly large proportion of oncoproteins have been found to act in the cytoplasm.

What do we know about the cytoplasmic oncogene products? A seminal discovery here was that pp60$^{v\text{-}src}$ had an associated protein kinase activity that could transfer phosphate from the γ position of ATP to protein (Collett and Erikson 1978; Levinson et al. 1978). This revelation was exciting because there were many precedents for protein phosphorylation changing the activity of proteins. For instance, phosphorylation of glycogen phosphorylase by phosphorylase kinase increases its activity severalfold. Thus, it appeared that pp60$^{v\text{-}src}$ could transform cells through the unregulated phosphorylation of cellular proteins whose activity would be changed upon phosphorylation. Since most protein kinases are pleiotropic, one would anticipate that pp60$^{v\text{-}src}$ would be able to phosphorylate many distinct target proteins, altering the activity of each one. In this way, the multifaceted nature of the transformed phenotype could be explained by the existence of target proteins in many different cellular pathways, each of which would be affected by pp60$^{v\text{-}src}$-mediated phosphorylation. In particular, activation of a signal pathway leading to the nucleus, which induces gene expression, would neatly explain how a cytoplasmic oncoprotein could influence nuclear events. We will see later to what extent these ideas have been borne out in the discussion of the substrates for the oncogenic protein kinases.

At the outset, pp60$^{v\text{-}src}$ was thought to be a typical protein kinase that phosphorylates the hydroxyl groups of serine or threonine in its target proteins. Shortly after its discovery, however, it was shown that pp60$^{v\text{-}src}$ phosphorylates proteins exclusively on the hydroxyl group of tyrosine and is therefore a protein tyrosine kinase (Hunter and Sefton 1980). Simultaneously, the transforming protein of Abelson murine leukemia virus (the v-*abl* protein) was found to have protein tyrosine kinase activity (Witte et al. 1980). Within a year, several additional retroviral oncogene products had been shown to phosphorylate proteins on tyrosine. This implied that aberrant tyrosine phosphorylation could be a common mechanism of transformation.

At that time, no cellular protein kinase had been reported to phosphorylate tyrosine, so the next step was to find out if there are cellular enzymes with this specificity. The natural starting point was with the products of the proto-oncogenes, which gave rise to the oncogenic protein kinases. The first to be examined was pp60$^{c\text{-}src}$, the cellular progenitor of pp60$^{v\text{-}src}$ (by convention viral oncogenes are given the prefix "v-," and the cellular oncogenes from which they originated are given the prefix "c-"), and it too was found to have protein tyrosine kinase activity (Hunter and Sefton 1980). Subsequently, each one of the cellular counterparts of the oncogenic protein tyrosine kinases has proved to be a protein tyrosine kinase.

The third cellular protein tyrosine kinase to be identified did not come from an examination of proto-oncogene products, but from another direction. At the time pp60$^{v\text{-}src}$ was reported to be a protein tyrosine kinase, the receptor for epidermal growth factor (EGF), which is a mitogen for a wide variety of cell types, was already known to be a protein kinase whose activity was stimulated severalfold upon binding EGF. With the realization that protein kinases could phosphorylate tyrosine, the specificity of the EGF receptor was reexamined, and it was found to be a protein tyrosine kinase as well (Ushiro and Cohen 1980). This immediately suggested that there might be a normal mitogenic signal pathway that uses tyrosine phosphorylation. The subsequent discovery that several other growth factor receptors are ligand-stimulated protein tyrosine kinases strongly supports this notion. The existence of a mitogen-activated tyrosine phosphorylation signal pathway raises the possibility that oncogenic protein tyrosine kinases might usurp this pathway and thus incite the unregulated growth characteristic of transformed cells. Since mitogens activate nuclear signal pathways leading to gene induction, the usurpation of such a pathway could be the means by which the oncogenic cytoplasmic protein tyrosine kinases perturb gene expression.

The number of distinct cellular protein tyrosine kinase genes has now risen to more than 30 (Table 1) (for review, see Hunter and Cooper 1985; Hunter 1987b), but despite the plethora of such enzymes, tyrosine phosphorylation only accounts for a very small fraction of protein phosphorylation events in normal cells. The majority of phosphate linked to protein is in the form of phosphoserine (~90%) and phosphothreonine (~9%), with phosphotyrosine contributing less than 0.1% (Hunter and Sefton 1980). The discrepancy between the number of enzymes and the level of

Table 1 Vertebrate cellular protein kinases

Protein tyrosine kinases	
src family	
$pp60^{c\text{-}src}$ (two forms generated by alternate splicing)	
c-*yes* protein	
lck protein	
c-*fgr* protein	
fyn protein	
lyn protein	
hck protein	
tkl protein (possibly chicken *lck*)	
fps/*fes* family	
$p92^{c\text{-}fes}/p98^{c\text{-}fps}$	
NCP94 (FER protein)	
abl family	
$p150^{c\text{-}abl}$ (2 different amino termini generated by alternate splicing)	
arg protein	
growth factor receptors	
EGF receptor	PDGF receptor (α and β forms)
neu (*erbB2*) protein	CSF-1 receptor
	c-*kit* protein
insulin receptor	*ret* protein
IGF-1 receptor	FGF receptor (*flg* protein)
met protein	
trk protein	*eph* protein
c-*ros* protein	*eck* protein
c-*sea* protein	*elk* protein
others	
p75	
ltk protein	
flt protein	

(*Continued on following page.*)

Table 1 (continued).

Protein serine kinases
cyclic nucleotide regulated
cAMP-dependent protein kinase (α and β forms)
cGMP-dependent protein kinase
Ca^{++}/calmodulin regulated
myosin light chain kinase (skeletal and smooth muscle forms)
calmodulin-dependent protein kinase I
calmodulin-dependent protein kinase II (α and β forms)
calmodulin-dependent protein kinase III
phosphorylase kinase γ subunit
PSK-C3
diacylglycerol regulated
protein kinase C (α, βI, βII, γ, δ, ϵ, and ζ forms)
raf family
c-*raf* protein
A-*raf* protein
B-*raf* protein
others
casein kinases I and II
proteinase-activated kinase I
glycogen synthase kinases 3 and 4
double-stranded RNA and double-stranded DNA regulated protein kinases
heme-regulated protein kinase
S6 protein kinases
β-adrenergic receptor and rhodopsin protein kinases
MAP-2 protein kinase
HMGCoA reductase protein kinase
pyruvate dehydrogenase protein kinase
c-*mos* protein
pim-1 protein
CDC2Hs protein (catalytic subunit of maturation promoting factor [MPF] and histone H1 growth-associated protein kinase)
PSK-J3

phosphotyrosine indicates that cellular protein tyrosine kinases are normally under strict negative control. As we will see, it is often this negative control that is abrogated when an oncogenic protein tyrosine kinase arises. The currently ascribed functions of the protein tyrosine kinases suggest that tyrosine phosphorylation is largely reserved for signal transduction and regulatory systems involved in cell growth, cell–cell interaction, and differentiation. Perturbation of such functions could readily lead to cellular transformation. Indeed, it may well prove that every cellular protein tyrosine kinase gene has the potential to be converted into an oncogene.

One should not get the impression, however, that all the oncogenic protein kinases are protein tyrosine kinases. Oncogenic protein kinases with specificity for serine and threonine are known (Table 2). This is not totally unexpected since serine and threonine phosphorylation events, although commonly used for metabolic regulation, are clearly important in some signal transduction pathways. For instance, the protein serine kinase, protein kinase C, is activated by diacylglycerol (DAG) that is produced as a result of hormonal activation of phospholipase C. The same arguments advanced earlier about the ability of an unregulated protein tyrosine kinase to perturb cellular regulation hold true for such protein serine kinases as well.

All known protein tyrosine kinases are related structurally in their catalytic domains. From the molecular cloning and sequencing of the oncogenes encoding protein kinases, it emerges that each one has a region of homology spanning about 300 amino acids (Hanks et al. 1988). This region was originally identified as the catalytic domain by comparison with the sequence of the catalytic subunit of the cAMP-dependent protein kinase, which is a protein serine kinase (Barker and Dayhoff 1982). Examination of the catalytic domain sequences from over 60 protein tyrosine and protein serine kinases shows that there are a number of highly

Table 2 Oncogenic protein kinases

Protein tyrosine kinases
membrane-associated
growth factor receptor-related
v-*erbB* (derived from EGF receptor)
neu (*erbB2*) protein
v-*fms* protein (derived from CSF-1 receptor)
v-*kit* protein
trk protein
met protein
ret protein
v-*ros* protein
v-*sea* protein
src family
v-*src* protein ($pp60^{v\text{-}src}$)
v-*yes* protein
v-*fgr* protein
lck protein
cytoplasmic
v-*fps* (v-*fes*) protein
v-*abl* protein
Protein-serine kinases
v-*mos* protein
v-*raf* (v-*mil*) protein
pim-1 protein

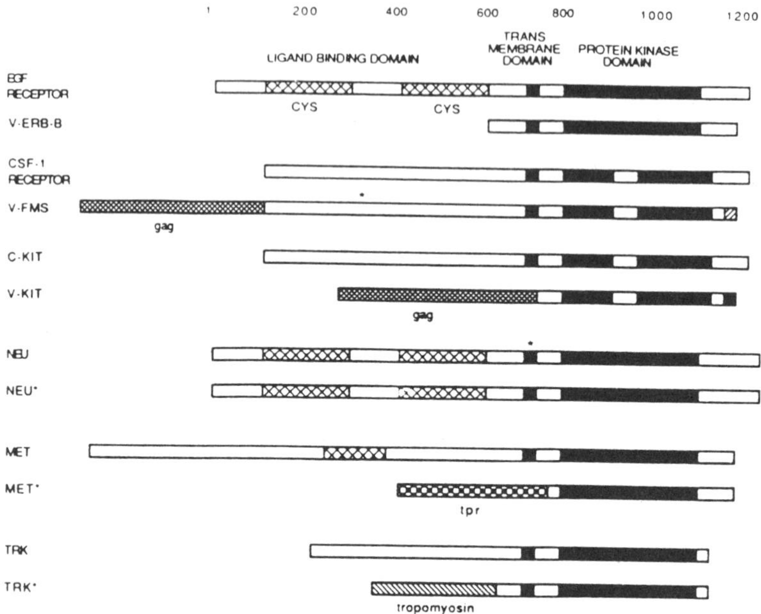

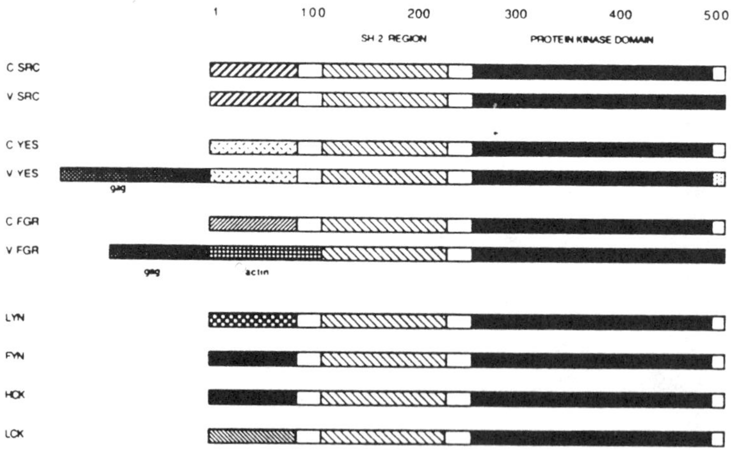

Figure 1 (*Continued on facing page.*)

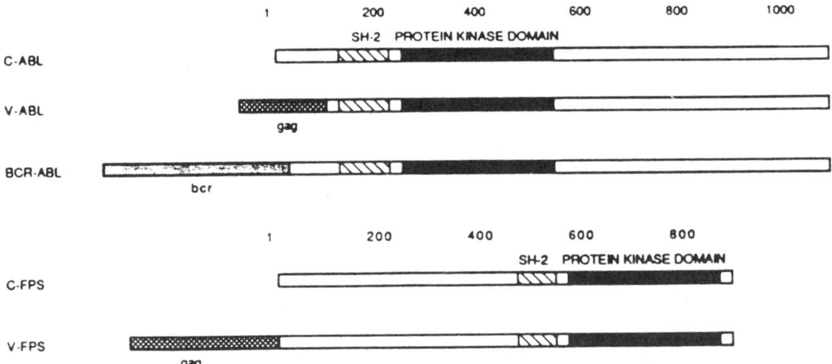

Figure 1 Structures of oncogenic protein tyrosine kinases and their cellular progenitors. The structures of the various protein kinases are depicted as boxes whose approximate size in numbers of amino acids is indicated above the first protein in each section with the amino terminal being on the left. The protein kinase domain is indicated by a black filled box in each case (the catalytic domain is interrupted in the case of the CSF-1 receptor and c-*kit* protein). Where there are sequence differences between the cellular protein tyrosine kinase and its oncogenic derivative, these are indicated by a box with a different fill. An asterisk above the box indicates single amino acid differences that are essential for oncogenic activity. In the growth factor receptor protein kinases, cysteine-rich regions in the ligand-binding domains are indicated as cross-hatched boxes and the transmembrane domains as stippled boxes. The identities of the new amino termini for oncogenic derivatives are given under the relevant boxes. The oncogenic derivatives of *neu, met,* and *trk* are designated NEU*, etc. In the *src* protein kinase family, the unique amino-terminal sequence of each member is indicated by a box with a different fill. The SH-2 region is shown as a hatched box. The same conventions are used for the *abl* and *fps* protein kinases.

conserved groups of residues spread over a region of about 300 amino acids (Hanks et al. 1988). These conserved structural features permit one to diagnose whether any novel protein sequence is likely to be a protein kinase. In addition, there are distinguishing differences in some of these conserved regions, which allow one to deduce whether the sequence in question is that of a protein tyrosine or a protein serine kinase. This has been particularly useful in predicting the function of oncogene products. In several instances, oncoprotein sequences decoded from cloned DNA sequences have been found to possess putative protein kinase domains, and upon isolation, these oncoproteins are indeed found to be protein kinases.

The oncogenic protein kinases are derived from normal cellular enzymes that do not have transforming properties. The key question then is what are the differences between the oncogenic protein kinases and their normal cellular counterparts that account for their oncogenic properties. The fact that the corresponding proto-oncogenic protein kinases are also specific for tyrosine rules out the unlikely possibility that an alteration in amino acid specificity might be important for the transforming activity of the oncogenic protein kinases. Moreover, although it would be an attractive explanation, there is no evidence so far that the oncogenic protein kinases have altered protein substrate specificities, which would lead to the phosphorylation of proteins not phosphorylated by their normal cellular counterparts. What then is the basis for their oncogenic potential? In general, protein kinases are larger than the minimal catalytic domain (see Figs. 1 and 2), and in most cases, the additional sequences appear to be regulatory in nature. As we will see, the mutations that are responsible for converting normal protein kinase genes into transforming genes commonly abolish negative regulatory domains, thus turning these enzymes into protein kinases that can no longer be regulated by the cell and therefore act constitutively to phosphorylate their substrates.

A second important issue in understanding transformation by the oncogenic protein kinases is the exact nature of their protein substrates. A knowledge of these substrates and how phosphorylation affects their function is obviously essential for a molecular understanding of the process of transformation by oncogenic protein kinases. For instance, we need to know whether it is really true that the relevant substrates phosphorylated by these protein kinases are normally phosphorylated by their nononcogenic counterparts or whether, despite current evidence, the oncogenic

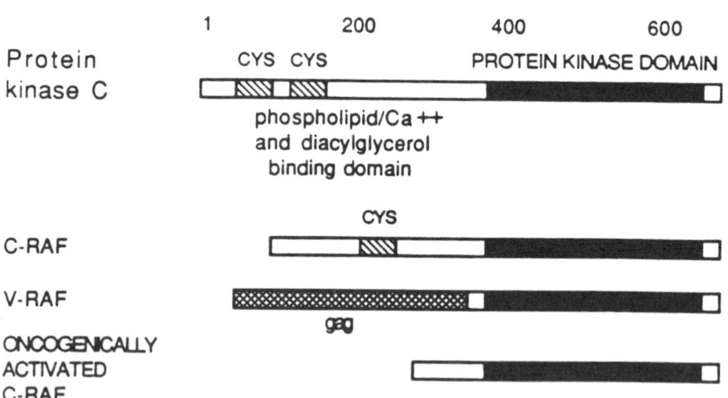

Figure 2 Structures of protein kinase C and *raf* protein kinases. The structures of protein kinase C and three different *raf* protein kinases are shown using the conventions described in Fig. 1. Two homologous cysteine-rich regions are shown as hatched boxes in protein kinase C. A cysteine-rich region related to those in protein kinase C is indicated in the c-*raf* protein.

protein kinases might have altered specificities. These points will be addressed later.

More than half of the approximately 30 known oncoproteins that act outside the nucleus have proved to be protein kinases. The majority of these are protein tyrosine kinases, but there are three oncogenes that encode protein serine kinases (Table 2). The oncogenes that encode protein tyrosine kinases will be discussed first, followed by a consideration of those encoding protein serine kinases. A few cytoplasmic oncoproteins are neither protein kinases nor *ras* proteins (see Chapter 5), and for completeness these will be summarized briefly at the end.

II. ONCOGENIC PROTEIN TYROSINE KINASES

It is convenient to classify the oncogenic protein tyrosine kinases on the basis of their specific cytoplasmic localization. Most of these enzymes are associated with cytoplasmic membranes either as transmembrane proteins or through a covalently attached lipid moiety. A minority are more diffusely distributed in the cytoplasm. One can further subdivide the membrane-associated oncogenic protein tyrosine kinases into growth-factor-receptor-related protein tyrosine kinases and *src*-related protein tyrosine kinases. The receptor protein tyrosine kinases span the membrane once, having a large amino-terminal ligand-binding domain on the outside and the protein kinase domain on the inside. In contrast, the *src*-related protein tyrosine kinases do not span the membrane, but rather are associated with the inner face of the membrane.

A. Growth-factor-receptor-related Oncogenes

The discovery that the v-*erbB* oncogene of avian erythroblastosis virus was derived from the chicken EGF receptor gene (Downward et al. 1984; Ullrich et al. 1984) foreshadowed a veritable explosion of oncogenes that are derived from genes for growth factor receptors with protein tyrosine kinase activity. Another example is the v-*fms* oncogene, which was derived from the gene for the receptor for colony-stimulating factor-1 (CSF-1), a myeloid cell growth factor (Sherr et al. 1985). The binding of growth factor to this type of receptor stimulates protein tyrosine kinase activity. In this way, the presence of bound growth factor is converted into an intracellular signal by the phosphorylation of cytoplasmic proteins on tyrosine, which in turn propagate the mitogenic signal to the nucleus.

There are several other oncogenes that were engendered by cellular genes that appear to be growth factor receptor protein tyrosine kinase genes (Table 2). This supposition is based on the similarities between the structures of their products and those of authentic growth factor receptor protein tyrosine kinases (i.e., the EGF, platelet-derived growth factor [PDGF], insulin-like growth factor-1 [IGF-I], insulin, fibroblast growth factor [FGF], and CSF-1 receptors). The canonical structure of this type of receptor consists of a large amino-terminal external domain, a single membrane-spanning region, a 50–70-amino-acid cytoplasmic spacer followed by a protein kinase catalytic domain, and then a carboxy-terminal tail of variable length (Fig. 1) (for review, see Yarden and Ullrich 1988). Recognizable remnants of such a structure are evident in the *neu*, *trk*, *met*, *kit*, *ros*, *sea*, and *ret* oncogene products. Most of them have at least a residual external domain, a transmembrane sequence, and a protein kinase catalytic domain. In those cases where the complete structure of the cellular homologs has been deduced from cDNA clones (i.e., for the *neu*, *trk*, *met*, and *kit* genes), they are indeed typical of the growth factor receptor protein tyrosine kinases. Nevertheless, it should be borne in mind that the identification of a ligand will be required to prove that these are bona fide receptors.

How is a normal growth factor receptor protein tyrosine kinase converted into a protein with oncogenic potential? In thinking about possible principles of oncogenic activation, an understanding of the mechanism through which the binding of ligand to the normal receptor stimulates its protein tyrosine kinase activity will clearly be important (see Chapter 3). The most widely accepted model of signal transduction proposes that ligand binding to the external domain induces a conformational change that leads to dimerization of the receptor in the plane of the plasma membrane (Yarden and Schlessinger 1987a,b).

The exact mechanism by which receptor protein kinase activity is increased is not known. The best guess is that an autophosphorylation reaction is involved, which results in the relief of an inhibitory constraint. Most receptors autophosphorylate at one or more tyrosines following ligand binding, and in some cases, this has been shown to result in an increase in protein kinase activity. Receptor autophosphorylation sites can lie within the catalytic domain or in a separate regulatory domain. In both cases, these autophosphorylation sites may exert a negative effect in their unphosphorylated state by competing with substrates at the active site. One plausible idea is that within a receptor dimer, one protein kinase domain can phosphorylate the other, thus leading to mutual activation.

In summary, there are two main levels of regulation of receptor protein tyrosine kinase activity, both of which ensure that the catalytic domain is normally in an inactive state. First, ligand binding is needed to provide a positive signal. Second, negative regulation of the protein kinase domain has to be nullified by autophosphorylation. Although these principles hold true for the studied receptor protein tyrosine kinases, one has to remember that the mechanisms of regulation differ in detail, and this is reflected in the ways in which receptor genes are activated into oncogenes.

Thus, when we examine the individual receptor-derived oncogenes, it becomes clear that there are several mechanisms of oncogenic activation, rather than a universal principle of activation. In some instances, simple overexpression of a normal receptor is sufficient to induce the transformed phenotype in a cultured cell line. For example, overexpression of either the EGF receptor in the presence of EGF or the closely related normal *neu* protein in NIH-3T3 cells leads to transformation (Di Fiore et al. 1987; Hudziak et al. 1987). In addition, there are human tumor types where either the EGF receptor gene or the *neu* gene is found to be amplified between 10- and 50-fold (Libermann et al. 1985; Slamon et al. 1987). This amplification is accompanied by a large increase in protein expression. However, it has not been shown that these amplifications are instrumental in tumorigenesis. The reason why overexpression of the *neu* protein induces transformation in culture is not well defined. Even though the protein tyrosine kinase activity of receptors is tightly negatively regulated, the extraordinarily high level of receptor may mean that the basal level of protein tyrosine kinase activity now exceeds the threshold required for mitogenic signaling. This tendency may be exacerbated by low levels of the cognate growth factor in the culture medium of these cells, which would normally be insufficient to induce mitogenesis.

Activation by overexpression does not require any change in the structure of the receptor protein. In contrast, the other mechanisms of receptor activation all involve mutations causing structural changes in the receptor that result in deregulation of protein kinase activity. The most common change is the loss of all or part of the amino-terminal external ligand-binding domain, including the signal peptide (Fig. 1). This has occurred in the v-*erbB* gene, which is derived from the EGF receptor gene, and in the *trk*, *met*, *kit*, *ros*, *sea*, and *ret* genes. In every instance except the v-*erbB* protein, the amino-terminal truncation has occurred through recombination with another sequence, which results in a chimeric protein. In most cases the foreign amino terminus contains a signal peptide or a lipid-attachment signal, and these oncoproteins are found to be membrane associated. Regardless of whether or not they span or simply affiliate with the membrane, the absence of the true receptor external domain will clearly preclude both ligand binding and ligand-dependent regulation of protein kinase activity.

The exact effect that the loss of the external domain will have on protein kinase activity is hard to predict. Given that this region normally transmits a positive signal, it is possible that the truncated receptors cannot achieve maximal activity unless the foreign amino terminus is in some manner able to promote dimerization. In the case of the v-*erbB* protein, sequences present in the EGF receptor at the carboxyl terminus containing one of the autophosphorylation sites have also been lost. This may partially activate the protein kinase by relieving the normal negative constraint of this region. The carboxyl termini of the v-*ros* and v-*kit* proteins are also altered, but those of the *trk, met,* v-*sea,* and *ret* receptor-derived oncoproteins are unchanged. We can generalize by concluding that the structural mutations in these receptors result in proteins that have constitutive unregulated kinase activity.

Two other receptor-derived oncogenes have distinct mutational activation mechanisms. Both of them are instructive. The activation of the *neu* gene (also known as c-*erbB2* or HER2 gene), which is closely related to the EGF receptor gene, requires only a point mutation (Bargmann et al. 1986). This mutation results in the conversion of a valine residue to a glutamic acid in the transmembrane domain. Transmembrane domains consist of 20–26 uncharged hydrophobic residues. In proteins with a single transmembrane domain, the presence of charged residues in a transmembrane domain is normally forbidden. Nevertheless, the *neu* oncoprotein is transported and displayed on the cell surface just like the normal *neu* protein. The location and charged nature of this activating mutation must provide an important clue to the normal mechanism of signal transduction by the *neu* protein and other receptors of this type. Site-directed mutational analysis shows that glutamine, which is hydrophilic but uncharged, as well as aspartic acid, can substitute for glutamic acid, but positively charged amino acids do not activate the *neu* gene (Bargmann and Weinberg 1988a). The oncogenic *neu* protein has greater protein tyrosine kinase activity both in vivo and in vitro than the normal *neu* protein, implying that the mutation leads to activation of the protein kinase domain (Bargmann and Weinberg 1988b). Exactly how the mutation in the transmembrane domain might do this is unclear, but one possibility is that it causes the protein to dimerize and thus adopt an active configuration.

A study of the v-*fms* oncogene indicates that two mutational events are required to convert the c-*fms* or CSF-1 receptor gene into an oncogene (Roussel et al. 1987; for review, see Sherr 1988). First, the carboxy-terminal region, which lies beyond the catalytic domain, has to be eliminated. This region contains a tyrosine six residues from the carboxyl terminus, which is suspected to have a negative regulatory function. Experimentally, activation of the carboxy-terminal region can be achieved by site-directed mutation of the tyrosine to a phenylalanine (Roussel et al. 1987). Second, a point mutation in the amino-terminal CSF-1-binding region is necessary for complete oncogenic activation. Interestingly, this mutation does not abolish CSF-1 binding, but in some undefined way makes the v-*fms* protein tyrosine kinase activity independent of ligand, and therefore considerably higher than that of the unstimulated CSF-1 receptor.

The protein kinase activity of these mutant receptors has been shown by site-directed mutation to be essential for transformation (for example, see Chen et al. 1987). Their activity is ligand-independent and constitutive, and cells transformed by these oncoproteins contain higher levels of phosphotyrosine in protein, which reflects the unregulated protein tyrosine kinase activity. The identities of the substrates that need to be phosphorylated to induce the transformed phenotype, however, have not been determined. It has been shown that the v-*erbB*, v-*fms*, *neu*, and v-*ros* proteins, all of which are transmembrane in nature, must reach the cell surface to transform, where they may truly mimic ligand-occupied growth factor receptors and phosphorylate proteins normally involved in the mitogenic pathway. However, even though their progenitors are transmembrane proteins, the *trk* (Mitra et al. 1987) and *met* oncogene products are soluble cytoplasmic proteins. Thus, a plasma membrane location is clearly not essential for transformation.

B. The *src* Family Oncogenes

The second class of membrane-associated oncogenic protein tyrosine kinases is typified by pp60$^{c\text{-}src}$, which is a member of a group of closely related protein tyrosine kinases with very similar structures, known as the *src* gene family (for review, see Cooper 1989). This family includes the *src*, *yes*, *fgr*, *fyn*, *lyn*, *lck*, and *hck* genes. All these protein kinases are about 500 amino acids in length and have the same general organization, with the 250-residue catalytic domain positioned near the carboxyl terminus, followed by a carboxy-terminal tail of about 15 residues (Fig. 1). Over the carboxy-terminal 420 amino acids, these proteins have about 75% identity, but, with the exception of the amino-terminal glycine residue, their amino-terminal 80 residues are almost completely divergent. This amino-terminal glycine is modified by covalent attachment of a myristyl group through an amide linkage. Although these proteins have neither a signal peptide nor a transmembrane domain, this fatty acid provides the means by which these proteins associate with membranes. Thus, the *src* family protein tyrosine kinases are localized to the inner face of the plasma and other cytoplasmic membranes, but, unlike the receptor protein tyrosine kinases, they do not span the membrane.

The physiological functions of the *src* family protein tyrosine kinases are not known. The pattern of expression of the genes in this family, however, gives some clues. Many of these genes are uniquely expressed in individual hematopoietic lineages. For instance, the *lck* protein is present nearly exclusively in cells of the T-cell lineage. In contrast, the *hck* gene is expressed predominantly in granulocytes. The expression of pp60$^{c\text{-}src}$ is regulated in a somewhat different manner. Although it is present in megakaryocytes and platelets at high levels, pp60$^{c\text{-}src}$ is found in nearly every cell type in the body. In particular, pp60$^{c\text{-}src}$ is found in abundance in neurons of the central nervous system, where an altered form of pp60$^{c\text{-}src}$ is expressed that contains six additional amino acids within the amino-terminal half of the protein. It is not yet known whether the different members of the *src* gene family play equivalent roles in the cell types in which they are expressed, or whether the unique amino-terminal sequence of each protein could dictate a unique activity.

Based on the patterns of expression and subcellular location, there have been a number of speculations about the function of these protein kinases. Even though mutant forms can incite continuous growth in transformed cells, the high levels of pp60$^{c\text{-}src}$ and other members of this family in terminally differentiated cells are incompatible with the simple model that these protein kinases function only to regulate cell growth. In differentiated cells, their submembranous location suggests that these protein kinases could regulate the activity of transmembrane proteins such as ion channels or receptors, which would influence the response of cells to their external enivronment. In keeping with this notion, there is evidence that the flux of Na^+ and K^+ is abnormal in RSV-transformed cells. pp60$^{v\text{-}src}$ also decreases intercellular communication through gap junctions, which might imply a regulatory role for pp60$^{c\text{-}src}$ in this system. Since pp60$^{c\text{-}src}$ is present at high levels in many cells that are active in secretion (e.g., neurons, platelets, and chromaffin granule cells, where at least some of the protein is associated with secretory granules), it has been proposed that pp60$^{c\text{-}src}$ may be involved in secretion. Another attractive possibility is that these proteins may act as subunits for surface receptors, which lack an intrinsic protein kinase domain. The reported association of the *lck* protein with the CD4 lymphocyte surface protein is consistent with this idea. As subunits of receptors, the *src* family protein tyrosine kinases could serve to transduce signals for a growth factor receptor in dividing cells, and a different receptor in differentiated cells. This dual role could explain the apparent paradox that these proteins can affect the growth of cells as well as being important in nondividing cells.

One essential feature of this family of protein tyrosine kinases is that their phosphotransferase activity is negatively regulated by phosphorylation. pp60$^{c\text{-}src}$, which is the best-studied member, is phosphorylated by a protein tyrosine kinase of unknown provenance at the most carboxy-terminal tyrosine, Tyr-527, which lies in the tail beyond the catalytic domain (Cooper et al. 1986). This phosphorylation suppresses the catalytic activity of pp60$^{c\text{-}src}$ by an as yet undefined mechanism (Courtneidge 1985; Cooper and King 1986). When isolated from the cell, pp60$^{c\text{-}src}$ is nearly fully phosphorylated at Tyr-527 and is therefore largely in an inactive state. Presumably, the stimulus that turns on pp60$^{c\text{-}src}$ either inhibits the Tyr-527 protein kinase or else activates the Tyr-527 phosphatase. A conserved tyrosine is present at this position in each of the *src* family protein kinases, and it seems likely that they are all negatively regulated by phosphorylation at this residue (Cooper 1989).

The regulation of these normal protein tyrosine kinases has an important bearing on their oncogenic activation. As an example, we can consider the conversion of pp60$^{c\text{-}src}$ into pp60$^{v\text{-}src}$ (for review, see Hunter 1987a). Although chicken pp60$^{c\text{-}src}$ and pp60$^{v\text{-}src}$ are very similar in structure over their amino-terminal 514 amino acids, apart from a few scattered point mutations, the two proteins diverge completely at their carboxyl termini. From residue 515, the carboxy-terminal 19 amino acids of pp60$^{c\text{-}src}$ have been replaced in pp60$^{v\text{-}src}$ by 12 unrelated amino acids. The obvious consequence of removal of the carboxyl terminus is the elimination of the regulatory tyrosine. Indeed, as predicted by the negative regulation model, pp60$^{v\text{-}src}$ has much greater protein kinase activity than pp60$^{c\text{-}src}$. Conversion of pp60$^{c\text{-}src}$ into a transforming protein can be achieved by simply mutating Tyr-527 to the nonphosphorylatable residue phenylalanine. This confirms that the major effect of the deletion of the carboxyl terminus is the removal of this phosphorylation site. Although some of the other point mutations in the body of the v-*src* gene have been shown to be sufficient to induce transforming activity in their own right, it seems likely that the primary event in the conversion of the c-*src* gene into a transforming gene is the inactivation through deletion or mutation of the critical regulatory residues at the carboxyl terminus.

Two other members of the *src* gene family have been isolated as retroviral oncogenes, v-*yes* and v-*fgr*. In both cases, the viral proteins are missing the carboxyl terminus of the normal cellular protein, including the putative regulatory tyrosine (Fig. 1). Furthermore, the *lck* gene can be activated for fibroblast transformation by mutation of Tyr-505 to phenylalanine. Thus, one suspects that all the members of the *src* gene family can be oncogenically activated by this means. However, it should be noted that elevated expression of the normal *lck* protein in certain Moloney murine leukemia virus-derived murine thymomas may be responsible for transformation. In this particular cell type, overexpression may be sufficient to overwhelm the normal negative regulation of the *lck* protein, resulting in a transformed phenotype.

Site-directed mutation of Lys-295 in pp60$^{v\text{-}src}$, which corresponds to a conserved lysine residue in the ATP-binding site of the catalytic domain of all protein kinases, coordinately abolishes protein kinase activity and transforming ability, thus proving that transformation requires tyrosine phosphorylation. A membrane localization has also been shown to be essential for transformation by site-directed mutagenesis of the amino-terminal glycine to alanine in pp60$^{v\text{-}src}$, which prevents myristoylation and renders pp60$^{v\text{-}src}$ soluble in the cell, and concomitantly abrogates transforming activity. This suggests that certain critical substrates are present exclusively in the membrane locale. Until such substrates are identified, however, we will not know whether transformation by pp60$^{v\text{-}src}$ requires the phosphorylation of novel substrates or whether unscheduled phosphorylation of the substrates for pp60$^{c\text{-}src}$ itself and/or for other normal protein tyrosine kinases is sufficient (see below).

C. Other Cytoplasmic Protein Tyrosine Kinases

There are two oncogenic protein tyrosine kinases derived from normal cellular enzymes, which themselves are not exclusively membrane associated. These are the *abl* and *fps* oncoproteins.

Activation of the c-*abl* gene can occur through incorporation into a retrovirus and by a chromosomal translocation (for review, see Rosenberg and Witte 1988). In both cases the *abl* oncogene is expressed as a chimeric protein with foreign sequences at its amino terminus (Fig. 1). For the viral oncogene, v-*abl*, the amino-terminal *gag* sequences provide a myristoylation signal, so that the resultant *gag-abl* protein is membrane associated. In addition, v-*abl* is missing the amino-terminal exon (one of two possible amino-terminal exons is chosen by alternate splicing), the first common exon, and part of the second common exon of the c-*abl* protein. Activation of the c-*abl* gene also occurs in chronic myelogenous leukemias that possess the Philadelphia chromosome. This marker chromosome arises from a translocation that links the 3′ half of the c-*abl* gene on chromosome 9 with the 5′ half of the *bcr* locus on chromosome 22. A chimeric *bcr-abl* protein is produced in which a segment from the amino terminus of the *bcr* protein is joined to the first c-*abl* common exon, replacing the variable first exon. The good correlation between the presence of the *bcr-abl* protein and the leukemic state implies that its protein tyrosine kinase activity plays a role either in the maintenance or onset of this disease.

Truncation of the amino terminus of the c-*abl* protein appears to be essential for oncogenic activation. A complete c-*abl* cDNA, which lacks transforming activity, can be activated for transformation by truncation and fusion to the *gag* gene at the same position as in the v-*abl* protein. Presumably, the amino terminus of the c-*abl* protein acts as a negative regulator of protein kinase activity. Simple elimination of the variable exon from the c-*abl* protein, however, is not sufficient for oncogenic activation. Therefore, the appended amino-terminal *bcr* sequence may provide a critical function for the *bcr-abl* protein.

Although rather little is known about the regulation of *abl* phosphotransferase activity, the v-*abl* and *bcr-abl* proteins are phosphorylated on tyrosine when isolated from the cell, whereas the c-*abl* protein is not. This implies that the c-*abl* protein is less active in vivo than the oncogenic *abl* proteins, and that the nature of the regulation is unlike that of other protein tyrosine kinases such as pp60$^{c\text{-}src}$, which requires tyrosine phosphorylation. The v-*abl* protein is found in the cytoplasm, where it partitions in both the membrane and soluble fractions. The amino terminus of the v-*abl* protein is modified by a myristyl group, which may explain its membrane localization. Site-directed mutation at the amino terminus of the v-*abl* protein indicates that the myristyl group is essential for fibroblast transforming activity. Since most cells that can be transformed by the v-*abl* gene express the c-*abl* protein, transformation may involve deregulation and relocalization of the *abl* protein tyrosine kinase rather than inappropriate expression.

In the case of the *fps* gene, a transforming protein can be generated by simply adding foreign amino-terminal sequences to the amino terminus of the intact c-*fps* protein (Foster et al. 1985). However, deletion analysis of the transforming v-*fps* protein of Fujinami sarcoma virus, which has its amino-terminal sequences provided by the viral structural protein *gag* (Fig. 1), has shown that the *gag* sequences are not required for its transforming activity (Foster et al. 1985). There are several single amino acid differences between the v-*fps* and c-*fps* proteins, and one or more of these mutations must be responsible for its transforming activity. Thus, as we learned for the c-*src* gene, the c-*fps* gene can be oncogenically activated in multiple independent ways, and these are often found to occur in combination.

Exactly how either type of activating change in the c-*fps* protein works is unclear, but both result in higher protein kinase activity. Little is known about the regulation of the protein tyrosine kinase activity of the c-*fps* protein or its true subcellular location. The carboxyl terminus of the c-*fps* protein is unrelated to that of the *src* family. Moreover, unlike the v-*fps* protein, the c-*fps* protein is not phosphorylated on tyrosine when isolated from the cell. Thus, the c-*fps* protein is not negatively regulated in the same manner as the *src* family protein kinases. In contrast to the c-*fps* protein, which is predominantly soluble, the v-*fps* protein is associated in part with the particulate cytoskeletal fraction of the cell, and this location may be important for transformation. Since the c-*fps* gene is expressed only in myeloid cells and can be activated simply by appending *gag* sequences, transformation of fibroblasts could then be a result of ectopic expression in an inappropriate cell type that is unable to regulate *fps* protein kinase activity properly.

D. Targets for Oncogenic Protein Tyrosine Kinases

Although it is relatively easy to show that the oncogenic protein tyrosine kinases are active in cells they transform, it has proved difficult to identify the critical target proteins whose phosphorylation leads to the transformed phenotype. In part, this stems from the very fact that the oncogenic enzymes are deregulated, which results in a wholesale increase in tyrosine phosphorylation of many different cellular proteins. The problem is to sort out which of these phosphorylations are relevant and which are gratuitous. This difficulty is compounded by the fact that we know little about what processes are normally controlled by tyrosine phosphorylation. Clearly, the fact that six bona fide growth factor receptors are protein tyrosine kinases implies that there is at least one mitogenic pathway whose first step is regulated by tyrosine phosphorylation. Although a number of substrates for the growth factor receptor protein tyrosine kinases have recently been identified through the use of antiphosphotyrosine antibodies, so far none of them has been shown to be critical for mitogenesis.

A plethora of phosphotyrosine-containing proteins have been found in cells transformed by acutely transforming retroviruses encoding protein tyrosine kinases, such as RSV (for example, see Kamps and Sefton 1988). Among these proteins are several whose phosphorylation is clearly gratuitous. These include the three glycolytic enzymes, enolase, lactate dehydrogenase, and phosphoglycerate mutase (Cooper et al. 1983). In all three cases, the stoichiometry of tyrosine phosphorylation is low, and there is no measurable difference in the activities of these enzymes in RSV-transformed cells. Furthermore, none of these enzymes is rate-limiting in glycolysis, so that even if their activity were to change, this would not lead to an alteration in the rate of glycolysis.

Another set of substrates form part of the cytoplasmic submembranous skeleton. These include p36 (also known as calpactin I or lipocortin II) (Radke and Martin 1979), a Ca^{++}-dependent phospholipid-binding protein, p81, a component of the microvillar core (Gould et al. 1986), and three elements of the focal contact structure, vinculin (Sefton et al. 1981), talin (Pasquale et al. 1986), and the fibronectin receptor β subunit (Hirst et al. 1986). Since most of the oncogenic protein kinases are themselves associated with either the membrane or the cortical skeleton, they are in an ideal position to phosphorylate these proteins. The question is whether these proteins are phosphorylated adventitiously due to a physical juxtaposition, or whether their phosphorylation has functional consequences. In the case of the fibronectin receptor β subunit, there is evidence that tyrosine phosphorylation leads to a decreased affinity for talin and for fibronectin. Thus, phosphorylations in the focal contact structure could result in diminished cellular adhesiveness and could cause cell rounding, both of which are characteristic of transformed cells.

More recently, the availability of the antiphosphotyrosine antibodies for use in immunoblotting has revealed the existence of many more phosphotyrosine-containing proteins in transformed cells. Up to 50 proteins can be detected in RSV-transformed cells, and many of these are also found in cells transformed by other oncogenic protein tyrosine kinases (Kamps and Sefton 1988). Fewer phosphotyrosine-containing proteins are detected by immunoblotting in cells transformed by oncogenes derived from growth factor receptor protein tyrosine kinases, which generally show smaller increases in the level of phosphotyrosine in cellular protein than those elicited by oncogenes derived from the *src* family. The fact that there are such a large number of substrates for the oncogenic protein tyrosine kinases makes it even more difficult to discern the critical targets. There is increasing evidence that these critical targets are minor cellular proteins, such as regulatory proteins, which are very hard to detect by global screening methods. As antibodies to essential regulatory proteins become available, it will be possible to take a more directed approach and ask which of these proteins are substrates for either oncogenic or normal protein tyrosine kinases. Among the proteins in the submembranous environment that would make reasonable targets are ion channels, transport proteins, G proteins, and the enzymes of phosphatidylinositol (PtdIns) turnover, including phospholipases C and A_2 and the PtdIns kinases.

There is recent evidence that a search among these proteins may be fruitful. The type I PtdIns kinase appears to be activated by tyrosine phosphorylation (Courtneidge and Heber 1987; Kaplan et al. 1987). Normally, PtdIns is phosphorylated in two steps to PtdIns-1,4-diphosphate ($PtdInsP_2$), which is then hydrolyzed by phospholipase C, releasing the second messengers, inositol trisphosphate ($InsP_3$) and diacylglyerol. Although PtdIns-3-phosphate, the product of the type I PtdIns kinase (Whitman et al. 1988), does not lie directly on this pathway, it may itself be a second messenger or give rise to one. Second, the PtdIns-specific phospholipase C-γ is rapidly phosphorylated on tyrosine when cells are treated with PDGF. The type I PtdIns kinase and phospholipase C-γ may prove to be the first examples of critical substrates.

III. ONCOGENIC PROTEIN SERINE KINASES

Compared to the oncogenic protein tyrosine kinases, there are considerably fewer known oncogenes that encode protein serine kinases. Whether this reflects an inherent difference in the physiological functions of protein serine kinases or is due to the type of assay currently employed to detect oncogenes is unclear. It is true that many of the known protein serine kinases have functions in regulating metabolism, and one might not expect such protein serine kinases to have transforming potential. However, there are other protein serine kinases, such as protein kinase C, with cardinal roles in signal transduction, which one might anticipate would have oncogenic potential.

Protein kinase C is a family of isozymes, with at least six members, all of which have Ca^{++}- and phospholipid-dependent protein kinase activity that is stimulated by DAG (Nishizuka 1988). As discussed earlier, agonist-induced phospholipase C hydrolysis of $PtdInsP_2$ leads to production of $InsP_3$, which causes the release of intracellular Ca^{++}, and DAG. In consequence, both the second messengers of the phospholipase-C-dependent PtdIns turnover pathway are activators of protein kinase C. Many mitogens activate phospholipase C and thus stimulate protein kinase C.

Indeed, for mitogens such as bombesin, this may be the main mitogenic signal pathway.

An important connection between carcinogenesis and protein kinase C was established when it was shown that tumor promoters, such as the phorbol esters, also bind to and activate protein kinase C by substituting for DAG. For some cell types, phorbol esters are mitogens, which reinforces the notion that activation of a protein kinase C signal pathway is sufficient for mitogenesis. Little is known about protein kinase C substrates that are critical for mitogenesis, but because of its phospholipid requirement, the active form of protein kinase C is membrane associated, and its substrates are therefore likely to be membrane associated. One candidate is the Na^+/H^+ antiporter, which is activated by mitogens and phorbol esters and is responsible for the alkalinization of the cytoplasm that is required for subsequent DNA synthesis.

On the basis of these properties, one might suspect that a constitutively activated form of protein kinase C would be oncogenic. In support of this idea, overexpression of a normal protein kinase C isozyme leads to a partially transformed phenotype (Housey et al. 1988; Persons et al. 1988). Mutant deregulated forms of protein kinase C might have potent oncogenic activity. One would also expect protein serine kinases that are part of mitogenic signal pathways to be oncogenic. The *raf* protein may be a case in point.

The v-*raf* protein transforms fibroblasts and has protein serine kinase activity. The v-*raf* and c-*raf* proteins are diffusely distributed in the cytoplasm, although a small fraction appears to be membrane associated. Clues to the mechanism of oncogenic activation of the c-*raf* gene come from the structures of the oncogenic *raf* genes that arise frequently during transfection of human DNA into NIH-3T3 cells (for review, see Rapp et al. 1988). In every case, at least the first 5 exons, and commonly the first 7, are missing from the oncogene, which results in an amino-terminally truncated *raf* protein, retaining an intact protein kinase catalytic domain at the carboxyl terminus (Fig. 2). From this we can deduce that the amino terminus of the c-*raf* protein normally plays a negative regulatory role, suppressing its protein kinase activity. Given the similarity of the structure of the c-*raf* protein with protein kinase C, which has an amino-terminal regulatory activator-binding domain, there may be a regulatory molecule that interacts with this amino-terminal domain (Fig. 2). The c-*raf* protein kinase is rapidly activated following mitogen treatment of fibroblasts, and could therefore lie on a mitogenic signal pathway. Constitutive activation of the c-*raf* kinase protein by deletion of the negative regulatory domain may be sufficient to account for the transforming activity of the v-*raf* protein.

The v-*mos* protein has homology with other protein serine kinases and autophosphorylates on serine in vitro. Although a mutation of the essential lysine in the ATP-binding site abolishes both autophosphorylating activity and transforming ability, so far the v-*mos* protein has not been shown capable of phosphorylating any protein other than itself. There are several hundred phosphoserine-containing proteins in normal cells, and most transformed cells evince changes in serine phosphorylation. Thus, it will be very difficult to identify substrates for the v-*mos* protein or any other protein serine kinase-derived oncoprotein and show that it transforms through aberrant serine phosphorylation. The v-*mos* protein is localized to the cytoplasm and fractionates as a soluble protein, which unfortunately reveals little about its likely targets.

There is a paucity of information on the products of the c-*mos* gene, but it has recently been shown that the c-*mos* gene is expressed primarily in developing gametes (Propst et al. 1987) and is required for meiotic division. When expressed at high levels from a retroviral long terminal repeat (LTR), the c-*mos* protein transforms fibroblasts efficiently. Like the v-*mos* protein, the c-*mos* protein is extremely potent, and a few thousand molecules per cell are sufficient for transformation of NIH-3T3 mouse fibroblasts. Thus, in one sense v-*mos* is an exceptional protein kinase oncogene, since expression of the normal cellular protein is sufficient to transform. However, since the c-*mos* gene is not normally expressed in fibroblasts, this is not a simple case of overexpression leading to transformation. Rather, oncogenic activation may require ectopic expression in an inappropriate cell type.

The *pim-1* gene is a locus identified as a frequent site of proviral integration in Moloney murine leukemia virus-induced thymomas in certain mouse strains (Selten et al. 1986; see Chapter 1). Although there is no formal proof that the *pim-1* gene has oncogenic activity, other genes that are preferred sites of leukemia virus proviral integration have proved to be oncogenes. Little is known about the *pim-1* protein, but it is autophosphorylated on serine in an immune complex kinase assay, suggesting that the *pim-1* protein is a protein serine kinase. All the proviral insertions that have been examined occur in the 3′-untranslated region of the *pim-1* transcription unit, leaving the coding region unaffected. In this position, not only does the proviral LTR provide a transcriptional enhancer for the *pim-1* gene, but it also eliminates an mRNA instability sequence. Thus, the level of expression of the *pim-1* protein is elevated by two separate mechanisms. Since *pim-1* RNA is normally present at low levels in T cells, transformation by the *pim-1* gene may involve overexpression of the normal *pim-1* protein.

So far, no generalizations can be made about the mechanisms of activation of protein serine kinase genes into oncogenes. It appears likely that there will be many regulatory cytoplasmic protein serine kinases that propagate signals initiated by the membrane-associated protein tyrosine kinases. Such protein serine kinases are likely candidates for oncogenic activation, and these may provide some general principles of oncogenic activation. Indeed, it has already been shown that the A-*raf* gene, which is closely related to the c-*raf* gene, is readily converted into an oncogene.

IV. OTHER CYTOPLASMIC ONCOGENE PRODUCTS

Not all oncoproteins localized in the cytoplasm are either protein kinases or *ras* proteins (Table 3). Less is known about the functions of such oncoproteins, but there are some intriguing hints. The recently described v-*crk* oncogene encodes a protein that has short stretches of homology with the phospholipase C-γ isozyme (Mayer et al. 1988; Stahl et al. 1988). This same region of v-*crk* is also related to a domain present in a subset of the protein tyrosine kinases, including the *src* family and the *abl* and *fps* proteins. However, this homology does not lie in the catalytic domain of the protein tyrosine kinases, but instead within a region about 100 residues in length lying amino-terminal to the catalytic domain, which has been termed the SH-2 domain (Fig. 3) (Sadowski et al. 1986). Analysis of the SH-2 region in the v-*src* and v-*fps* genes has shown that it has a regulatory role and may be involved in interactions with other cellular proteins. Finally, there is also a region of SH-2 homology in the GTPase activator protein (GAP) that stimulates the GTPase activity of normal c-*ras* proteins (see Chapter 5). This raises the intriguing possibility that there is a regulatory protein(s) capable of interacting with all four types of proteins, i.e., the protein tyrosine kinases, phospholipase C, *crk*, and GAP, and thus coordinating the activity of discrete signaling pathways. In keeping with this idea, v-*crk*-transformed cells are found to have elevated levels of phosphotyrosine in cellular proteins, even though the v-*crk* protein itself lacks protein tyrosine kinase activity (Mayer et al. 1988). One explanation for this increase in phosphotyrosine is that the high level of v-*crk* protein can titrate out a negative regulatory protein, thus relieving the constraints on one or more normal cellular protein tyrosine kinases.

It should also be borne in mind that other cytoplasmic oncogene products indirectly activate protein tyrosine kinases. For instance, the middle T

Table 3 Cytoplasmic oncoproteins that are not protein kinases

ras protein
v-*crk* protein
mas protein
bcl-2 protein
dbl protein
v-*sis* protein (PDGF-related)
hst protein (fibroblast growth-factor-related)
Polyomavirus middle T antigen

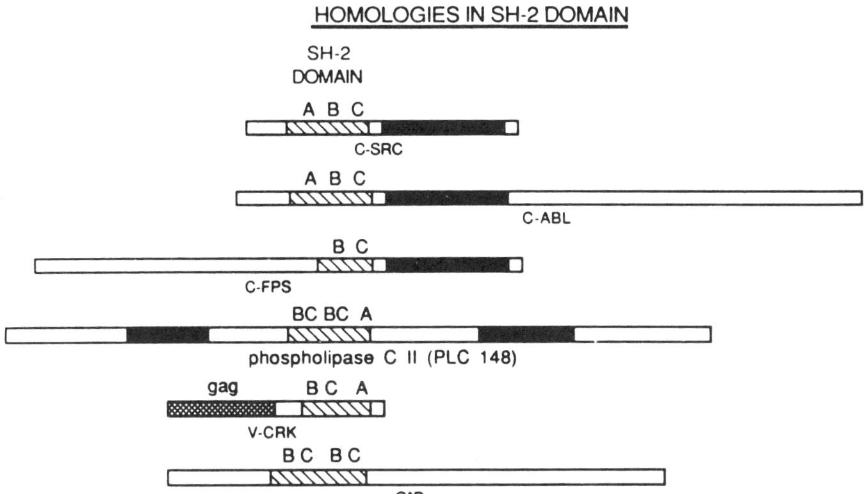

Figure 3 Homologies between cytoplasmic proteins in the SH-2 domain. The structures of the c-*src*, c-*abl*, and c-*fps* protein tyrosine kinases, phospholipase C-γ (also known as PLC 148), the v-*crk* protein, and the c-*ras* GTPase activator protein (GAP) are shown using the conventions described in Fig. 1. The SH-2 domain is divided into three parts (A, B, and C), which are the most highly conserved regions. The order of these three regions differs in some of the proteins. Regions of phospholipase C-γ related to sequences in phospholipases β and δ are shown as filled boxes and may correspond to catalytic domains.

antigen of polyomavirus binds to and activates pp60$^{c\text{-}src}$ and at least two other members of the *src* gene family (see Chapter 8). This activation appears to be critical for transformation by middle T antigen and leads to increased tyrosine phosphorylation of cellular proteins. On a historical note, the phosphorylation of middle T antigen on tyrosine in vitro, which results from this association, led to the initial report of tyrosine phosphorylation (Eckhart et al. 1979). Oncogenes, such as the v-*sis* gene, encode growth factors that can also interact with and activate growth factor receptors with protein tyrosine kinase activity. Thus, the secreted v-*sis* protein binds to and activates the PDGF receptor and promotes growth in an autocrine fashion.

Of the other three cytoplasmic oncoproteins, two are localized to the membrane, *mas* and *bcl-2*. The *mas* protein has a structure with seven potential transmembrane domains similar to the β-adrenergic and muscarinic acetylcholine receptors and is therefore postulated to be a receptor. Recent evidence suggests it may be an angiotensin receptor. The *bcl-2* protein is not homologous to any known protein but is apparently localized to the cytoplasmic face of the membrane, where it may have a role in signal transduction. The *dbl* oncoprotein also lacks strong homology with any known protein. The normal *dbl* protein has a region with a predicted helical structure similar to cytoskeletal proteins, like vimentin, but this amino-terminal region is missing in the *dbl* oncoprotein.

V. CONCLUSIONS

The frequent occurrence of oncogenes encoding protein kinases underscores the importance of protein phosphorylation in cellular regulatory networks. Among the oncogenic protein kinases, we find enzymes that work at the plasma membrane, others that function in the submembrane environment, and yet others that are either soluble in the cytoplasm or else associated with the cytoskeleton. Presumably, all of these locations are usually occupied by normal cellular protein kinases, and the oncogenic enzymes home to these positions. In some cases, the transforming protein kinases reside in their appropriate locations and simply act in an unregulated fashion. A good example is that of the growth-factor-receptor-derived oncogenes, whose products mimic ligand-occupied receptors at the cell surface in activating a mitogenic pathway. In other instances, such as the *trk* and *met* oncoproteins, the oncogene products adopt abnormal locations and may compete with the enzymes that normally fill these sites.

We are sorely lacking in an understanding of the targets for the oncogenic protein kinases, or, for that matter, their normal counterparts. For this reason, it is not clear whether the substrate specificities of the transforming protein kinases are altered, or whether the oncogenic mutations result in an inability of the cell to regulate their protein kinase activity without any change in their substrate specificity. Since in most cases that have been analyzed in detail, oncogenic activation is accomplished by mutations that abrogate negative regulation of protein kinase activity, it seems likely that deregulation rather than a change in substrate specificity is the cardinal event. However, there may also be changes in subcellular distribution that give access to new substrates. In the near future, progress will undoubtedly be made in identifying critical substrates for the protein tyrosine kinases, which will allow a better appreciation of the molecular bases for transformation by oncogenic protein kinases.

It seems likely that among the substrates for these oncogenic protein kinases will be other protein kinases. Evidence is mounting that there is a network of regulatory protein kinases in which protein kinases can function in series to propagate signals (Hunter 1987b). There is already a solid precedent for the existence of a protein kinase "cascade" in the phosphorylation of the ribosomal protein S6. One aspect of such a network that may be tractable to experimental analysis is the nature of pathways by which cytoplasmic protein kinases induce gene expression. The recent characterization of growth-factor-inducible genes and the transcription factors that regulate them allows one to approach protein kinase signal pathways from both ends with the hope of meeting in the middle. In this regard, although all oncogenic protein kinases known to date are cytoplasmic, it seems likely that there will be oncogenes encoding nuclear protein kinases. The recent identification of the v-*jun* oncogene product as a transcription factor, coupled with the indications that the activities of transcription factors may be modulated by phosphorylation, suggests that nuclear protein kinases, which are able to phosphorylate and activate transcription factors, could have oncogenic potential.

It has been speculated that there may be as many as 1000 protein kinase genes in the mammalian genome. If this is true, then we can anticipate that there are a lot more protein kinase oncogenes waiting to be discovered and that many of these will function in the cytoplasm.

REFERENCES

Bargmann, C.I. and R.A. Weinberg. 1988a. Oncogenic activation of the *neu*-encoded receptor protein by point mutation and deletion. *EMBO J.* **7:** 2043–2052.

———. 1988b. Increased tyrosine kinase activity associated with the protein encoded by the activated *neu* oncogene. *Proc. Natl. Acad. Sci.* **85:** 5394–5398.

Bargmann, C.I., M.C. Hung, and R.A. Weinberg. 1986. Multiple independent activations of the *neu* oncogene by a point mutation altering the transmembrane domain of p185. *Cell* **45:** 649–657.

Barker, W.C. and M.O. Dayhoff. 1982. Viral *src* gene products are related to the catalytic chain of the mammalian cAMP-dependent protein kinase. *Proc. Natl. Acad. Sci.* **79:** 2836–2839.

Chen, W.S., C.S. Lazar, M. Poenie, R. Tsien, G.N. Gill, and M.G. Rosenfeld. 1987. Requirement for intrinsic protein kinase in the immediate and late actions of the EGF receptor. *Nature* **328:** 820–823.

Collett, M.S. and R.L. Erikson. 1978. Protein kinase activity associated with the avian sarcoma virus *src* gene product. *Proc. Natl. Acad. Sci.* **75:** 2021–2024.

Cooper, J.A. 1989. The *src*-family of protein-tyrosine kinases. In *Peptides and protein phosphorylation* (ed. B. Kemp and P. Alewood). CRC Press, Boca Raton. (In press.)

Cooper, J.A. and C.S. King. 1986. Dephosphorylation or antibody binding to the carboxy terminus stimulates pp60$^{c\text{-}src}$. *Mol. Cell. Biol.* **6:** 4467–4477.

Cooper, J.A., K.L. Gould, C.A. Cartwright, and T. Hunter. 1986. Tyr^{527} is phosphorylated in pp60$^{c\text{-}src}$: Implications for regulation. *Science* **231:** 1431–1433.

Cooper, J.A., N.A. Reiss, R.J. Schwartz, and T. Hunter. 1983. Three glycolytic enzymes are phosphorylated at tyrosine in cells transformed by Rous sarcoma virus. *Nature* **302:** 218–223.

Courtneidge, S.A. 1985. Activation of pp60$^{c\text{-}src}$ kinase by middle T antigen binding or by dephosphorylation. *EMBO J.* **4:** 1471–1477.

Courtneidge, S.A. and A. Heber. 1987. An 81 kd protein complexed with middle T antigen and pp60$^{c\text{-}src}$: A possible phosphatidylinositol kinase. *Cell* **50:** 1031–1037.

Di Fiore, P.P., J.H. Pierce, T.P. Fleming, R. Hazan, A. Ullrich, C.R. King, J. Schlessinger, and S.A. Aaronson. 1987. Overexpression of the human EGF receptor confers an EGF-dependent transformed phenotype to NIH 3T3 cells. *Cell* **51:** 1063–1070.

Downward, J., Y. Yarden, E. Mayes, G. Scrace, N. Totty, P. Stockwell, A. Ullrich, and M.D. Waterfield. 1984. Close similarity of epidermal growth factor receptor and v-*erb*B oncogene protein sequences. *Nature* **307:** 521–527.

Eckhart, W., M.A. Hutchinson, and T. Hunter. 1979. An activity phosphorylating tyrosine in polyoma T antigen immunoprecipitates. *Cell* **18:** 925–933.

Foster, D.A., M. Shibuya, and H. Hanafusa. 1985. Activation of the transforming potential of the cellular *fps* gene. *Cell* **42:** 105–115.

Gould, K.L., J.A. Cooper, A. Bretscher, and T. Hunter. 1986. The protein-tyrosine kinase substrate, p81, is homologous to a chicken microvillar core protein. *J. Cell Biol.* **102:** 660–669.

Hanks, S.K., A.M. Quinn, and T. Hunter. 1988. The protein kinase family: Conserved features and deduced phylogeny of the catalytic domains. *Science* **241:** 42–52.

Hirst, R., A. Horwitz, C. Buck, and L. Rohrschneider. 1986. Phosphorylation of the fibronectin receptor complex in cells transformed by oncogenes that encode tyrosine kinases. *Proc. Natl. Acad. Sci.* **83:** 6470–6474.

Housey, G.M., M.D. Johnson, W.L.W. Hsiao, C.A. O'Brian, J.P. Murphy, P. Kirschmeier, and I.B. Weinstein. 1988. Overproduction of protein kinase C causes disordered growth control in rat fibroblasts. *Cell* **52:** 343–354.

Hudziak, R.M., J. Schlessinger, and A. Ullrich. 1987. Increased expression of the putative growth factor receptor $p185^{HER2}$ causes transformation and tumorigenesis of NIH 3T3 cells. *Proc. Natl. Acad. Sci.* **84:** 7159–7163.

Hunter, T. 1987a. A tail of two *src*'s: Mutatis mutandis. *Cell* **49:** 1–4.

———. 1987b. A thousand and one protein kinases. *Cell* **50:** 823–829.

Hunter, T. and J.A. Cooper. 1985. Protein-tyrosine kinases. *Annu. Rev. Biochem.* **54:** 897–930.

Hunter, T. and B.M. Sefton. 1980. The transforming gene product of Rous sarcoma virus phosphorylates tyrosine. *Proc. Natl. Acad. Sci.* **77:** 1311–1315.

Kamps, M.P. and B.M. Sefton. 1988. Identification of multiple novel polypeptide substrates of the v-*src*, v-*fps*, v-*ros*, and v-*erb*-B oncogenic tyrosine protein kinases utilizing antisera against phosphotyrosine. *Oncogene* **2:** 305–315.

Kaplan, D.R., M. Whitman, B. Schaffhausen, D.C. Pallas, M. White, L. Cantley, and T.M. Roberts. 1987. Common elements in growth factor stimulation and oncogenic transformation: 85 kd phosphoprotein and phosphatidylinositol kinase activity. *Cell* **50:** 1021–1029.

Levinson, A.D., H. Oppermann, L. Levintow, H.E. Varmus, and J.M. Bishop. 1978. Evidence that the transforming gene of avian sarcoma virus encodes a protein kinase associated with a phosphoprotein. *Cell* **15:** 561–572.

Libermann, T.A., H.R. Nusbaum, N. Razon, R. Kris, I. Lax, H. Soreq, N. Whittle, M.D. Waterfield, A. Ullrich, and J. Schlessinger. 1985. Amplification and possible rearrangement of EGF receptor gene in primary human brain tumors of glial origin. *Nature* **313:** 144–146.

Mayer, B.J., M. Hamaguchi, and H. Hanafusa. 1988. A novel viral oncogene with structural similarity to phospholipase C. *Nature* **332:** 272–275.

Mitra, G., D. Martin-Zanca, and M. Barbacid. 1987. Identification and biochemical characterization of $p70^{TRK}$, product of the human *TRK* oncogene. *Proc. Natl. Acad. Sci.* **84:** 6707–6711.

Nishizuka, Y. 1988. The molecular heterogeneity of protein kinase C and its implications for cellular regulation. *Nature* **334:** 661–665.

Pasquale, E.B., P.A. Maher, and S.J. Singer. 1986. Talin is phosphorylated on tyrosine in chicken embryo fibroblasts transformed by Rous sarcoma virus. *Proc. Natl. Acad. Sci.* **83:** 5507–5511.

Persons, D.A., W.O. Wilkison, R.M. Bell, and O.J. Finn. 1988. Altered growth regulation and enhanced tumorigenicity of NIH 3T3 fibroblasts transfected with protein kinase C-I cDNA. *Cell* **52:** 447–458.

Propst, F., M.P. Rosenberg, A. Iyer, K. Kaul, and G. Vande Woude. 1987. c-*mos* proto-oncogene RNA transcripts in mouse tissues: Structural features, developmental regulation and localization in specific cell types. *Mol. Cell. Biol.* **7:** 1629–1637.

Radke, K. and G.S. Martin. 1979. Transformation by Rous sarcoma virus: Effects of *src* gene on the synthesis and phosphorylation of cellular polypeptides. *Proc. Natl. Acad. Sci.* **76:** 5212–5216.

Rapp, U.R., J.L. Cleveland, and T.I. Bonner. 1988. The *raf* oncogene family. In *The oncogene handbook* (ed. E.P. Reddy et al.), pp. 213–253. Elsevier, Amsterdam.

Rosenberg, N. and O.N. Witte. 1988. The viral and cellular forms of the *abl* oncogene. *Adv. Virus. Res.* **35:** 39–81.

Roussel, M.F., T.J. Dull, C.W. Rettenmeier, P. Ralph, A. Ullrich, and C.J. Sherr. 1987. Transforming potential of the c-*fms* proto-oncogene (CSF-1 receptor). *Nature* **325:** 549–552.

Sadowski, I., J.C. Stone, and T. Pawson. 1986. A non-catalytic domain conserved among cytoplasmic protein-tyrosine kinases modifies the kinase function and transforming action of Fujinami sarcoma virus P130$^{gag\text{-}fps}$. *Mol. Cell. Biol.* **6:** 4396–4408.

Sefton, B.M., T. Hunter, E.H. Ball, and S.J. Singer. 1981. Vinculin: A cytoskeletal target of the transforming protein of Rous sarcoma virus. *Cell* **24:** 165–174.

Selten, G., H.T. Cuypers, W. Boelens, E. Robanus-Maandag, J. Verbeek, J. Domen, C. Van Beveren, and A. Berns. 1986. The primary structure of the putative oncogene *pim*-1 shows extensive homology with protein kinases. *Cell* **43:** 603–611.

Sherr, C.J. 1988. The *fms* oncogene. *BBA Rev. Cancer* **948:** 225–243.

Sherr, C.J., C.W. Rettenmeier, R. Sacca, M.F. Roussel, A.T. Look, and E.R. Stanley. 1985. The c-*fms* proto-oncogene product is related to the receptor for the mononuclear phagocyte growth factor, CSF-1. *Cell* **41:** 665–676.

Slamon, D.J., G.M. Clark, S.G. Wong, W.J. Levin, A. Ullrich, and W.L. McGuire. 1987. Human breast cancer: Correlation of relapse and survival with amplification of the HER-2/*neu* oncogene. *Science* **235:** 177–182.

Stahl, M.L., C.R. Ferenz, K.L. Kelleher, R.W. Kriz, and J.L. Knopf. 1988. Sequence similarity of phospholipase C with the non-catalytic region of *src*. *Nature* **332:** 269–272.

Ullrich, A., L. Coussens, J.S. Hayflick, T.J. Dull, A. Gray, A. Tam, J. Lee, Y. Yarden, T.A. Libermann, J. Schlessinger, J. Downward, E.L.V. Mayes, N. Whittle, M.D. Waterfield, and P.H. Seeburg. 1984. Human epidermal growth factor receptor cDNA sequence and aberrant expression of the amplified gene in A431 epidermoid carcinoma cells. *Nature* **309:** 418–425.

Ushiro, H. and S. Cohen. 1980. Identification of phosphotyrosine as a product of epidermal growth factor-activated protein kinase in A-431 cell membranes. *J. Biol. Chem.* **255:** 8363–8365.

Whitman, M., C.P. Downes, M. Keeler, T. Keller, and L. Cantley. 1988. Type I phosphatidylinositol kinase makes a novel inositol phospholipid, phosphatidylinositol-3-phosphate. *Nature* **332:** 644–646.

Witte, O.N., A. Dasgupta, and D. Baltimore. 1980. The Abelson murine leukemia virus protein is phosphorylated in vitro to form phosphotyrosine. *Nature* **283:** 826–831.

Yarden, Y. and J. Schlessinger. 1987a. Self-phosphorylation of EGF receptor; evidence for a model of intermolecular allosteric association. *Biochemistry* **26:** 1434–1442.

———. 1987b. EGF induces rapid reversible aggregation of the purified EGF receptor. *Biochemistry* **26:** 1443–1451.

Yarden, Y. and A. Ullrich. 1988. Growth factor receptor tyrosine kinases. *Annu. Rev. Biochem.* **57:** 443–478.

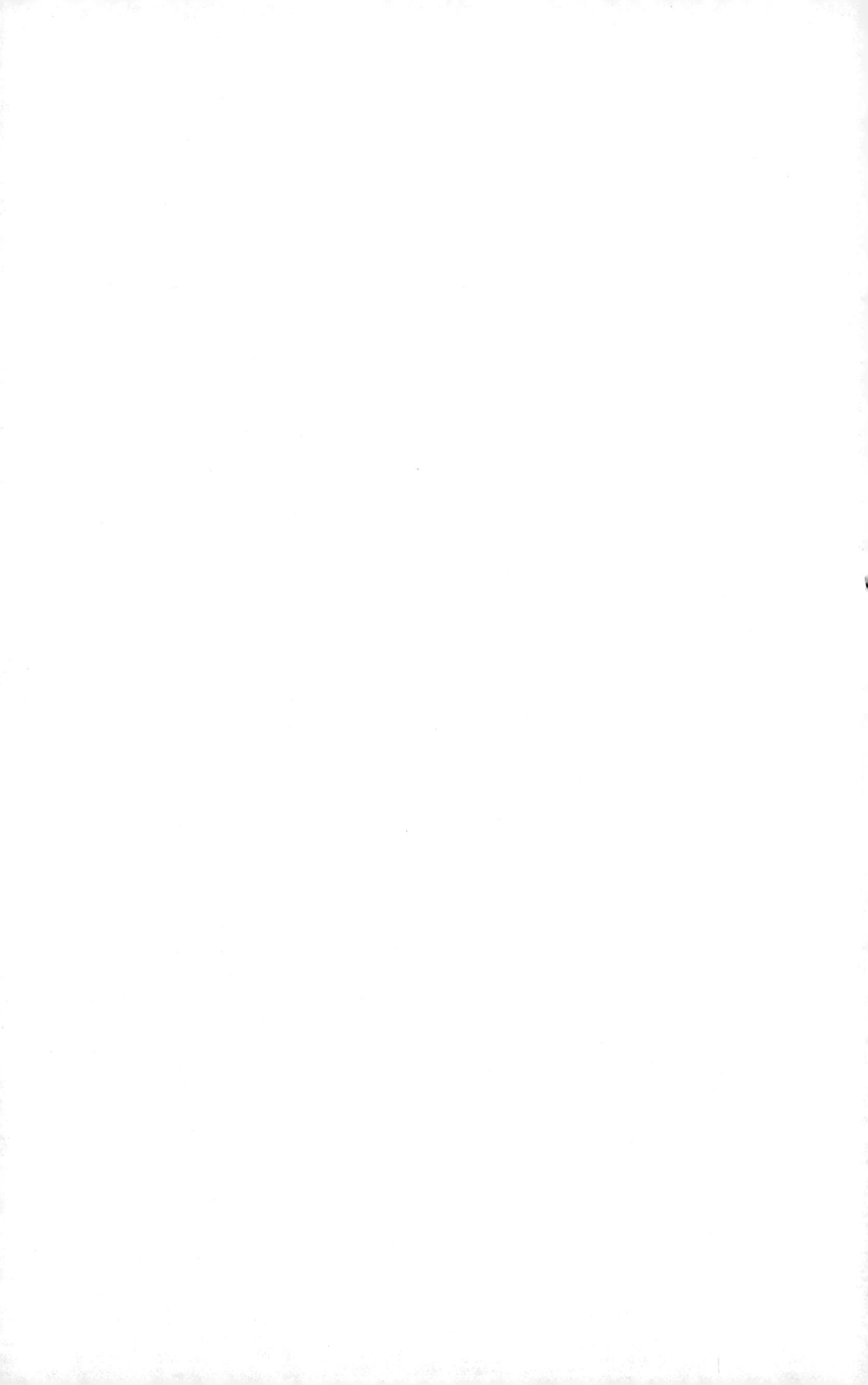

7

Nuclear Oncogenes

Robert N. Eisenman
Division of Basic Sciences
Fred Hutchinson Cancer Research Center
Seattle, Washington 98104

Oncogenes and the Molecular Origins of Cancer.

I. INTRODUCTION: THE IMPORTANCE OF BEING NUCLEAR

A. Final Steps in the Mitogenic Pathway

The early work on papovavirus tumor antigens taught us that the cell nucleus was likely to be the stage upon which proteins involved in cell transformation acted. It was something of a surprise when the first wave of studies on retroviral oncogenes and their cellular counterparts produced a picture of oncoprotein action as largely confined to the cytoplasm and the plasma membrane. Indeed, experiments using enucleated cells suggested that at least the multiple morphological alterations induced by one well-studied oncogene (v-*src*) could occur in the absence of a nucleus (Beug et al. 1978). Thus, for many workers involved in the initial characterization of retroviral oncoproteins, the subcellular fraction containing nuclei was usually discarded when cells were lysed for studies on oncogene function. This picture has changed dramatically in recent years, since it has become apparent that an important set of proto-oncogenes encode proteins that are predominantly localized in the nucleus. These include the *myc* family, *fos*, *myb*, *erbA*, *jun*, *p53*, the less-studied *ski*, and probably *rel* and *ets*. These genes, their human chromosome locations, and some of their general properties are listed in Table 1. In addition, the protein product of the retinoblastoma "anti-oncogene," recently found to be mutated in several types of tumors, is also nuclear (see Chapter 11).

The nuclear localization of this group of cellular oncoproteins indicated a functionally distinct class of oncogenes and suggested as much diversity in oncoprotein function as in oncoprotein localization. As it became clear that cytoplasmic and plasma-membrane-localized oncoproteins were components of mitogenic signal transduction pathways (see preceding chapters), it seemed plausible to also consider the nuclear oncoproteins as part of such a signaling system. In this scenario, the nuclear oncoproteins might well be thought of as potential mediators of the final steps in signal transduction, conveying information from the cytoplasm to the nucleus, with the possibility that, once in the nucleus, they might have a direct role in control of gene expression. More specifically, these oncoproteins might act as *trans*-acting factors interacting with DNA elements that stimulate or repress transcription. Such activities could in turn underlie the ability of these oncoproteins to act as central regulators of important cellular functions, such as proliferation and differentiation. In fact, the notion that nuclear oncoproteins are gene regulatory proteins has recently begun to be experimentally substantiated.

At present, our knowledge of the nuclear oncoproteins resembles a lopsided patchwork quilt: For a few of these proteins, such as Myc,[1] Myb,

[1]I will adhere to the convention of denoting the protein product of a gene by capitalizing the first letter of the gene designation: Hence, Myc is the protein encoded by the *myc* gene.

Table 1 Properties of nuclear oncoproteins

Oncoprotein	Human chromosome	Family members	DNA binding		Molecular associations	Function
			random	specific		
c-Myc	8q24	P-, N-, L-, R-, B-Myc	+	?	?	?
c-Myb	6q22-24	A-, B-Myb	+	+	?	transcription
c-Fos	14q21-31	Fra-1 other related antigens	+	?	Jun	transcription regulation
c-ErbA	17	THRβ; tissue-specific receptors	+	+	T3/T4 thyroid hormone	thyroid hormone receptor
c-Jun	1p31-32	JunB, JunD	+	+	Fos and homodimer	transcription regulation
p53	17p13	?	+	?	adenovirus E1B hsc70 SV40 large T	suppressor of transformation
c-Ski	1q22-24	Sno	?	?	?	?
c-Ets-2	21q22.3	c-Ets-1	?	?	?	?
c-Rel	1p12-13	?	?	?	several cellular proteins	?

and p53, a great deal of descriptive information has been acquired concerning potential biological roles, whereas little is known about how they might function biochemically; for others, such as Jun, Fos, and ErbA, information relating to molecular mechanisms of action and to possible physiological roles are just beginning to merge to create a coherent picture. In the following sections, I discuss specific genes as exemplars of some of the most intriguing aspects of nuclear oncogenes: regulation of expression by sets of complex external stimuli, involvement in cell proliferation and differentiation, oncogenic activation, macromolecular interactions, and function in the control of gene expression.

B. Retroviral Origins

Many of the genes encoding the nuclear oncoproteins were first identified as transforming genes in avian and murine retroviruses isolated from experimentally induced or spontaneous tumors. The transduced oncogenes interrupt and replace portions of the retroviral structural genes required for virus multiplication. The oncogene sequences are thus expressed under the control of the viral promoter and utilize viral RNA processing and translation signals to achieve relatively high levels of expression. This association with retroviral promoters removes these genes from sequences that normally modulate their expression in the cell in response to physiological stimuli and places them under control of viral sequences that usually force high, steady levels of expression. That such cellular oncogenes can be studied in their guise as transduced retroviral genes has aided greatly in elucidating the nature of their protein products as well as their structure and expression (for review, see Bister and Jansen 1986).

II. THE *MYC* GENE FAMILY

Of all the nuclear oncogenes, *myc* has probably been the most intensively studied. Much of this attention stems from the fact that rearrangements of the normal cellular *myc* gene (c-*myc*) locus have been shown to be associated with diverse neoplasms in a wide range of species. The diversity itself suggests that *myc* function may be linked to some regulatory mechanisms so fundamental to cell behavior that its alteration can underlie the genesis of neoplasia in many different cell types. This idea has been bolstered by findings relating *myc* expression to differentiation and proliferation. In addition, c-*myc* turns out to be only one member of a family of structurally and functionally related genes, some of which have also been implicated in neoplasia (for recent reviews, see Cole 1986; Cory 1986; Eisenman and Thompson 1986; DePinho et al. 1987b).

A. Retroviral Transduction of *myc*

myc first came to light as a retroviral transforming gene (v-*myc*) discovered as a novel sequence in the genomes of four independent isolates of avian acute leukemia viruses. These are highly oncogenic retroviruses capable of inducing a wide range of tumors in chickens (primarily myelocytomatosis, but also endotheliomas and liver and kidney carcinomas) and transforming hematopoietic cells of the macrophage lineage as well as embryonic fibroblasts in tissue culture. Molecular analyses revealed that these four viruses share, in addition to the well-characterized set of viral replication genes, a genetic region not found in any other retroviruses. This segment was termed *myc* (for *my*elo*c*ytomatosis) and was later demonstrated to be a gene of cellular origin (c-*myc*) that had been transduced by these retroviruses (Roussel et al. 1979; Sheiness and Bishop 1979). Interestingly, although tissue culture fibroblasts infected with the v-*myc*-containing viruses share many of the transformed phenotypes of cells infected by retroviruses possessing other oncogenes, they are different in at least one property: Their growth rate is nearly double that of other transformants (Palmieri et al. 1983). This finding, coupled with the observations that the v-*myc* proteins lacked kinase activity and were located in the nucleus, led to the notion that *myc* may represent a class of oncogene, functionally distinct from the cytoplasmic and membrane-localized kinases, whose action directly impinges on cell proliferation.

B. c-*myc* Structure and Conservation

Molecular cloning of the retrovirus-transduced v-*myc* region provided a probe that permitted analysis of the cellular progenitor of v-*myc*: the c-*myc* gene. The structure of c-*myc* was found to be relatively simple when compared with many of the other proto-oncogenes, in that it consists of only three exons with a large protein-coding region beginning with the first ATG translational initiation codon near the 5′ end of exon 2 and extending through about two-thirds of exon 3 (Fig. 1, center; open boxes indicate the open reading frame). Thus, as observed for many proto-oncogenes, the protein-coding region of the c-*myc* mRNA is framed by long leader and trailer sequences. As we shall see, these sequences are involved in the regulation of expression and stability of c-*myc* RNA. c-*myc* is unusual in that it also appears to make low amounts of a longer form of its major protein product by initiating translation at a nonstandard initiation codon located upstream of and in the same reading frame as the major ATG initiator (Hann et al. 1988).

c-*myc* has been highly conserved throughout vertebrate evolution with homologs identified in mammals, birds, amphibians, and fish. Develop-

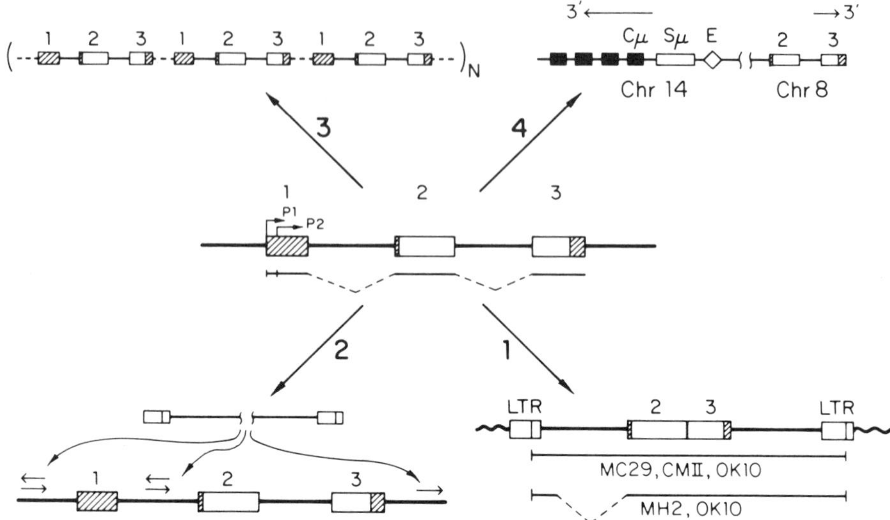

Figure 1 Genetic alterations associated with the c-*myc* locus. The exon-intron structure of the normal c-*myc* gene is shown in the center (not to scale) with the three exons, two RNA initiation sites (P1 and P2; arrows showing direction of transcription), open reading frame (open boxes), untranslated regions (hatched boxes), and RNA splicing pattern (below the gene structure) indicated. Large arrows point to schematized genetic alterations of c-*myc*: (1) Retroviral transduction. An integrated provirus contains the two transduced exons of c-*myc* between two LTRs flanked by host sequences (wavy lines). The avian viruses MC29, CMII, and OK10 express v-*myc* as part of a genomic length RNA initiated from the 5′ LTR. MH2 and OK10 also express v-*myc* as a spliced subgenomic RNA (indicated below the provirus). c-*myc* has also been found to be transduced by feline leukemia viruses. (2) Retroviral insertions proximal to c-*myc*. In avian bursal lymphomas and mouse, cat, and rat thymomas, retroviruses integrate in the vicinity of the c-*myc* locus. Integration occurs frequently between exons 1 and 2 but has also been detected both upstream and downstream, often at great distance from the c-*myc* locus. The horizontal arrows indicate directions of transcription observed from the integrated viral LTRs. The LTR can act as an enhancer and/or a direct promoter of c-*myc* transcription. (3) Amplification of the c-*myc* locus. All three exons are shown amplified, as in HL60 cells. In some tumors, amplification of only exons 2–3 has been observed. (4) Chromosomal translocation. In many murine plasmacytomas, rat immunocytomas, and human Burkitt's lymphomas, the chromosomal region containing the c-*myc* locus (human chromosome 8; mouse chromosome 15) is translocated in the vicinity of an immunoglobulin gene. In many endemic (African) Burkitt's lymphomas, the translocation breakpoint occurs upstream or downstream from c-*myc*, leaving all three translocated exons intact. In sporadic (Western) Burkitt's lymphomas, exon 1 is frequently lost, as the translocation breakpoint lies between exons 1 and 2. Shown here is the truncated c-*myc* allele in the Burkitt's lymphoma cell line Manca that has been translocated to the immunoglobulin heavy-chain locus on chromosome 14. The horizontal arrows indicate the direction of transcription of the two genes.

mental studies in several of these organisms have shown that c-*myc* is expressed at a relatively low level, compared to the virally transduced v-*myc* gene, in many proliferating cell types throughout development. However, the possibility of eludicating *myc* function through genetic analysis in *Drosophila* or yeast, as was carried out for *ras* (see Chapter 5), has been stymied by the failure to detect closely related *myc* homologs in any invertebrates. This suggests that the functions of *myc* in vertebrate cells are either served in lower organisms by a very divergent gene, are carried out by an altogether different mechanism, or are simply not required. Interestingly, the *Drosophila achaete-scute* gene product, which is involved in neuronal differentiation, has been shown to have limited similarity to a small segment of the c-*myc* protein (Villares and Cabrera 1987; see Section X.B).

C. The *myc* Multigene Family

The c-*myc* gene is but one member of a multigene family whose members are related in terms of both structure and function (DePinho et al. 1987b). Thus far, five loci, in addition to c-*myc*, have been defined by low-stringency hybridization: N-*myc*, L-*myc* (and an L-*myc* pseudogene), P-*myc*, R-*myc*, and B-*myc*. These *myc* family genes are dispersed on different chromosomes. Recent reports suggest that yet other family members may exist.

The N-*myc* and L-*myc* genes appear to be the most highly related to c-*myc*, and these have also been examined in the most detail. N-*myc* and L-*myc* possess the same 3-exon–2-intron structure characteristic of c-*myc* genes. All three *myc* family genes have substantial regions of high amino acid sequence homology scattered throughout the protein-coding regions of the second and third exons, with the most extensive homology region at the carboxyl termini of the proteins. Such homologies hint at functionally important domains, an idea given some credence by deletion-mapping studies and by the existence of common sequence motifs that may participate in DNA binding and the formation of protein:protein complexes (see Section X). The regions of greatest divergence are located in the 5′- and 3′-untranslated portions of the mRNAs. If these can be considered as control regions, then their lack of homology may reflect the different tissue- and stage-specific expression patterns observed for these genes.

Experiments demonstrating that N-*myc*, L-*myc*, and c-*myc* can cooperate with an activated *ras* oncogene to transform rat embryo fibroblasts suggest that the *myc* family genes are functionally as well as structurally related (Land et al. 1983; Schwab et al. 1985; DePinho et al. 1987a; see Chapter 12). Furthermore, both the recently identified N-*myc* and L-*myc* proteins have been found in the nucleus, and it is likely that the other related proteins will also be nuclear.

D. *myc* Family Gene Expression

The c-*myc* gene is expressed in virtually all proliferating cells in embryonic and adult tissues. The absolute levels of c-*myc* mRNA and protein can vary considerably in different tissues, being lowest in quiescent and differentiated cells and highest in rapidly proliferating cells. Some of these differences are probably dependent on the presence of growth factors or other mitogens (see below).

The nearly universal expression of c-*myc* stands in contrast to the more restricted expression of N-*myc* and L-*myc*. Studies in human and mouse development have revealed N-*myc* and L-*myc* expression to be dependent both on the cell lineage and on its stage of development. N-*myc* and L-*myc* expression levels tend to be higher in more primitive tissues (i.e., from fetal or newborn animals). For example, all three *myc* family genes were expressed in newborn kidney, but only c-*myc* expression persisted into the adult stage. On the other hand, pre-B cells expressed N-*myc* and c-*myc*, but not L-*myc*, whereas more mature B cells expressed only c-*myc*. These complex expression patterns may represent integrated sets of responses to multiple environmental stimuli. The different temporal combinations of *myc* family gene expression may be linked in some manner to specific developmental pathways (Zimmerman et al. 1986; for review, see DePinho et al. 1987b).

E. c-*myc* Expression during Proliferation and Differentiation

The idea that c-*myc* function is linked to cellular proliferation has received strong support from experiments showing that dramatic changes in c-*myc* expression accompany alterations in the growth and differentiation state of many cell types. A good example of this for c-*myc* involves the mitogenic stimulation of quiescent lymphoid cells. Small resting T or B cells do not express significant amounts of c-*myc* gene products. When such cells are stimulated to enter the G_1 phase of the cell cycle by treatment with one of a wide variety of mitogenic agents, a transient increase in c-*myc* RNA and protein is observed within 1–3 hours (Kelly et al. 1983). Such bursts of c-*myc* expression upon mitogenic stimulation are not confined to lymphoid cells but have been observed after growth factor stimulation (for example, with platelet-derived growth factor, PDGF) of growth-arrested fibroblasts, as well as neuronal and muscle cells. Furthermore, a transient increase in c-*myc* expression occurs immediately following the wounding of liver tissue and thus is an early event in the growth-stimulated changes leading to tissue regeneration (Makino et al. 1984). As discussed below, even more dramatic modulations of expression have been observed for other nuclear oncogenes like c-*fos*.

The high level of c-*myc* expression observed following mitogenic stimulation is maintained for only a few hours. Expression then declines to a basal level that remains constant throughout the cell cycle as the activated cell continues to proliferate (Hann et al. 1985). This basal, cell-cycle-independent expression of c-*myc* is probably a characteristic of all proliferating cells.

It is tempting to assume that the correlations between mitogenic activation and bursts of c-*myc* expression reflect a requirement for high levels of c-*myc* protein in order for cells to enter the cell cycle. However, there is some evidence that this straightforward idea needs to be considered with some caution. For example, it has been demonstrated that c-*myc* expression can also be up-regulated by agents that are weak inducers or noninducers of proliferation. Thus, an increase in c-*myc* expression is not invariably connected to proliferation. Furthermore, under certain conditions, quiescent cells can be made to enter the cell cycle after PDGF treatment without a significant augmentation in levels of c-*myc* RNA. These observations suggest that the transient increases in c-*myc* expression observed after mitogenic stimulation can be uncoupled from entry into the cell cycle (Coughlin et al. 1985).

A much more difficult question is whether any c-*myc* expression is required for mitogenesis. A recent attempt to test this has been made using the "antisense" method. This strategy is aimed at inhibiting synthesis of specific gene products by expressing or introducing nucleotide sequences complementary (i.e., in the antisense orientation) to regions of the target mRNA (which is in the "sense" orientation). The partially or wholly double-stranded molecules thus formed are not properly processed or translated, resulting in a specific block to synthesis of the protein. Treatment of human T lymphocytes with c-*myc* antisense oligonucleotides prior to mitogenic activation prevented entry of the cells into S phase and blocked expression of the c-*myc* protein, although certain G_1-specific genes were expressed (Heikkila et al. 1987). Together, these results suggest that c-*myc* is indeed likely to function as part of a pathway in which its expression is necessary but not sufficient for full entry into the cell cycle.

In contrast to the situation with proliferating cells, many terminally differentiated cell types do not express c-*myc*. In fact, the down-regulation of c-*myc* expression appears to be an early event in a number of hematopoietic and nonhematopoietic cell types that have been induced to differentiate (Westin et al. 1982a,b; Lachman and Skoultchi 1984; Dony et al. 1985; Sejersen et al. 1985). In at least some cases, this down-regulation appears complex. For example, in mouse erythroleukemia cells treated with certain differentiation inducers, c-*myc* RNA levels undergo a rapid decline followed by a transient period of reexpression that precedes the final shutoff characteristic of the terminally differentiated erythrocytes (Lachman and Skoultchi 1984).

It is important to understand whether the decrease in c-*myc* expression is a driving force of differentiation or simply a by-product of changes in growth status. Indeed, it has been observed that undifferentiated and differentiated keratinocytes express equivalent levels of c-*myc* (Dotto et al. 1986) and that c-*myc* can be reinduced in differentiated muscle cells by serum stimulation (Endo and Nadal-Ginard 1986). At the very least, such observations suggest that expression of c-*myc* is not incompatible with terminal differentiation. Nonetheless, the potential role of c-*myc* during differentiation has begun to be examined, with interesting results. It has now been shown that murine erythroleukemia cells, in which an introduced c-*myc* is strongly and constitutively expressed under the control of a viral promoter, cannot be induced to differentiate (Coppola and Cole 1986). In the converse experiment, it was demonstrated that the HL60 promyelocytic leukemia cell line could be induced to differentiate after inhibition of endogenous c-*myc* expression by addition of antisense oligonucleotides (Holt et al. 1988). Such experiments point to down-regulation of c-*myc* expression as being a critical determinant of differentiation in at least these cell types. In this regard, it is intriguing that one region of Myc has been found to be conserved in the *Drosophila achaete-scute* and *daughterless* as well as in the mouse MyoD proteins, all of which have been linked to differentiation (Davis et al. 1987; Villares and Cabrera 1987; Caudy et al. 1988; Murre et al. 1989).

F. Control of c-*myc* Expression

The degree to which c-*myc* gene products are allowed to accumulate in the cell is subject to an extraordinarily complex set of controls. The transcriptional regulatory regions preceding the first exon of c-*myc* appear to be unusually complex, consisting of a mosaic of sequences that produce both positive and negative effects on transcription (Hay et al. 1987). There are examples of regulation at nearly every possible level of c-*myc* expression: transcription initiation, elongation of nascent RNA transcripts, RNA processing, mRNA stability, translational initiation, and protein turnover.

One particularly interesting control mechanism for c-*myc* appears to operate at the level of elongation of nascent RNA transcripts. Under normal conditions, a high percentage of transcripts initiated at the c-*myc* promoters at the 5′ end of exon 1 fail to elongate past the end of the exon. This premature termination of transcription appears to be significantly increased during the period when c-*myc* levels decline upon differentiation of HL60 and mouse erythroleukemia cells (Bentley and Groudine 1986; Nepveu et al. 1987). This suggests that the elongation block is a regulatory mechanism normally used to modulate c-*myc* expression levels. In striking contrast, this transcriptional block appears to be alleviated in a class of Burkitt's lymphomas that have sustained mutations in exon 1, leading to deregulation of normal c-*myc* transcription (Cesarman et al. 1987) and possibly to suppression of an alternative translational initiation site as well (Hann et al. 1988). Although transcriptional attenuation of the type observed for c-*myc* has also been detected in L-*myc*, the N-*myc* gene does not appear to have any block to transcript elongation once RNA molecules have been initiated (Krystal et al. 1988).

Another mechanism for ensuring tight control over *myc* expression is reflected in the extremely short half-lives of c-*myc* mRNA and protein relative to most cell proteins (also characteristic of c-*myb* and c-*fos* gene products). Even small fluctuations in the rates of oncogene transcription or RNA metabolism are mirrored by rapid adjustments in the steady-state levels of protein. In general, the oncoproteins are present at relatively low levels. Only a few hundred molecules of c-*myc* protein exist at steady state in normal proliferating nonestablished cells. Higher levels are attained in established cell lines, whereas the highest amounts (on the order of 10^5 molecules per cell) are observed in tumors carrying *myc* gene amplifications (see below). Stabilization of c-*myc* mRNA, possibly in concert with increased transcription, plays an important role in the rapid increases in c-*myc* RNA levels following growth factor stimulation of quiescent cells and after inhibition of protein synthesis (Blanchard et al. 1985). The decreases in c-*myc* RNA levels after differentiation or interferon treatment have also been at least partly ascribed to increased mRNA turnover (Dani et al. 1985; Dony et al. 1985).

It now seems likely that the multiple controls over c-*myc* can be exerted coordinately and at several levels of c-*myc* expression. Thus, whereas the decline in c-*myc* mRNA immediately after induction of mouse erythroleukemia cell differentiation appears due to the block to transcriptional elongation, the final shutoff of c-*myc* after terminal differentiation is a result of increased message turnover (Nepveu et al. 1987). Recent evidence also suggests that different cell types may regulate c-*myc* expression at different levels in response to the same stimuli. The multiple levels of c-*myc* control underscore the notion of c-*myc* as an important regulatory entity whose accumulation must be kept in check.

G. Oncogenic Activation of c-*myc*

One of the most crucial problems facing those who study oncogenes concerns the mechanism(s) of proto-oncogene activation. Put simply, the question is how can gene products that presumably play critical roles in normal cellular processes have their functions subverted in such a manner that they now lead the cell toward neoplasia? The answer to this question is important, since it must be closely tied to oncogene function and could potentially provide new strategies for diagnosis and intervention. In principle, oncogenic activation could occur through two mechanisms: (1) Deregulation of expression through mutation or rearrangement of the nucleotide sequences that constitute signals for control of transcription, mRNA processing and stability, or translation could lead to inappropriate expression of the gene product with regard to cell type, differentiation pathway, or timing within the cell cycle. It could also lead to abnormally high levels of expression. (2) Mutation or rearrangement of the protein coding region of the oncogene could lead to alteration of function.

Elucidation of the mechanism by which *myc* is oncogenically activated is especially challenging in light of the diverse alterations detected at the c-*myc* locus in human, rodent, avian, and feline neoplasms (as outlined in Fig. 1). These alterations include retroviral transduction, gene amplification, insertional mutagenesis, and chromosome translocation; additionally, point mutations are often found in the rearranged c-*myc* genes. Given this bewildering plethora of c-*myc* alterations, it appears difficult to discern whether there is a single underlying event common to all these changes or whether there are different routes leading to activation in different cell types or stages. Nonetheless, although much still remains to be learned about *myc* activation, it is increasingly apparent that the fundamental result of these *myc* rearrangements is deregulation of expression, often, but not always, linked to overproduction of the *myc* protein.

To understand how c-*myc* expression could be deregulated through gene rearrangement, it is worthwhile briefly examining specific examples of c-*myc* alterations (see Fig. 1; see also Chapter 13).

1. *Retrovirus transduction and insertional mutagenesis*: As discussed above, retroviral "capture" of c-*myc* invariably results in complete loss of upstream promoter regulatory sequences and the normal mRNA initiation sites. High-level transcription of v-*myc* is imposed by the retroviral promoter and is quite clearly divorced from normal cellular control. The imposition of a retroviral promoter/regulator is also observed in avian bursal lymphomas and murine and feline T-cell lymphomas, where nontransforming retroviruses integrate in the vicinity of the c-*myc* locus. In some cases, the result of the integration is to directly displace c-*myc* exon 1 and other regulatory sequences by the retroviral promoter, effectively turning c-*myc* into a viral gene (which, in some cases, has actually been observed to be encapsidated, as RNA, into viral particles). In other instances, the viral integration event does not disrupt the exon-intron structure of c-*myc* but rather influences c-*myc* transcription through the retroviral enhancer. Both forms of "insertional mutagenesis" are likely to result in loss of normal transcriptional regulation (Hayward et al. 1982; Bister and Jansen 1986).
2. *Gene amplification*: Examples of overexpression can be found in human tumors in which *myc* family gene amplifications have occurred (for review, see Alitalo and Schwab 1985). N-*myc* amplifications have been found in neuroblastomas, small cell lung carcinomas, and retinoblastomas; L-*myc* has been amplified in a specific subset of small cell lung carcinomas; and c-*myc* amplifications have been detected in lung car-

cinomas, neuroblastomas, and certain tumor cell lines. The N-*myc* amplifications correlate strongly with high metastatic potential and poor prognosis in primary neuroblastomas (Brodeur et al. 1984). The common thread here is that these amplifications result in high-level expression of the gene. Greatly elevated levels of N-*myc* expression, in the absence of gene amplification, have also been observed in some small cell lung carcinomas and in Wilms' tumors, suggesting that the amplification itself may be less important than elevated expression.

3. *Chromosomal translocations*: Invariably associated with human Burkitt's lymphomas, mouse plasmacytomas, and rat immunocytomas are chromosomal translocations involving the c-*myc* locus (for review, see Cory 1986). Although individual tumors can differ with regard to exact chromosomal breakpoints and stage of B-cell differentiation, the common theme in all this chromosomal reshuffling is that c-*myc* is removed from its normal environment. In many tumors, c-*myc* transcription appears to be driven by an immunoglobulin enhancer located near the translocation breakpoint of the recipient chromosome. In most cases, the displaced c-*myc* has either suffered mutations within, or completely lost, its first exon. This region contains sequences that normally regulate transcriptional initiation and elongation. The resulting levels of c-*myc* expression are not exceptionally high when compared to nontransformed lymphoid cells, suggesting that deregulated expression rather than overexpression is more likely to be responsible for transformation.

The loss or alteration of critical control sequences observed in the diverse neoplasms described above apparently acts to uncouple expression of c-*myc* from its normal physiological regulators. This results in an inability to modulate expression of the c-*myc* gene in response to intracellular and extracellular signals that normally govern such events as exit from the cell cycle and terminal differentiation.

That deregulation of c-*myc* expression can have profound consequences on cell physiology has been amply demonstrated by experiments entailing the introduction of different c-*myc* DNA constructs into cells. Constitutive, high-level c-*myc* expression decreases the requirement for multiple growth factors for both continued cell proliferation and entry into the cell cycle (Armelin et al. 1984; Sorrentino et al. 1986; Stern et al. 1986). Unregulated *myc* expression also induces immortalization of certain cell types and blocks differentiation of others. At the organismic level, the effects of deregulation are perhaps best exhibited by transgenic mice carrying the c-*myc* gene driven by an immunoglobulin enhancer, so that deregulated expression of *myc* is targeted to B cells (Adams et al. 1985). Such mice possess a significantly expanded population of apparently normal progenitor B cells compared to mice not carrying the c-*myc* transgene. Expression of c-*myc* is constitutive in these cells. Since all the mice carrying the transgene eventually develop clonal B-cell lymphomas, there is a good possibility that the expanded, highly proliferative pre-B-cell population serves as a pool within which other genetic alterations may occur, leading to frank disease (Langdon et al. 1986; for review of oncogenes in transgenic mice, see Compere et al. 1988).

Other genetic alterations of *myc* may well include further changes such as point mutations (which have been shown to positively affect v-*myc*-induced transformation) and overexpression (as a consequence of the events leading to deregulation). These may well be strong secondary contributors to tumorigenesis. Probably more important are the synergistic effects of deregulated *myc* acting together with other activated oncogenes (Land et al. 1983). Cotransfection of activated *myc* and *ras* results in transformation of cell types that neither gene alone can transform. More importantly, a synergistic increase in tumor formation has also been shown by mating of separate strains of transgenic mice containing either c-*myc* or activated *ras* under control of a retroviral promoter. This demonstrates that cooperative transformation by oncogenes can occur in vivo (Sinn et al. 1987; see Chapter 12).

The c-*myc* rearrangements and the results of many biological experiments all point to *myc* as an important regulator of cell growth and differentiation. At various times, it has been proposed that c-*myc* might function as a transcriptional regulator (Kaddurah-Daouk et al. 1987; Onclercq et al. 1988), a regulator of DNA synthesis (Classon et al. 1987; Iguchi-Ariga et al. 1988), a component of the RNA processing machinery (Spector et al. 1987), a controller of other posttranscriptional events (Prendergast and Cole 1989), or a component of the nuclear substructure (Eisenman et al. 1985). A major problem is interpreting which effects are a *direct* result of the action of the Myc protein and which represent secondary or later events. These diverse proposals also reflect both the belief in the importance of *myc* and the difficulties inherent in precisely defining its physiological functions. At present, we lack decisive evidence concerning how this protein functions in the nucleus. However, the fact that Myc contains structural elements analogous to those found in several DNA-binding transcriptional regulators (see Section X.B) suggests that Myc is also likely to exert its effects through gene-specific regulation.

III. THE *myb* ONCOGENE

Although both the *myc* and *myb* oncogenes were first discovered as retroviral genes implicated in transformation of myeloid cells, they differ not only in nucleotide sequence, but also in two other important characteristics. First, whereas *myc* is expressed and oncogenically activated in a wide variety of tissues, *myb* has a rather restricted tissue specificity. Second, oncogenic activation of *myc* is primarily caused by deregulation, whereas in *myb*, structural changes in the protein as well as unregulated expression appear to be responsible for activation.

c-*myb* expression appears to be largely restricted to cells of hematopoietic origin. Highest levels are detected in early T- and B-lymphoid cells as well as in myeloid and erythroid cells. *c-myb* has also been found to be expressed in certain non-hematopoietic tumor cell lines (Thiele et al. 1988), and two *myb*-related mRNAs have recently been identified that appear to be more broadly expressed than c-*myb* (Nomura et al. 1988). As with *myc*, cell differentiation correlates with down-regulation of c-*myb* expression (Gonda et al. 1982; Westin et al. 1982a; Sheiness and Gardinier 1984), and enforced expression of c-*myb* blocks the differentiation of murine erythroleukemia cells (Clarke et al. 1988). The restricted action of *myb* is also reflected in the relatively narrow range of tumor types associated with *myb* oncogenesis. In contrast to the wide spectrum of tumors induced by the *myc*-containing retroviruses discussed above, avian myeloblastosis virus (AMV), a v-*myb*-containing acute leukemia virus, induces myelomonocytic leukemias in young chicks and transforms only myeloid precursors and mature macrophages in vitro. Transformation is thought to involve dedifferentiation of more mature cells into immature blastlike cells (Ness et al. 1987). When an AMV-transformed myeloid cell line is chemically induced to differentiate, a redistribution of the v-Myb protein from the nucleus to the cytoplasm is observed, suggesting that the presence of nuclear v-Myb protein may be blocking the normal signals for differentiation of these cells (Klempnauer et al. 1984).

The E26 retrovirus, by virtue of the fact that it contains, in addition to v-*myb*, the putative oncogene *ets*, has an expanded oncogenic potential, producing both myeloid and erythroid leukemias in vivo and transforming erythroid, myeloid, and fibroblast cells in vitro (Golay et al. 1988). The predominantly myeloid character of v-*myb*-related tumors is also manifested in the myeloid leukemias induced in mice by murine leukemia virus proviral integrations within the c-*myb* locus (Shen-Ong et al. 1984).

The viral *myb* oncogenes of E26 and AMV have both undergone loss of substantial amino-terminal and carboxy-terminal coding regions compared to their c-*myb* cellular progenitor. It is intriguing, then, that in the myeloid leukemias induced in mice by murine leukemia virus, the proviral insertions into c-*myb* interrupt nearly the same amino- or carboxy-terminal regions as in E26 and AMV (Fig. 2) (Shen-Ong et al. 1984; Rosson and Reddy 1986). All oncogenically activated *myb* genes contain substantial deletions of their protein-coding regions, suggesting, in contrast to what has been observed for c-*myc*, that *myb* is activated by changes in both its regulation and its protein structure.

In contrast to c-*myc* and c-*fos*, which are induced very early following mitogenic stimulation, c-*myb* expression occurs late, near the G_1/S border (Thompson et al. 1986; Lipsick and Boyle 1987). In addition, during the

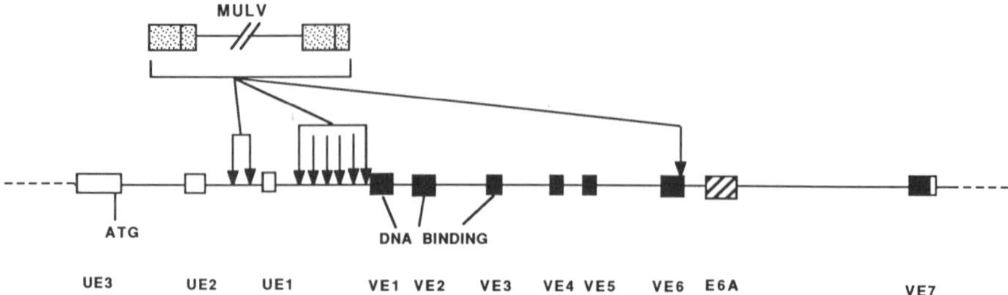

Figure 2 Structure and oncogenic activation of c-*myb*. Ten coding exons of the c-*myb* locus are shown as boxes separated by introns (not to scale) spread out over ~ 35 kb of DNA. Additional exons probably exist at either end but have not been defined. ATG indicates the probable translational initiation site for the 75-kD c-*myb*-encoded protein. Black boxes indicate the exons (viral exons VE1–VE7) included in the v-*myb* gene of AMV; the E26 virus lacks VE7 and the 3′ end of VE6. Vertical arrows indicate the approximate integration sites for murine leukemia virus (MuLV) detected in a series of murine myeloid tumors. These remove some of the same exons (upstream exons UE1–UE3) that are absent in v-*myb*. All the oncogenically activated *myb* genes retain the DNA-binding region in VE1–VE3. The cross-hatched exon (E6A) is present in only a fraction of c-*myb* mRNAs, due to alternative splicing (Shen-Ong 1987).

cell cycle of some cell types, c-*myb* expression increases transiently during S phase (Thompson et al. 1986). The correlation between c-*myb* expression and the onset of S phase may hint at a role for Myb in the replication or organization of chromatin.

myb proteins are DNA-binding proteins with affinity for random DNA sequences. Preferential binding to a specific sequence of nucleotides has very recently been detected, but it is unclear whether or not this sequence is a component of a regulatory element (Biedenkapp et al. 1988). The region of the *myb* protein responsible for interaction with DNA has been mapped to a threefold, imperfect repeat of 53 amino acids in the amino-terminal portion of the protein (Klempnauer and Sippel 1987; Peters et al. 1987). This segment is found essentially intact in the oncogenically activated *myb* genes noted above, suggesting that it is important for both normal and transforming *myb* function (Ibanez and Lipsick 1988). Also striking is the high degree of evolutionary conservation of the DNA-binding region: In addition to its presence in vertebrate *myb* genes, it appears to be expressed in both *Drosophila* and the plant *Zea Mays* as a domain within proteins that otherwise bear little or no homology with c-*myb* (Paz-Ares et al. 1987; Peters et al. 1987), somewhat reminiscent of the conserved homeobox domains. The plant gene containing the *myb* DNA-binding domain is a regulatory locus affecting localized pigment production, a fact consistent with the idea that the conserved DNA-binding region may have a biological function.

Very recent experiments strongly suggest that both v- and c-Myb can function as transcriptional activators. First, when Myb is linked to the DNA-binding domain of a yeast activator protein, it specifically stimulates expression of a reporter gene containing the binding site (Weston and Bishop 1989). Second, Myb also appears to stimulate transcription from promoters containing the Myb-specific DNA-binding sequence referred to above (Sakura et al. 1989; Weston and Bishop 1989). In addition, these studies have begun to define a region within Myb, distinct from the DNA-binding domain, that is required for the transcriptional activation. Furthermore, another Myb region, also downstream of the DNA-binding domain, appears to negatively affect Myb's ability to activate transcription, since its deletion appears to lead to increased Myb transcriptional activity. This negative regulator is contained within the segment that is lost in the oncogenic v-Myb proteins. Thus, it is possible that oncogenic activation may involve loss of a region of the Myb protein that can modulate transcription from promoters containing the Myb DNA-binding site. It will be important to now determine which cellular gene promoters are affected by Myb. Since myelomonocytic cells expressing a temperature-sensitive v-Myb can be converted by temperature shift from a mature, non-dividing, differentiated phenotype to an immature proliferating state, it seems likely that Myb will interact directly with genes that play a role in the choice between differentiation and proliferation in hematopoietic cells (Beug et al. 1987).

IV. THE *p53* ONCOGENE

The *p53* oncogene was discovered not through its transduction by oncogenic retroviruses nor through genetic analysis, but rather through the direct association of the p53 protein with two important DNA tumor virus nuclear proteins: SV40 large T antigen (Lane and Crawford 1979; Linzer and Levine 1979) and the adenovirus type 5 E1B 55-kD protein (Sarnow et al. 1982). The participation of the p53 protein in noncovalent oligomeric complexes with these DNA tumor virus proteins in transformed cells has a profound effect on p53 metabolism. In normal cells, p53 is present at low levels and has a very short half-life (from 6 to 30 min.). Complex formation, following adenovirus or SV40 infection, results in a 100-fold increase in half-life and a concomitant increase in the level of p53 (Reich et al. 1983). Of particular interest is the fact that stabilization and elevated levels of p53 are not confined to virally transformed cells, but are also observed in chemically transformed and tumor cell lines (Crawford et al. 1981; Dippold et al. 1981).

If elevated levels of p53 can be attained by stabilization of the protein through association with DNA tumor virus proteins, then might p53 be stabilized in nonvirally transformed cells by association with a cellular protein? Examination of rat embryo cells transformed by cotransfection with *p53* and activated *ras*, as well as other transformed lines containing high levels of p53, revealed that p53 is indeed complexed with a known cellular protein: hsc70, a constitutively expressed member of the heat-shock protein family (Hinds et al. 1987). Evidence now indicates that the ability of p53 protein to bind hsc70 can be conferred by point mutation within the middle third of the *p53* protein-coding region (Finlay et al. 1988). Transfection of the mutated *p53* gene into primary rodent cells results in immortalization (Jenkins et al. 1984). In addition, the mutant, but not the wild-type *p53* gene can collaborate with an activated *ras* oncogene to transform primary rat embryo fibroblasts (Parada et al. 1984; Finlay et al. 1988).

Little is known concerning the function of p53. As is the case with c-*myc*, cell differentiation appears to correlate with decreased levels of p53 expression. For example, the induction of endodermal differentiation of F9 embryonal carcinoma cells results in a significant drop in *p53* RNA levels due to increased RNA turnover. This occurs much later after induction than the immediate decrease in c-*myc* RNA levels (Dony et al. 1985). Expression of p53 in normal cells appears to be regulated during cell growth with an increase in the abundance of its mRNA occurring in late G_1 or early S phase following mitogen stimulation of quiescent cells. Since direct injection of anti-p53 antibodies into nuclei early in G_1 prevents entry of cells into S phase, it would seem that p53 function may in some way be required for DNA replication (Mercer et al. 1982). Further support for this idea comes from the finding that DNA polymerase α and p53 bind to the same region of SV40 T antigen (Gannon and Lane 1987). Indeed, overexpression of p53 appears to specifically inhibit T-antigen-dependent replication of SV40 DNA (Braithwaite et al. 1987). Since cells lacking any detectable p53 expression are viable, it would appear that p53 does not have an essential activator function (Wolf et al. 1984).

In one model, p53 is thought to act essentially as an anti-oncogene (see Chapter 11). Loss of function could occur either through transcriptional inactivation of the gene (as observed in a tumor cell line with a proviral integration in p53), sequestration of p53 protein by viral proteins (T antigen, E1B), or mutation leading to binding of p53 protein by heat-shock protein.

If this anti-oncogene model for p53 is correct, then cellular transformation occurring through loss of normal p53 function should in principle be reversed by introduction of wild-type p53. Very recent experiments have now shown this to be the case by demonstrating that wild-type p53 can block the cotransformation of rat embryo cells by mutant p53 plus activated *ras* (Finlay et al. 1989). The results are also consistent with the notion that excess mutant p53 can act in a dominant fashion to transform cells by interfering with the proliferation-limiting function of normal p53, probably by forming complexes with the normal protein and hsc70. Whether normal p53 functions to regulate the cell cycle or other critical cellular functions remains to be determined.

V. THE *fos* ONCOGENE

The thesis that nuclear oncoproteins act to control specific gene expression as an integrated response to transmembrane signals is beginning to be substantiated by studies on the *fos* oncogene. On the one hand, a great deal of past work has demonstrated that c-*fos* gene expression is induced by an extraordinarily diverse group of agents that promote growth and/or differentiation in a wide range of cell types (for reviews, see Verma and Sassone-Corsi 1987; Curran 1988). On the other hand, a series of recent experiments has directly demonstrated that the c-*fos*-encoded protein is a component of a nucleoprotein complex that specifically associates with gene regulatory sequences (see Section VIII). Thus, two major areas of research in signal transduction are converging on *fos*.

A. v-*fos* and c-*fos*

The v-*fos* oncogene was first identified in two murine retroviruses (FBJ-MSV and FBR-MSV), which possess the unusual ability to rapidly induce osteogenic sarcomas in mice. Molecular cloning and sequencing of c-*fos* and the testing of c-*fos*/v-*fos* chimeric genes in fibroblast transformation assays demonstrated that c-*fos* can be oncogenically activated (1) by emplacement of a transcriptional enhancer leading to constitutive expression and (2) by altering sequences at the 3′ end of the noncoding sequence in the c-*fos* mRNA that act normally as signals for the rapid degradation of this RNA (Miller et al. 1984; Lee et al. 1988). These alterations, which are incorporated into the structures of the v-*fos* genes of FBR and FBJ viruses, have the net effect of greatly increasing the abundance of *fos* mRNA and encoded protein while overriding the normal ability to regulate expression (for review, see Verma 1986). Transgenic mice expressing a c-*fos* gene that has been altered in this way develop hyperplastic abnormalities in long bone formation and, at later times, osteogenic sarcomas reminiscent of, but distinct from, the invasive osteogenic sarcomas produced by the FBR and FBJ viruses (Ruther et al. 1987).

Point mutations within the c-*fos*-coding sequence can also profoundly contribute to the transformed phenotype, since a substitution of glutamic acid for valine at residue 138 is crucial for the ability of FBR v-*fos* to immortalize cells. In addition, v-Fos proteins contain a truncated and substituted carboxyl terminus compared to the c-Fos protein (Fig. 3). These changes appear to block the ability of Fos to down-regulate transcription of the c-*fos* gene (Wilson and Treisman 1988 and see below).

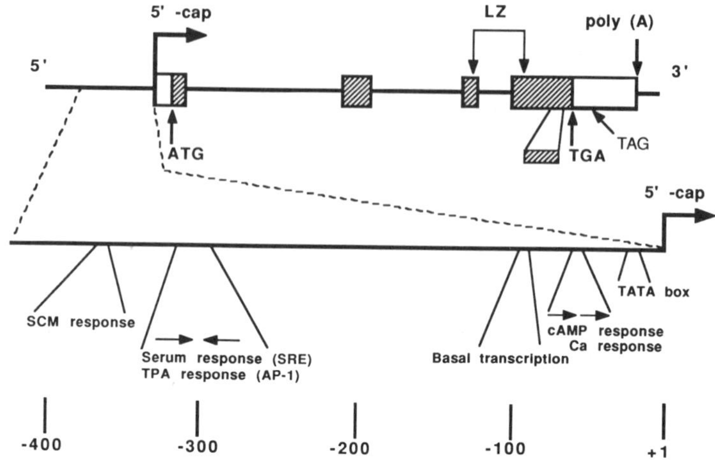

Figure 3 Organization of the c-*fos* gene and its regulatory regions. The top line depicts the arrangement of c-*fos* exons over a region of ~ 3.5 kb of DNA. Hatched boxes show the extent of the protein-coding region with the ATG initiator and TGA terminator for the 55-kD c-*fos*-encoded protein. (LZ) Leucine zipper region, a periodic array of leucines apparently involved in dimerization and DNA binding (see text). The small segment of the protein-coding region in the last c-*fos* exon that is shown expanded is the portion that is deleted in the v-*fos* of the FBJ-MSV retrovirus. Loss of this 104-nucleotide region results in a reading frame shift and termination of the v-*fos* protein at a TAG codon located in a normally untranslated region of the last exon (see Verma 1986). The bottom line is an expanded view of the 400-nucleotide region upstream of the c-*fos* transcriptional initiation site (5′-cap). Approximate locations of important regulatory sequences are indicated. Elements located between +1 and −100 are also required for basal level expression. The two arrows indicate direct repeats or palindromes. SCM response refers to the sequence element that controls the transcriptional activation of c-*fos* response to conditioned medium from cells transformed by the v-*sis* oncogene (see text; for review, see Verma and Sassone-Corsi 1987).

c-*fos* is normally expressed at very low basal levels in most growing cells. The higher levels of c-*fos* produced in some embryonic and bone marrow cell types are probably due to the presence of certain growth factors. Striking transient increases in c-*fos* expression occur in different cell types following stimulation with serum, specific growth factors (e.g., PDGF, fibroblast growth factor, epidermal growth factor, colony-stimulating factor 1, interleukin-3, and nerve growth factor), or after trauma (Greenberg and Ziff 1984; for review, see Curran 1988). In some cases, addition of mitogen leads within minutes to a more than 100-fold increase in the levels of *fos* mRNA, followed by a return to prestimulation levels within 30–60 minutes. This rapid and dramatic induction of c-*fos* expression can be made to occur when protein synthesis is blocked, indicating that the components mediating the c-*fos* transcriptional activation are already present in the cell (Greenberg et al. 1986). A number of other genes, including *myc*, *jun*, and the newly characterized Fos-related proteins (see below), appear to be similarly poised for rapid activation by mitogens. Such "early response" genes very likely encode proteins that play critical roles in early cell-cycle events. Since expression of antisense c-*fos* appears to block cell proliferation (Holt et al. 1986), it would seem that c-*fos* is also intimately involved in growth-related processes.

It is becoming clear that c-*fos* is a member of a larger gene family. A number of proteins with related antigenicity (Fos-related antigens or Fras) have been described. At least some are highly related to c-*fos* (Cohen and Curran 1988).

B. Sequences Controlling c-*fos* Gene Expression

As described above, the expression of both c-*fos* and c-*myc* is dramatically increased by a wide variety of agents known to affect cell growth and behavior. The extent and duration of c-*fos* expression is determined by transcriptional and posttranscriptional controls (particularly mRNA degradation), much as described above for *myc*. The mechanism of induction at the transcriptional level has attracted much interest because it promises to link transmembrane signal transduction with specific regions on DNA that mediate transcription. For c-*myc*, this has led to an interesting but highly complex picture of interspersed positive and negative control elements both inside and outside the c-*myc*-coding regions. Some of these are likely to be primarily involved in posttranscriptional rather than transcriptional regulation. However, in c-*fos*, small sequence elements have been rather precisely defined that mediate the transcriptional response of the gene to specific stimuli. Some of these are involved in regulating the basal levels of c-*fos* transcription, whereas others seem likely to play roles in specific responses to transmembrane signals (Fig. 3). One of these, the serum response element (SRE), was initially identified as a 60-bp region lying approximately 300 nucleotides upstream of the start site for c-*fos* transcription. The SRE is essential for the induction of c-*fos* RNA in response to stimulation of cells by serum growth factors (Treisman 1985, 1986; Gilman et al. 1986).

Molecular dissection of the SRE revealed that only a small region within it was both necessary and sufficient for growth factor response: a 20-bp imperfect palindrome or dyad symmetry element (DSE). Since this sequence is also required for c-*fos* induction by the phorbol ester TPA, the DSE may mediate the transcriptional response to multiple signals, possibly through association with Jun and Fos itself (see Sections VII and VIII). A sequence highly related to the DSE has also been detected upstream of the actin gene promoter, which is also known to be serum inducible (Mohun et al. 1987). Thus, the DSE may function in the coordinate expression of subsets of genes in response to multiple signals of extracellular origin.

The c-*fos* DSE serves as a highly specific binding site for a protein, the serum response factor (SRF) (Treisman 1987). Interaction between the SRF and the DSE is required for the c-*fos* response to serum. In addition, the SRF appears to play a role as a regulator of serum-induced as well as constitutive c-*fos* transcription (Norman et al. 1988). Similar specific DNA–protein interactions probably also govern the response of c-*fos* to other agents, since sequences required for induction of c-*fos* following treatment with cAMP, calcium, and conditioned media have also been identified (Fig. 3) (Verma and Sassone-Corsi 1987; Sheng et al. 1988). Since the expression of c-*fos* in response to serum is only transient, it seems likely that c-*fos* transcription can also be down-regulated. Sequences upstream of the promoter also appear to be involved in repression of c-*fos* transcription, probably through interaction with the Fos protein itself (Wilson and Treisman 1988 and see Section VIII). It is not difficult to envision how the induction of c-*fos* by a large number of diverse agents could be integrated through the interaction of preexisting protein transcription factors with specific sequence elements that influence the c-*fos* promoter.

Thus far, we have viewed *fos* from the perspective of gene regulation through growth factors and other mitogens, leaving open the question of what the *fos*-encoded protein (Fos) might actually do once it is so forcefully induced by such stimuli. The notion that Fos acts to regulate expression of other genes will be discussed in the later section on the interaction of Fos with the Jun transcription factor (Section VIII).

VI. ErbA: AN ONCOGENIC HORMONE RECEPTOR

A. The v-erbA Oncogene

v-*erbA* and v-*erbB* were originally identified as the two cellular genes cotransduced by avian erythroblastosis virus (AEV) (Vennstrom and Bishop 1982). AEV rapidly induces erythroleukemias in young chicks and transforms erythroblasts and fibroblasts in tissue culture. *erbA* was somewhat overshadowed by *erbB* when it was shown that the latter was a truncated homolog of the epidermal growth factor receptor (localized in the plasma membrane, see Chapter 3) and was the only oncogene required by AEV for erythroblast and fibroblast transformation (Frykberg et al. 1983).

More detailed studies proved the biological effects of *erbA* to be more subtle but no less interesting than those of v-*erbB*. Molecularly altered constructs of AEV that lacked v-*erbA* were indeed capable of transforming erythroid cells, but such cells displayed a high rate of spontaneous terminal differentiation and could only be propagated under a narrow range of ion concentrations and pH. Introduction of v-*erbA* into the v-*erbB*-transformed erythroblasts allowed proliferation under a considerably expanded range of growth conditions and blocked the spontaneous differentiation characteristic of the v-*erbA*$^-$ cells (Kahn et al. 1986; Damm et al. 1987). Moreover, v-*erbA* can enhance the transformation of erythroid progenitor cells by cooperating with the v-*src*, v-*fps*, v-*sea*, and v-*fms* tyrosine kinases as well as with v-Ha-*ras* in a similar manner as with v-*erbB* (Kahn et al. 1986).

The v-*erbA* gene thus posed an intriguing question: What sort of function would one expect for a gene product that is not in itself capable of overt transformation but which has subtle effects on growth and differentiation and, in addition, collaborates with a wide variety of other oncogenes to enhance transformation? The finding that v-*erbA* is a modified intracellular hormone receptor has provided some new ways of thinking about this problem.

B. A Superfamily of Intracellular Receptors

The most well characterized eukaryotic signal-response pathways are those mediated by the intracellular hormone receptors. These receptors are members of a superfamily of intracellular regulatory proteins capable of binding to small, usually lipid-soluble ligands that enter the cell by diffusing through the plasma membrane. Ligand binding elicits a structural change in the receptor that promotes interaction of the ligand-receptor complex with a defined set of DNA "response elements" located in the vicinity of transcriptional promoters. Binding of the complex to the response element results in activation or repression of specific gene expression by influencing RNA polymerase II transcription (for review, see Yamamoto 1985).

This receptor superfamily comprises proteins that bind the steroid hormones (glucocorticoid, testosterone, progesterone, estrogen, and aldosterone hormones, as well as vitamin D_3), thyroid hormones, and retinoic acid. Molecular analysis of the steroid hormone receptors has allowed the definition of distinct structural and functional domains (for review, see Evans 1988). A very similar domain organization has been revealed for the other members of the receptor family and is diagramed in Figure 4. A large carboxy-terminal region of the receptor that binds ligand is connected through a flexible "hinge" to the DNA-binding domain. The specific association between hormone receptor and the DNA response sequence element of the target gene is thought to be brought about by the folding of a segment of the receptor's DNA-binding domain into two fingerlike structures that interact with DNA. This finger structure, which forms through bonding between metal ions and pairs of histidines and cysteines

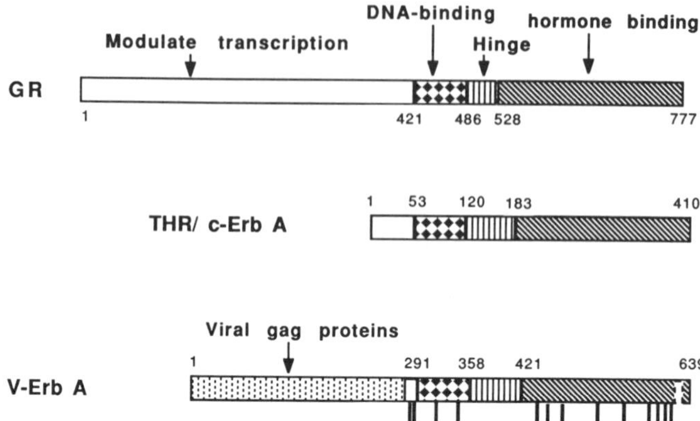

Figure 4 Organization of hormone receptors. Domain structures of the glucocorticoid receptor (GR) and of the cellular and retroviral forms of the thyroid hormone receptor (THR/c-ErbA and v-ErbA, respectively) are depicted. Numbers indicate amino acid position at the domain boundaries. Although the overall domain organization as shown is the same between GR and THR, there is considerable sequence divergence between them (the human GR and THR proteins are 17% and 47% homologous in the hormone-binding and DNA-binding regions, respectively; Evans 1988). v-ErbA, in comparison to c-ErbA, contains retroviral structural (gag) protein at its amino terminus; lacks the first 12 amino acids of its putative transcriptional modulatory region; contains 13 amino acid substitutions scattered throughout (vertical bars); and contains a deletion of 9 amino acids near the carboxyl terminus. These changes prevent hormone binding and probably affect transcriptional activation (Munoz et al. 1988).

uniquely positioned at the base of the fingers, has been found in other eukaryotic transcription factors and may mediate metal-coordinated protein–protein as well as protein–DNA interactions (Evans and Hollenberg 1988; Freedman et al. 1988). The amino-terminal segment of the receptor is presumed to be involved in activation or repression of transcription, although recent evidence indicates that the ligand-binding domain may also be critical for transcriptional regulation, whereas the amino-terminal domain modulates activity (Webster et al. 1988). Signals for nuclear transport of the receptor also exist in the vicinity of the DNA-binding and hormone-binding regions.

Elucidation of the structural organization of the receptors has led to ideas about how they might be regulated. In the absence of hormone, the ligand-binding domain is thought to shield the DNA-binding region. In this state, the receptor is localized in the cytoplasm or loosely retained in the nucleus. Binding to hormone alters the conformation of the ligand-binding region, thus unmasking the nuclear transport signals and the DNA-binding domain. The receptor, thus activated, would now associate with its specific target gene response sequence and promote transcription of the gene.

Support for this model comes from experiments demonstrating that removal of the ligand-binding domain results in constitutive activation of the receptor (Godowski et al. 1987; Hollenberg et al. 1987).

C. The c-*erbA* Oncoprotein is a Thyroid Hormone Receptor

One might imagine the hormone receptors to be ideal candidates for cellular oncoproteins. However, none of the nuclear or cytoplasmic oncogenes previously described exhibited any homology or even organizational similarity to the known hormone receptors. It was somewhat of a surprise, then, when the relatively obscure *erbA* oncogene was shown by sequence comparison to be a member of the family, although not a member that had previously been identified (Fig. 4). Its relationship became clear when it was shown that the c-*erbA* protein was capable of specific high-affinity binding of the T3 and T4 forms of thyroid hormone (Sap et al. 1986; Weinberger et al. 1986).

Thyroid hormone is present in all chordates and exerts profound and complex effects on cell metabolism, differentiation, and development. In amphibians, the multitude of biochemical and morphological events that accompany metamorphosis of the aquatic larval tadpole into an amphibious adult are largely driven by thyroid hormone. Furthermore, thyroid hormone regulates dynamic homeostatic processes in numerous adult tissues and influences differentiation of muscle and erythroid precursors. Many of these events are likely to be due to specific gene activations by the thyroid hormone receptor after thyroid hormone binding. For example, growth hormone gene transcription in rat pituitary cells is stimulated after thyroid hormone treatment. c-*erbA* can directly bind to a transcriptional response element located upstream of the rat growth hormone gene promoter (Glass et al. 1987). Thus, both the structure and the initial characterization of c-*erbA* suggest that it functions in a similar manner to the steroid hormone receptors.

How does the ability of v-*erbA* to arrest erythroid differentiation relate to the function of c-*erbA* as a thyroid hormone receptor, especially when thyroid hormone is thought to potentiate erythropoiesis? When compared to c-*erbA*, the v-*erbA* gene was found to be fused to the retroviral structural protein gene (*gag*) and to contain deletions and mutations, several of which, clustered near the carboxyl terminus, appear to cooperate to prevent v-*erbA* from binding thyroid hormone (Fig. 4) (Munoz et al. 1988). Although incapable of binding hormone, v-*erbA* is nonetheless found in the nucleus and binds DNA (Boucher et al. 1988). One of the key events in erythroid differentiation is the expression of the band 3 anion transporter gene. The transporter protein is not only an important regulator of intracellular pH, but also serves a structural role as an anchor of the red cell cytoskeleton to the membrane. It is intriguing, then, that band

3 gene expression (and, to a lesser extent, other differentiation markers) is efficiently blocked at the transcriptional level in a manner that correlates rather directly with v-*erbA* expression (Zenke et al. 1988). One possibility is that, whereas c-*erbA* might be expected to activate band 3, the over-expressed, mutated, and hormone-unresponsive v-ErbA may bind to band 3 and physically block its gene transcription, an event that may contribute

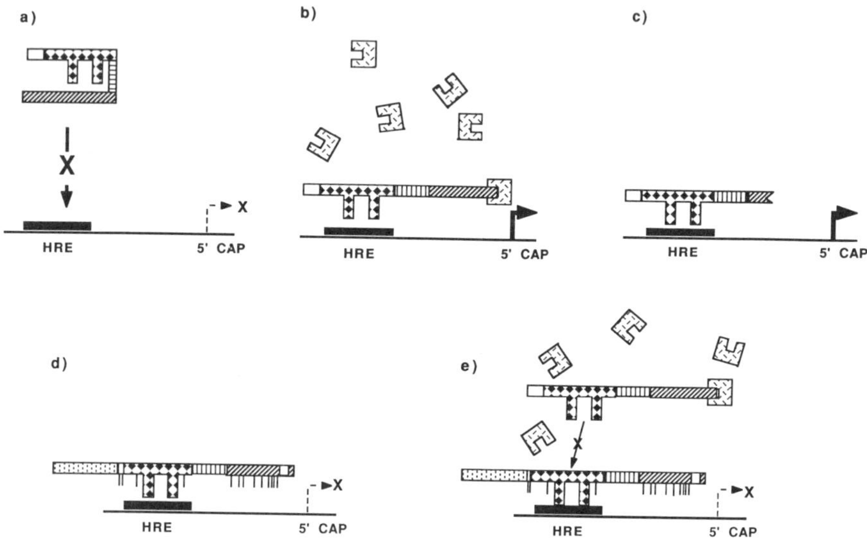

Figure 5 Hypothetical scheme for thyroid hormone receptor action. The thyroid hormone receptor/c-ErbA is shown with the domains coded as in Fig. 4, except for protrusions in the DNA-binding domain that represent the "zinc finger" structures (see text). (*a*) A normal c-ErbA is shown. In the absence of ligand, the hormone-binding domain shields the DNA-binding region, preventing binding to the DNA hormone response element (HRE). This might result in either a low basal level, or a complete lack, of transcription of the structural region of the gene located downstream from the HRE (indicated by weak arrow at the 5′ cap site). (*b*) Thyroid hormone is present. Its interaction with the ligand-binding domain frees the DNA-binding region to interact with the HRE. This might allow RNA polymerase and other accessory factors (not shown) to initiate high-level transcription (strong arrow at the 5′ cap site). (*c*) Truncation or mutation of the ligand-binding domain permits binding and high-level transcription even in the absence of hormone. (*d*) v-ErbA not only binds the HRE in a hormone-independent manner, but also fails to activate the gene due to both mutations and deletions. (*e*) The presence of high levels of v-ErbA leads to permanent occupation of the HRE and the subsequent inability of normal endogenous receptor to regulate the gene in response to hormone. In the scheme shown here, the normal hormone receptor is portrayed as a positive regulator; however, it is becoming increasingly clear that hormone receptors can frequently function to negatively regulate expression of many genes.

to the inability of these cells to terminally differentiate (Fig. 5). Strong support for this model has recently come from experiments demonstrating that v-ErbA prevents thyroid hormone-induced transcriptional activation by c-ErbA (Damm et al. 1989; Sap et al. 1989). More detailed studies on the mutant receptor and its interaction with DNA hold the promise not only of elucidating the mechanism of v-*erbA*-induced transformation, but also of understanding how differentiation is regulated (see also Chapter 11).

VII. JUN: AN ONCOGENIC TRANSCRIPTION FACTOR

The finding that c-*erbA* encodes an intracellular hormone receptor involved in regulation of transcription raises the issue of whether other nuclear oncoproteins also participate in transcriptional control. This appears to be the case, since the product of the *jun* oncogene has been shown to function as a transcriptional regulator. It appears to do this as part of a nucleoprotein complex that can also contain, as an additional component, the c-Fos protein, thus raising the possibility that two nuclear oncoproteins may interact to regulate gene expression (see below).

The work on *jun* provides a good example of how research from several apparently unrelated fields, in this case virology, yeast genetics, and transcription factor biochemistry, can converge in often surprising ways to rapidly elucidate an important function. *jun* was initially encountered as the transforming gene of avian sarcoma virus 17 (ASV 17), a retrovirus recently isolated from a spontaneous sarcoma in an adult chicken. ASV 17 induces fibrosarcomas in chickens and converts tissue culture fibroblast cells into densely packed, spindle-shaped transformants (a morphological phenotype quite distinguishable from cells transformed by v-*src* and other viral oncogenes). Cloning and sequencing demonstrated that ASV 17 carried a unique oncogene, dubbed *jun* (a contraction of ju-nana, Japanese for seventeen), and also led to the surprising finding of a significant degree of amino acid sequence homology between the carboxy-terminal region of *jun* and the well-studied yeast transcriptional activator protein GCN4 (Maki et al. 1987; Vogt et al. 1987).

In *Saccharomyces cerevisiae*, GCN4 mRNA is constitutively expressed but is only translated as a rapid response to amino acid starvation. The GCN4 protein functions to coordinately induce the transcription of genes involved in amino acid biosynthesis by directly binding, as a dimer, to a palindromic regulatory sequence located upstream of the promoters of the 15 genes under GCN4 control (Hope and Struhl 1985, 1986). Both a central acidic region responsible for transcriptional activation and a carboxy-terminal-specific DNA-binding region have been defined for GCN4, and it is this latter domain that is homologous to the carboxy-terminal quarter of v-Jun (Hope and Struhl 1986; Vogt et al. 1987). When the carboxy-terminal region of GCN4 was replaced by the homologous region of v-Jun, the chimeric gene was found to be functional in yeast and to bind to the same DNA sequences as GCN4. This result suggested that v-Jun may well be derived from a normal transcription factor (Struhl 1987). Some clue as to the nature of this normal transcription factor came from the realization that the palindromic GCN4-binding sequence, ATGA(C/G)TCAT, is related to the recognition sequence for activator protein-1 (AP-1), a recently characterized mammalian transcription factor involved in the cellular response to phorbol esters (Angel et al. 1987; Lee et al. 1987).

A series of biochemical analyses confirmed that the c-Jun and AP-1 proteins are highly related and probably identical (Bohmann et al. 1987; Angel et al. 1988b). The relationship between Jun and AP-1 is especially intriguing, given that AP-1 has been implicated in the transcriptional induction of a number of genes by phorbol esters (such as TPA). Since phorbol ester induction can occur in the absence of protein synthesis, it has been proposed that preexisting Jun/AP-1 may be posttranslationally activated through protein modification or by increased interaction with another protein (such as Fos, see below). Either of these potentially activating events might be mediated or enhanced by phosphorylations initiated by protein kinase C, which is the phorbol ester receptor.

The expression of c-*jun* itself also appears to be positively regulated through a high-affinity AP-1-binding site in its own promoter. One model would be that c-Jun, normally present at low basal levels, is functionally activated by inducer, causing rapid effects on responsive genes and up-regulating its own expression. Thus, two modes of c-*jun*/AP-1 activation, posttranslational and autoregulation, may account for both the immediate and the prolonged transcriptional responses to protein kinase C stimulation (Angel et al. 1988a). Two other genes have been identified (*junB* and *junD*) that possess a high degree of structural similarity to c-*jun* (Nakabeppu et al. 1988; Ryder et al. 1988). All three *jun* family members are rapidly expressed in response to mitogenic stimuli (Lamph et al. 1988; Ryder et al. 1988; Ryseck et al. 1988) and appear to be capable of self-associating to form dimers and binding to AP-1 sequences (Nakabeppu et al. 1988). Thus, c-*jun* belongs to a group of proteins that appear to act to regulate transcription in response to different stimuli.

We have followed the trail from an avian retroviral oncoprotein to yeast and human transcriptional regulatory factors. Once again we are faced with the question of oncogenic activation: What is it about v-*jun* that results in transformation? The v-*jun* and c-*jun* proteins differ substantially at their amino termini by virtue of the fact that v-Jun is fused to the retroviral *gag* protein and also lacks a 27-amino-acid region present in c-Jun (Bohmann et al. 1987; Vogt and Tjian 1988). In addition, v-Jun has several point mutations in its DNA-binding domain, although both c-Jun and v-Jun have similar binding specificities. Such changes may result in the v-Jun protein acting as a permanently "switched on" form of AP-1 that, when overexpressed in the context of retroviral infection, may lead to inappropriate gene expression and possibly to uncontrolled cell proliferation. Certainly, the wealth of information so rapidly gleaned from the work on v-*jun* indicates that the continued study of oncogenic retroviruses still has much to offer us in the way of insight into the genesis of neoplastic disease.

VIII. JUN AND FOS ASSOCIATE TO FORM A NUCLEOPROTEIN TRANSCRIPTION COMPLEX

Molecular biologists usually attach a great deal of significance to associations between important cellular components, since such interactions hold the promise of defining new pathways and merging different areas of study. Thus, the detection of associations between SV40 large T antigen and p53, polyomavirus middle T antigen and c-Src, and adenovirus E1A and the Rb protein have elicited much excitement, although the functional significance of these interactions is not always clear. The recent finding that the c-Fos and v-Fos proteins exist in a complex with the c-Jun/AP-1 transcription factor promises to reveal information both on oncogene function and on the regulation of transcription.

The uncovering of the interaction between Fos and Jun resulted from work involving what, at first glance, might seem to be a system rather remote from molecular oncogenesis: the differentiation of a preadipocyte cell line into adipocytes. Adipocyte differentiation is accompanied by the transcriptional activation of specific sets of genes achieved through shared regulatory sequences known as fat-specific elements (FSEs) upstream of the transcription initiation sites. One of these elements, a 21-bp region called FSE2, acts as a negative regulator of gene expression in preadipocytes. FSE2 contains an AP-1-binding motif and, not unexpectedly, associates with a protein complex that includes Jun. The surprising result was that antibodies against Fos were capable of specifically disrupting this complex (Distel et al. 1987; Rauscher et al. 1988a). Fos also associated with other consensus AP-1-binding sites, including primate retrovirus LTRs and the collagenase and metallothionein genes (Franza et al. 1988).

These findings highlighted important questions concerning the manner in which Fos and Jun might associate with the same DNA sequence motif. Since Fos possesses weak DNA-binding activity on its own, it seemed possible that Fos and Jun might either compete for, or bind cooperatively to, the AP-1 DNA site. An additional possibility is that Fos interacts with Jun and associates with DNA through direct binding of Jun to its consensus binding site. Several lines of evidence suggest that this latter mechanism is correct. First, Fos had long been known to be present in a complex with a protein of 39 kD, which recently has been demonstrated to be Jun (Chiu et al. 1988; Rauscher et al. 1988b; Sassone-Corsi et al. 1988a). Indeed, it appears that most cellular Fos is associated with Jun. In addition, Fos and Jun can form a complex in vitro after cell-free translation. Formation of the Fos–Jun complex appears to occur through the region in both proteins that is homologous to the DNA-binding domain of GCN4 (see Section VII) and that also comprises the "leucine zipper" (a structure postulated to mediate protein–protein interactions; see Section X). Jun itself is capable of forming a homodimer, whereas Fos apparently cannot (Halazonetis et al. 1988; Nakabeppu et al. 1988). Second, although Fos by itself does not bind to the AP-1 DNA sequence, the Jun-Fos heterodimer binds with high affinity and the Jun-Jun homodimer binds with relatively low affinity (Fig. 6) (Halazonetis et al. 1988; Kouzarides and Ziff 1988; Nakabeppu et al. 1988; Sassone-Corsi et al. 1988b). The formation and specific DNA binding of such Fos-Jun dimers is likely to be functional in vivo, since their presence correlates with increased transcription from promoters regulated by AP-1-binding sites (Chiu et al. 1988). However, binding of the Fos complex may not always result in transcriptional activation, since mounting evidence indicates that Fos can function as both an activator and a repressor (Schonthal et al. 1988; Wilson and Treisman 1988). In fact, a recent study has revealed that Fos/Jun appears to bind to a region of the c-*myc* promoter that negatively regulates c-*myc* gene transcription, raising the possibility that Fos may participate in the regulation of Myc expression (Hay et al. 1989). Indeed, the induction of Myc expression following the decrease in Fos levels during the "early response" to mitogen stimulation could perhaps be explained in terms of the alleviation of the negative regulatory effects of Fos on c-*myc* transcription.

The results of the binding experiments suggest a scenario in which the Jun-Fos complex would interact with the AP-1 DNA sequence motif primarily through the Jun DNA-binding domain. In such a complex, Fos may serve to modulate Jun binding to DNA or possibly to mediate interactions with other proteins in the transcription apparatus. In principle, there is the potential for enormous complexity in such a control system. Both c-*fos* and c-*jun* are members of gene families, and both the Fos and Jun proteins are highly modified by phosphorylation (Barber and Verma 1987; Cohen and Curran 1988; Nakabeppu et al. 1988). The multiple forms of these proteins and their relatives are rapidly induced by mitogens and must abound in proliferating cells. In addition, as discussed above (Section VII), expression of Jun may be autoregulated. This constellation of interacting protein forms might provide a gradient of affinities leading to the extraordinarily fine temporal regulation of sets and subsets of genes that has long been predicted to account for the flexibility and wide diversity of cellular responses to the environment. It is easy to imagine how overproduction and/or mutation of one of these key regulatory proteins could lock the control system into a single mode. A cell thus refractory to the

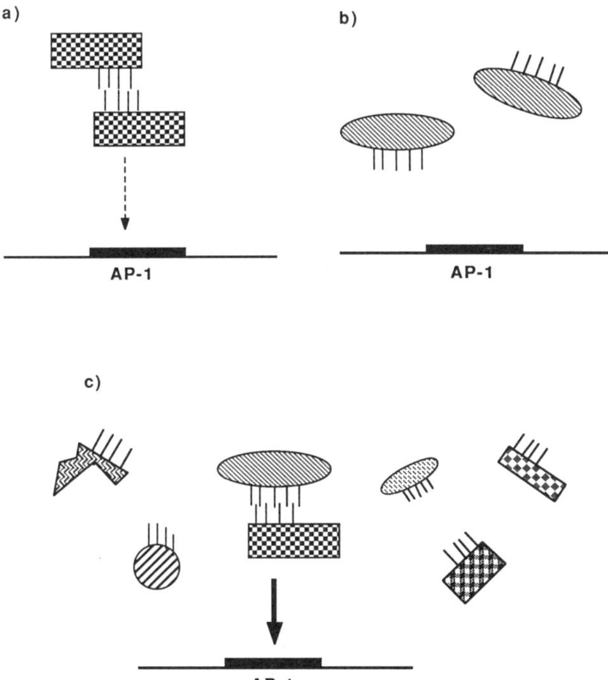

Figure 6 Dimerization involving Fos and Jun. The figure illustrates the types of interactions observed after cell-free translation of Fos and Jun. (*a*) Two molecules of Jun (rectangles) interact to form a dimer mediated by the periodic array of leucines known as a "leucine zipper" (indicated by the protruding spikes). This complex has detectable but weak affinity for binding to AP-1 sites on DNA. (*b*) Two molecules of Fos (ellipses) do not form stable dimers, although both proteins contain leucine zippers. No specific binding to AP-1 sites is observed. (*c*) Dimerization between Fos and Jun and significantly increased binding to AP-1 DNA are detected. The other structures in the figure represent Fos-related proteins (Fras) and Jun-related proteins (e.g., JunB and JunD). These and other proteins that contain zipper-like structures could potentially interact with each other, and subsequently with DNA, with different affinities. Changes in the active concentration of any of the components might lead to coordinate changes in the expression of genes linked to AP-1 control elements.

normal signals for growth arrest and differentiation would be well on the track to neoplasia.

IX. SKI, REL, AND ETS

The *ski*, *rel*, and *ets-2* genes have frequently been classified as nuclear oncogenes. For *ski* this is warranted, although the amount of information is limited. On the other hand, it is unclear whether *rel* actually functions in the nucleus and uncertain whether *ets-2* even directly participates in oncogenesis. In this section, I very briefly summarize recent information on these genes.

A. Ski

The Sloan-Kettering retroviruses (SKV) were originally isolated as transforming viruses present in a stock of avian leukosis virus (Stavnezer et al. 1981; for review, see Stavnezer 1988). A unique sequence present in the SKV genome, v-*ski*, was characterized as the SKV transforming gene and was shown to be a conserved cellular gene (c-*ski*) expressed in many tissues (Li et al. 1986; Stavnezer et al. 1986). The c-*ski* gene consists of at least seven exons, although exons 2 and 6 are subject to alternative splicing. The transduced v-*ski* contains 5′ and 3′ truncations that result in small amino-terminal and large carboxy-terminal deletions in the v-*ski*-encoded protein. c-*ski* can be oncogenically activated simply by overexpression of the exon-2-containing form of the *ski* mRNA, suggesting that the v-*ski* truncations are not critical (S. Hughes et al., pers. comm.).

Both v-Ski and c-Ski proteins are localized to the nucleus (Barkas et al. 1986; E. Stavnezer, pers. comm.). Infection of quail fibroblasts with v-*ski*-containing viruses results in an increase in the rate of proliferation (reminiscent of v-*myc* transformants) and in anchorage-independent growth. Surprisingly, a high percentage of the transformed cells terminally differentiate into cells having many of the characteristics of muscle cells. Thus, v-*ski* would appear to be unique among the oncogenes in its ability to induce a specific terminal differentiation. Preliminary evidence suggests that *ski* might activate, either directly or indirectly, muscle-specific gene expression (F. Stavnezer, pers. comm.).

B. Rel

The highly oncogenic reticuloendotheliosis virus strain T (REV-T) is an acute avian retrovirus that transforms lymphoid stem cells in vitro and in vivo but does not transform avian fibroblasts (Hoelzer et al. 1980; Gilmore and Temin 1986). In REV-T-transformed early lymphoid cells, the v-Rel protein is found in the cytoplasm, whereas in nonsusceptible, more differentiated, lymphoid cells and in nontransformed fibroblasts, v-Rel is localized predominantly in the nucleus (Gilmore and Temin 1986). The differences in subcellular localization that were apparently dependent on cell differentiation stage are reminiscent of the shift from nucleus to cytoplasm of v-Myb following induction of myeloid differentiation (Klempnauer et al. 1984; see Section III). Perhaps more importantly, the data suggested that only cytoplasmically localized v-Rel could transform cells.

Further study revealed that the v-Rel protein contains a region responsible for efficient nuclear transport and retention (Gilmore and Temin

1988). Removal of the nuclear localization signal altered neither the transforming activity nor the transformation-target-specificity of v-Rel. Furthermore, if v-Rel was forced into the nucleus of lymphoid cells by inserting an SV40 large T antigen nuclear localization signal into the v-*rel* coding sequence, it was still capable of fully inducing transformation. Thus, v-Rel localized to either nucleus or cytoplasm is capable of transforming lymphoid cells (Gilmore and Temin 1988).

The c-Rel protein has also been identified and localized to the cytoplasm of lymphoid cells. In contrast to v-Rel, which has an intrinsic or associated kinase activity, c-Rel is not phosphorylated (Walro et al. 1987; Simek and Rice 1988a). Recent evidence indicates that v-Rel can serve as a transcriptional *trans*-activator or repressor in a promoter-dependent and cell-type-dependent manner (Gelinas and Temin 1988). As is the case for Myc, it is uncertain whether the oncoprotein is directly interacting with promoter regulatory elements or whether the effect is indirect. In fact, v-Rel has been found to be stably complexed with several host cell proteins (Simek and Rice 1988b).

C. Ets

The avian acute leukemia virus E26 contains two oncogenes, v-*myb* and v-*ets*, which are expressed together as a large fusion protein predominantly localized in the nucleus (Klempnauer et al. 1984). The v-*ets* region permits E26 to transform erythroid cells and also influences its myeloid transformation (Golay et al. 1988). In chickens, c-*ets* exists at a single locus and encodes a protein that is cytoplasmic but probably also resides in the nucleus (Ghysdael et al. 1986; Fujiwara et al. 1988). In humans, however, v-*ets* sequences are divided into two separate nonlinked loci: c-*ets-1* and c-*ets-2*. Whereas the c-Ets-1 protein is cytoplasmic, c-Ets-2 (which corresponds to the 3′ region of v-Ets) is nuclear (Fujiwara et al. 1988). Expression of c-*ets-2* has been detected in many cell types, and its induction during hepatic regeneration and after treatment with protein synthesis inhibitors is reminiscent of the "early response" nuclear oncogenes (Bhat et al. 1987). However, *ets-2* has not been directly demonstrated to act as an oncogene. Nonetheless, it is likely to be of continued interest, since *ets-2* resides at a chromosomal locus (22q22.3) found to be translocated in some human leukemias and implicated in Down's syndrome.

X. STRUCTURAL AND FUNCTIONAL RELATIONSHIPS AMONG NUCLEAR ONCOPROTEINS

A priori, there would seem to be scant reason to expect nuclear oncoproteins to possess common characteristics aside from their gross localization. Nonetheless, various members of this group do share certain features, and some of these are worth considering in the context of what is known about nuclear oncogene function.

A. Sequence Relationships

Although certain limited structural motifs may be shared, there is little or no overall sequence homology between the nuclear oncoproteins. In other words, they are clearly not members of the same family. However, *myc*, *fos*, *erbA*, and *jun* are each representatives of larger gene families, each of whose members are related in terms of structure and, frequently, pattern of expression (summarized in Table 1). It seems likely that the members of each family are also functionally related, although probably not functionally redundant. The related family members might be expected to mediate either diverse responses to the same signal or a common response to different signals. The former probably applies to the different ErbA/thyroid hormone receptors expressed in a tissue-specific manner, whereas the latter might be exemplified by the *myc* family members. Recently, two distinct mRNAs containing regions highly related to human c-*myb* have been isolated (Nomura et al. 1988). *p53* does not appear to belong to a larger gene family.

All of the nuclear oncogenes, and indeed all of the proto-oncogenes, are highly conserved throughout vertebrate evolution. In some cases, the evolutionary conservation runs even deeper: The DNA-binding portions of *myb* and *jun* are preserved as domains in *Drosophila* and yeast proteins, respectively, and the nuclear oncogene *rel* is homologous to the *Drosophila* gene *dorsal*, a determinant of embryonic polarity (Peters et al. 1987; Struhl 1987; Steward 1987). There are also potential structural similarities between domains in *myc* family genes and genes critical for *Drosophila* embryogenesis (see Section X.B). Evolutionary conservation is often taken as an indication of a fundamental functional importance, consistent with the idea that these are key regulatory genes.

B. Structural Relationships: Fingers, Zippers, and Blobs

1. DNA Binding

Myc, Myb, Fos, ErbA, and Jun all have affinity for DNA (Table 1). For ErbA, Myb, and Jun, specific binding to DNA regulatory elements is clearly consonant with their functions as transcriptional activator proteins. Fos, although possessing homology with the AP-1-binding domain, does not directly bind the AP-1 DNA regulatory element (Halazonetis et al. 1988) and appears to act through protein–protein association. However, this does not necessarily mean that the weak affinity of Fos for DNA is irrelevant, since it may serve to bring Fos into the vicinity of chromatin (Renz et al. 1987), which would increase its chances of encountering Jun and forming a specific complex, or it might interact with DNA only when part of a Fos/Jun heterodimer. For Myc and Myb, it is not clear what role, if any, DNA binding might play. The Myb DNA-binding domain is well defined, highly conserved, and essential for v-*myb*-mediated transformation (Ibanez and Lipsick 1988) and for Myb transcriptional activity (Weston and Bishop 1989; Sakura et al. 1989).

Given that all of the nuclear oncoproteins, with the possible exception of p53, bind DNA, it is reasonable to ask whether they bind through a similar structural motif. They apparently do not. The DNA-binding domain of ErbA, like that of the other hormone receptors, is composed of DNA-binding fingers formed through chelation with zinc ions (see Evans and Hollenberg 1988). However, the DNA-binding regions of Myb and Jun do not appear to correspond to either the finger or the helical motifs previously thought to mediate protein–DNA interactions. Recently, a potential helix-loop-helix structure has been noted as a structural feature common to Myc, MyoD, immunoglobulin enhancer-binding proteins, and two critical genes in *Drosophila*: *achaete-scute*, which is involved in neuronal differentiation, and *daughterless*, which is essential for both neurogenesis and sex determination (Davis et al. 1987; Villares and Cabrera 1987; Caudy et al. 1988; Kouzarides and Ziff 1988; Murre et al. 1989). Since this region appears to govern dimerization and DNA binding for the enhancer-binding proteins, it may well serve a similar function for Myc and the others (Kouzarides and Ziff 1988; Murre et al. 1989).

2. Protein–Protein Interactions

It is well known that many enzymes and regulatory proteins function as dimers or as higher-order multimeric complexes. For DNA-binding proteins, the frequent requirement for formation of a symmetrical homodimeric subunit structure is thought to reflect the twofold symmetry of many DNA regulatory elements (e.g., the c-*fos* upstream DSE and the GCN4/Jun/AP-1 DNA-binding sites, both discussed above; for review, see Schleif 1988).

That nuclear oncoproteins can also act as subunits was clearly demonstrated by identification of the Fos-Jun complex. We have also discussed the potential importance of complex formation on the metabolism of p53. At present, it is not certain how prevalent complex formation is among the nuclear oncoproteins or which region(s) of the protein are involved in protein–protein interactions. Nevertheless, a provocative sequence motif, the leucine zipper, has recently been recognized in several transcriptional activator proteins and nuclear oncoproteins (Landschulz et al. 1988). The zipper is composed of an α-helical region of 20–30 amino acids with a leucine residue situated at every other helical turn. The resulting structure is predicted to be a "spine" of leucines with their extended hydrophobic side chains projecting from one face of the helix. Two proteins, each possessing the zipper structure, probably associate with each other by forming a dimer of parallel α helices in a coiled coil (O'Shea et al. 1989a). Leucine zipper sequence motifs have been found in GCN4 and a CAAT/

enhancer-binding protein as well as in c-Myc, N-Myc, L-Myc, Fos, and Jun. Recent evidence indicates that the zipper region is important for at least Fos-Jun association (Halazonetis et al. 1988; Kouzarides and Ziff 1988; Sassone-Corsi et al. 1988b). However, c-Myc, although possessing the zipper motif, does not associate with either Fos or Jun (Kouzarides and Ziff 1988), but the Myc zipper can apparently mediate formation of Myc homo-oligomers (Dang et al. 1989). These results suggest that zipper interactions can possess unique specificities. Indeed, studies using synthetic peptides have demonstrated that isolated zipper regions themselves are sufficient to determine the specificity of their interactions (O'Shea et al. 1989b).

3. Anionic Regions

Myc, Fos, Myb, and Jun all possess internal clusters of acidic amino acids. These so-called "acid blobs" have been found in some transcriptional activator proteins in yeast and larger eukaryotes, where they are thought to participate in the formation of transcription initiation complexes through hydrogen bonding with the highly extended hydrophilic carboxy-terminal "tail" of RNA polymerase II (for review, see Sigler 1988). Although it is far from certain that the anionic regions in Myc, Fos, and Myb also act in this manner, there is evidence that a region of Fos (and, to a much lesser extent, Myc) containing the acidic domain can promote transcription in yeast when fused to an appropriate DNA-binding region (Lech et al. 1988). The acidic regions also appear to serve as sites for phosphorylation by kinases (Lüscher et al. 1989). Such modifications might serve to regulate the degree of interaction with polymerase or other transcription factors. Point mutations within, or deletion of, the acid blobs affect the transforming potential of v-*myc* and v-*fos*, strengthening the possibility that these regions have functional importance.

4. Protein Half-lives

A common characteristic of Myc, Myb, Fos, and p53 is their rapid rate of degradation. Myc and p53 have half-lives of between 20 and 45 minutes, among the most rapidly degraded proteins known in higher eukaryotes, whereas Myb and Fos are degraded more slowly, but still very rapidly compared to most cellular proteins (Reich et al. 1983; Curran et al. 1984; Klempnauer et al. 1986; Lüscher and Eisenman 1988). In contrast, Jun and ErbA are stable. As described above, the stabilization of p53 occurs through protein–protein interaction and may play a role in p53-mediated oncogenesis. Rapid degradation probably reflects the tight control required for regulatory proteins. Increased stability of Myc has been reported in erythroleukemia differentiation in vitro (Wingrove et al. 1988) but has not been observed in many other situations and is unlikely to be generally important for Myc regulation. On the other hand, oncogenic activation of Fos results in increased stability and decreased phosphorylation, probably due to substitutions of the serine-rich carboxy-terminal region of c-Fos (Curran et al. 1984; Barber and Verma 1987). The stable Fos may tie up associated transcription factors in an inactive complex and prevent down-regulation of expression of c-*fos* and other genes (Wilson and Treisman 1988). Clearly, more needs to be learned about the relationship of oncoprotein turnover to function. Acidic regions as well as repeats of prolines, serines, and threonines common in Myc, Myb, and Fos have been suggested as possible targets for proteases (Rogers et al. 1986).

C. A Common Function for Nuclear Oncoproteins?

At this juncture, it is tempting to think of most of the nuclear oncoproteins as being involved in the regulation of transcription. ErbA, as a hormone receptor, is almost certainly involved in transcriptional activation. The rapidly accruing evidence on the relationship between the transcriptional activator AP-1 and Jun, on the association between Jun and Fos, and on Myb as a transcriptional activator brings three other oncoproteins into the circle. Finally, the constellation of structural and physiological similarities between Fos and the Myc family makes it difficult to avoid thinking of Myc in much the same way. Indeed, it seems possible that many nuclear oncoproteins might function as transducers of cytoplasmic and membrane-derived signals to specific nuclear targets. Nonetheless, simply because the nuclear oncoproteins are so diverse in terms of their structures and properties it is likely that, no matter what their generic function as transcriptional regulators, they will actually carry out their regulatory roles, and be themselves regulated, in quite different and unique ways. The plurality of DNA and protein interaction motifs, the presence of phosphorylation and other posttranslational modifications, and the fact that some transcription factors are also involved in DNA replication (for review, see DePamphilis 1988) all demonstrate that there is a great deal of functional heterogeneity even among the known transcription factors.

Another reason to avoid lumping most of the nuclear oncoproteins together simply stems from our ignorance concerning the structure and function of the nucleus. Although at one time it may have been sufficient to consider the nucleus as little more than a sack within which DNA and enzymes serenely floated, a great deal of recent research has made this view no longer tenable. Biochemical and microscopic analyses have revealed the presence of peripheral and internal structure as well as the preferential positioning of chromosomes (Agard and Sedat 1983; Mathog et al. 1984; Cook and Laskey 1985; Hutchison and Weintraub 1985). At least some of the arcane processes involved in mitosis, such as chromosome condensation and nuclear envelope disassembly and reassembly, can now be recreated in vitro using partially purified components (for review, see

Fisher 1987). Furthermore, the powerful tools of yeast genetics have defined a group of genes that act to control the cell cycle (for review, see Pringle and Hartwell 1981). Some of these encode protein kinases, which appear to act in a cascade to drive cells through mitosis and are functionally homologous in lower and higher eukaryotes (Dunphy et al. 1988; Gautier et al. 1988; for review, see Dunphy and Newport 1988). All of these studies point to a great deal of order underlying the organization and functions of the nucleus. Since transcription and replication occur within this structural context, it would not be surprising if the functions of both known and as yet undiscovered nuclear oncoproteins somehow impinged on the higher-order structure of the nucleus. Perhaps nuclear oncoproteins will teach us not only about signal transduction, transcription, and DNA replication, but also about the role of nuclear structure in integrating these events with other cellular processes.

ACKNOWLEDGMENTS

I am grateful to T. Curran, E. Harlow, P. Neiman, J. Roberts, P. Vogt, and V. Vogt for readings of the manuscript and to C. Finlay, A.J. Levine, N. Rice, G. Shen-Ong, E. Stavnezer, and I. Verma for advice and information. I also wish to thank the members of my laboratory for their critical comments on the manuscript and to thank J. Smith for secretarial assistance. This chapter is dedicated to my father, Sheldon M. Eisenman.

REFERENCES

Adams, J.M., A.W. Harris, C.A. Pinkert, L.M. Corcoran, W.S. Alexander, S. Cory, R.D. Palmiter, and R.L. Brinster. 1985. The c-*myc* oncogene driven by immunoglobin enhancers induces lymphoid malignancy in transgenic mice. *Nature* **318:** 533–538.

Agard, D. and J. Sedat. 1983. Three dimensional architecture of a polytene nucleus. *Nature* **302:** 676–681.

Alitalo, K. and M. Schwab. 1985. Oncogene amplification in tumor cells. A review. *Adv. Cancer Res.* **47:** 235–281.

Angel, P., K. Hattori, T. Smeal, and M. Karin. 1988a. The jun proto-oncogene is positively autoregulated by its product, Jun/AP-1. *Cell* **55:** 875–885.

Angel, P., E.A. Allegretto, S.T. Okino, K. Hattori, W.J. Boyle, T. Hunter, and M. Karin. 1988b. Oncogene *jun* encodes a sequence-specific *trans*-activator similar to AP-1. *Nature* **332:** 166–171.

Angel, P., M. Imagawa, R. Chiu, B. Stein, R.J. Imbra, H.J. Rahmsdorf, C. Jonat, P. Herrlich, and M. Karin. 1987. Phorbol ester-inducible genes contain a common *cis* element recognized by a TPA-modulated *trans*-acting factor. *Cell* **49:** 729–739.

Armelin, H.A., M.C.S. Armelin, K. Kelly, T. Stewart, P. Leder, B.H. Cochran, and C.D. Stiles. 1984. Functional role for c-*myc* in mitogenic response to platelet-derived growth factor. *Nature* **310:** 655–660.

Barber, J.R. and I.M. Verma. 1987. Modification of *fos* proteins: Phosphorylation of v-*fos* but not c-*fos*, is stimulated by 12-tetradecanoyl-phorbol-13-acetate and serum. *Mol. Cell. Biol.* **7:** 2201–2211.

Barkas, A.E., D. Brodeur, and E. Stavnezer. 1986. Polyproteins containing a domain encoded by the v-*ski* oncogene are located in the nuclei of SKV-transformed cells. *Virology* **151:** 131–138.

Bentley, D.L. and M. Groudine. 1986. A block to elongation is largely responsible for decreased transcription of c-*myc* in differentiated HL60 cells. *Nature* **321:** 702–706.

Beug, H., P.A. Blundell, and T. Graf. 1987. Reversibility of differentiation and proliferative capacity in avian myelomonocytic cells transformed by tsE26 leukemia virus. *Genes Dev.* **1:** 277–286.

Beug, H., M. Claviez, B.M. Jockusch, and T. Graf. 1978. Differential expression of Rous sarcoma virus-specific transformation parameters in enucleated cells. *Cell* **14:** 843–856.

Bhat, N.K., R.J. Fisher, S. Fujiwara, R. Ascione, and T.S. Papas. 1987. Temporal and tissue-specific expression of mouse *ets* genes. *Proc. Natl. Acad. Sci.* **84:** 3161–3165.

Biedenkapp, H., U. Borgmeyer, A.E. Sippel, and K.-H. Klempnauer. 1988. Viral *myb* oncogene encodes a sequence-specific DNA binding activity. *Nature* **335:** 835–837.

Bister, K. and H.W. Jansen. 1986. Oncogenes in retroviruses and cells: Biochemistry and molecular genetics. *Adv. Cancer Res.* **47:** 99–188.

Blanchard, J.-M., M. Piechaczyk, C. Dani, J.-C. Chambard, A. Franchi, J. Pouyssegur, and P. Jeanteur. 1985. c-*myc* gene is transcribed at high rate in Go-arrested fibroblasts and is post-transcriptionally regulated in response to growth factors. *Nature* **317:** 335–443.

Bohmann, D., T.J. Bos, A. Admon, T. Nishimura, P.K. Vogt, and R. Tjian. 1987. Human proto-oncogene c-*jun* encodes a DNA binding protein with structural and functional properties of transcription factor AP-1. *Science* **238:** 1386–1392.

Boucher, P., A. Koning, and M.L. Privalsky. 1988. The avian erythroblastosis virus *erbA* oncogene encodes a DNA-binding protein exhibiting distinct nuclear and cytoplasmic subcellular localizations. *J. Virol.* **62:** 534–544.

Braithwaite, A.W., H.-W. Sturzbecher, C. Addison, C. Palmer, K. Rudge, and J.R. Jenkins. 1987. Mouse p53 inhibits SV40 origin-dependent DNA replication. *Nature* **329:** 458–460.

Brodeur, G.M., R.C. Seeger, M. Schwab, and H.E. Varmus. 1984. Amplification of N-*myc* in untreated human neuroblastoma correlates with advanced disease stage. *Science* **224:** 1121–1124.

Caudy, M., H. Vassin, M. Brand, R. Yuma, L.Y. Jan, and Y.N. Jan. 1988. *daughterless*, a Drosophila gene essential for both neurogenesis and sex determination, has sequence similarities to *myc* and the *achaete-scute* complex. *Cell* **55:** 1061–1067.

Cesarman, E., R. Dalla-Favera, D. Bentley, and M. Groudine. 1987. Consistent mutations in a region of the first exon are associated with altered transcription of the c-*myc* oncogene in Burkitt lymphoma. *Science* **238:** 1272–1275.

Chiu, R., W.J. Boyle, J. Meek, T. Smeal, T. Hunter, and M. Karin. 1988. The c-*fos* protein interacts with c-Jun/AP-1 to stimulate transcription of AP-1 responsive genes. *Cell* **54:** 541–552.

Clarke, M.F., J.F. Kukowska-Latello, E. Westin, M. Smith, and E.V. Prochownik. 1988. Constitutive expression of a c-*myb* cDNA blocks Friend murine erythroleukemia cell differentiation. *Mol. Cell. Biol.* **8:** 884–892.

Classon, M., M. Henriksson, J. Sumegi, G. Klein, and M.-L. Hammarskjold. 1987. Elevated c-*myc* expression facilitates the replication of SV40 DNA in human lymphoma cells. *Nature* **330:** 272–274.

Cohen, D.R. and T. Curran. 1988. *fra*-1: A serum-inducible, cellular immediate-early gene that encodes a *fos*-related antigen. *Mol. Cell. Biol.* **8:** 2063–2069.

Cole, M.D. 1986. The *myc* oncogene: Its role in transformation and differentiation. *Annu. Rev. Genet.* **20:** 361–384.

Compere, S.J., P. Baldacci, and R. Jaenisch. 1988. Oncogenes in transgenic mice. *Biochim. Biophys. Acta.* **948:** 129–149.

Cook, P.R. and R.A. Laskey, eds. 1984. *Higher order structure in the nucleus.* The Company of Biologists Ltd., Cambridge, England.

Coppola, J.A. and M.D. Cole. 1986. Constitutive c-*myc* oncogene expression blocks mouse erythroleukemia cell differentiation but not commitment. *Nature* **320:** 760–763.

Cory, S. 1986. Activation of cellular oncogenes in hematopoietic cells by chromosome translocation. *Adv. Cancer Res.* **47:** 189–234.

Coughlin, S.R., W.M.F. Lee, P.W. Williams, G.M. Giels, and L.T. Williams. 1985. c-*myc* gene expression is stimulated by agents that activate protein kinase C and does not account for the mitogenic effect of PDGF. *Cell* **43:** 243–251.

Crawford, L.V., D.C. Pim, E.G. Gurney, P. Goodfellow, and J. Taylor-Papadimitriou. 1981. Detection of a common feature in several human tumor cell lines—a 53,000 dalton protein. *Proc. Natl. Acad. Sci.* **78:** 41–45.

Curran, T. 1988. *fos*. In *The oncogene handbook* (ed. E.P. Reddy et al.), pp. 307–326. Elsevier Science Publisher, The Netherlands.

Curran, T., A.D. Miller, L. Zokas, and I.M. Verma. 1984. Viral and cellular *fos* proteins: A comparative analysis. *Cell* **36:** 259–268.

Damm, K., C.C. Thompson, and R.M. Evans. 1989. Protein encoded by v-erbA functions as a thyroid hormone receptor antagonist. *Nature* **339:** 593–597.

Damm, K., H. Beug, T. Graf, and B. Vennstrom. 1987. A single point mutation in *erb*A restores the erythroid transforming potential of a mutant avian erythroblastosis virus (AEV) defective in both *erb*A and *erb*B oncogenes. *EMBO J.* **6:** 375–382.

Dang, C.V., M. McGuire, M. Buckmire, and W.M.F. Lee. 1989. Involvement of the "leucine zipper" region in the oligomerization and transforming activity of human c-*myc* protein. *Nature* **337**: 664–666.

Dani, C., N. Mechti, M. Piechaczyk, B. Lebleu, P. Jeanteur, and J.M. Blanchard. 1985. Increased rate of degradation of c-*myc* mRNA in interferon-treated Daudi cells. *Proc. Natl. Acad. Sci.* **82:** 4896–4899.

Davis, R.L., H. Weintraub, and A.B. Lassar. 1987. Expression of a single transfected cDNA converts fibroblasts to myoblasts. *Cell* **51:** 987–1000.

DePamphilis, M.L. 1988. Transcriptional elements as components of eukaryotic origins of DNA replication. *Cell* **52:** 635–638.

DePinho, R.A., K.S. Hatton, A. Tesfaye, G.D. Yancopoulos, and F.W. Alt. 1987a. The human myc gene family: Structure and activity of L-*myc* and an L-*myc* pseudogene. *Genes Dev.* **1:** 1311–1326.

DePinho, R., L. Mitsock, K. Hatton, P. Ferrier, K. Zimmerman, E. Legouy, A. Tesfaye, R. Collum, G. Yancopoulos, P. Nisen, R. Kriz, and F. Alt. 1987b. Myc family of cellular oncogenes. *J. Cell. Biochem.* **33:** 257–266.

Dippold, W.G., G. Jay, A.B. DeLeo, G. Khoury, and L.J. Old. 1981. p53 transformation-related protein: Detection by monoclonal antibody in mouse and human cells. *Proc. Natl. Acad. Sci.* **78:** 1695–1699.

Distel, R.J., H.-S. Ro, B.S. Rosen, D.L. Groves, and B.M. Spiegelman. 1987. Nucleoprotein complexes that regulate gene expression in adipocyte differentiation: Direct participation of c-*fos*. *Cell* **49:** 835–844.

Dony, C., M. Kessel, and P. Gruss. 1985. Post-transcriptional control of *myc* and p53 expression during differentiation of the embryonal carcinoma cell line F9. *Nature* **317:** 636–639.

Dotto, G.P., M.Z. Gilman, M. Maruyama, and R.A. Weinberg. 1986. c-*myc* and c-*fos* expression in differentiating mouse primary keratinocytes. *EMBO J.* **5:** 2853–2857.

Dunphy, W.G. and J.W. Newport. 1988. Unraveling of mitotic control mechanisms. *Cell* **55:** 925–928.

Dunphy, W.G., L. Brizuela, D. Beach, and J. Newport. 1988. The *Xenopus* homolog of cdc2 is a component of MPF, a cytoplasmic regulator of mitosis. *Cell* **54:** 423–431.

Eisenman, R.N. and C.B. Thompson. 1986. Oncogenes with potential nuclear function: *myc*, *myb* and *fos*. *Cancer Surv.* **5:** 309–327.

Eisenman, R.N., C.Y. Tachibana, H.D.Abrams, and S.R. Hann. 1985. v-*myc*- and c-*myc*-encoded proteins are associated with the nuclear matrix. *Mol. Cell. Biol.* **5:** 114–126.

Endo, T. and B. Nadal-Ginard. 1986. Transcriptional and posttranscriptional control of c-*myc* during myogenesis: Its mRNA remains inducible in differentiated cells and does not suppress the differentiated phenotype. *Mol. Cell. Biol.* **6:** 1412–1421.

Evans, R.M. 1988. The steroid and thyroid hormone receptor superfamily. *Science* **240:** 889–895.

Evans, R.M. and S.M. Hollenberg. 1988. Zinc fingers: Gilt by association. *Cell* **52:** 1–4.

Finlay, C.A., P.W. Hinds, and A.J. Levine. 1989. The p53 proto-oncogene can act as a suppressor of transformation. *Cell* **57:** 1083–1093.

Finlay, C.A., P.W. Hinds, T.-H. Tan, D. Eliyahu, M. Oren, and A.J. Levine. 1988. Activating mutations for transformation by p53 produce a gene product that forms an hsc70-p53 complex with an altered half-life. *Mol. Cell. Biol.* **8:** 531–539.

Fisher, P.A. 1987. Disassembly and reassembly of nuclei in cell-free systems. *Cell* **48:** 175–176.

Franza, R.B., F.R. Rauscher III, S.F. Josephs, and T. Curran. 1988. The Fos complex and Fos-related antigens recognize sequence elements that contain AP-1 binding sites. *Science* **239:** 1150–1153.

Freedman, L.P., B.F. Luisi, Z.R. Korszun, R. Basavappa, P.B. Sigler, and K.R. Yamamoto. 1988. The function and structure of the metal coordination sites within the glucocorticoid receptor DNA binding domain. *Nature* **334:** 543–546.

Frykberg, L., S. Palmieri, H. Beug, T. Graf, M.J. Hayman, and B. Vennstrom. 1983. Transforming capacities of avian erythroblastosis virus mutants deleted in the *erb*A and *erb*B oncogenes. *Cell* **32:** 227–238.

Fujiwara, S., R.J. Fisher, A. Seth, N.K. Bhat, S.D. Showalter, M. Zweig, and T.S. Papas. 1988. Characterization and localization of the products of the human homologs of the v-*ets* oncogene. *Oncogene* **2:** 99–103.

Gannon, J.V. and D.P. Lane. 1987. p53 and DNA polymerase alpha compete for binding to SV40 T antigen. *Nature* **329:** 456–458.

Gautier, J., C. Norbury, M. Lohka, P. Nurse, and J. Maller. 1988. Purified maturation-promoting factor contains the product of a *Xenopus* homolog of the fission yeast cell cycle control gene cdc2$^+$. *Cell* **54:** 433–439.

Gelinas, C. and H.M. Temin. 1988. The v-*rel* oncogene encodes a cell-specific transcriptional activator of certain promoters. *Oncogene* **3:** 349–355.

Ghysdael, J., A. Gegonne, P. Pognonec, D. Dernis, D. Leprince, and D. Stehelin. 1986. Identification and preferential expression in thymic and bursal lymphocytes of a c-*ets* oncogene encoded M_r 54,000 cytoplasmic protein. *Proc. Natl. Acad. Sci.* **83:** 1714–1718.

Gilman, M.Z., R.N. Wilson, and R.A. Weinberg. 1986. Multiple protein binding sites in the 5′-flanking region regulate c-*fos* expression. *Mol. Cell. Biol.* **6:** 4305–4316.

Gilmore, T.D. and H.M. Temin. 1986. Different localization of the product of the v-*rel* oncogene in chicken fibroblasts and spleen cells correlates with transformation by REV-T. *Cell* **44:** 791–800.

———. 1988. v-*rel* oncoproteins in the nucleus and in the cytoplasm transform chicken spleen cells. *J. Virol.* **62:** 703–714.

Glass, C.K., R. Franco, C. Weinberger, V.R. Albert, R.M. Evans, and M.G. Rosenfeld. 1987. A c-*erb*A binding site in rat growth hormone gene mediates *trans*-activation by thyroid hormone. *Nature* **329:** 738–741.

Godowski, P.J., S. Rusconi, R. Miesfield, and K.R. Yamamoto. 1987. Glucocorticoid receptor mutants that are constitutive activators of transcriptional enhancement. *Nature* **325:** 365–368.

Golay, J., M. Introna, and T. Graf. 1988. A single point mutation in the v-*ets* oncogene affects both erythroid and myelomonocytic cell differentiation. *Cell* **55:** 1147–1158.

Gonda, T.J., D.K. Sheiness, and J.M. Bishop. 1982. Transcripts from the cellular homologs of retroviral oncogenes: Distribution among chicken tissues. *Mol. Cell. Biol.* **2:** 617–624.

Greenberg, M.E. and E.B. Ziff. 1984. Stimulation of 3T3 cells induces transcription of the c-*fos* proto-oncogene. *Nature* **311:** 433–438.

Greenberg, M.E., A.L. Hermanowski, and E.B. Ziff. 1986. Effect of protein synthesis inhibitors on growth factor activation of c-*fos*, c-*myc*, and actin gene transcription. *Mol. Cell. Biol.* **6:** 1050–1057.

Halazonetis, T.D., K. Georgopoulos, M.E. Greenberg, and P. Leder. 1988. c-*Jun* dimerizes with itself and with c-Fos, forming complexes of different DNA binding affinities. *Cell* **55:** 917–924.

Hann, S.R., C.B. Thompson, and R.N. Eisenman. 1985. c-*myc* oncogene protein synthesis is independent of the cell cycle in human and avian cells. *Nature* **314:** 366–369.

Hann, S.R., M.W. King, D.L. Bentley, C.W. Anderson, and R.N. Eisenman. 1988. A non-AUG translational initiation in c-*myc* exon 1 generates an N-terminally distinct protein whose synthesis is disrupted in Burkitt's lymphomas. *Cell* **52:** 185–195.

Hay, N., J.M. Bishop, and D. Levens. 1987. Regulatory elements that modulate expression of human c-*myc*. *Genes Dev.* **1:** 659–671.

Hay, N., M. Takimoto, and J.M. Bishop. 1989. A fos protein is present in a complex that binds a negative regulator of myc. *Genes Dev.* **3:** 293–303.

Hayward, W.S., B.G. Neel, and S.M. Astrin. 1982. Avian leukosis viruses: Activation of cellular "oncogenes." *Adv. Viral Oncol.* **1:** 207–233.

Heikkila, R., G. Schwab, E. Wickstrom, S.L. Loke, D.H. Pluznik, R. Watt, and L.M. Neckers. 1987. A c-*myc* antisense oligodeoxynucleotide inhibits entry into S phase but not progress from Go to G1. *Nature* **328:** 445–449.

Hinds, P.W., C.A. Finlay, A.B. Frey, and A.J. Levine. 1987. Immunological evidence for the association of p53 with a heat-shock protein, hsc70, in p53-plus-ras-transformed cell lines. *Mol. Cell. Biol.* **7:** 2863–2869.

Hoelzer, J.D., R.B. Lewis, C.R. Wasmuth, and H.R. Bose. 1980. Hematopoietic cell transformation by reticuloendotheliosis virus: Characterization of the genetic defect. *Virology* **100:** 462–474.

Hollenberg, S.M., V. Giguere, P. Segui, and R.M. Evans. 1987. Colocalization of DNA binding and transcriptional activation functions of the human glucocorticoid receptor. *Cell* **49:** 39–46.

Holt, J.T., R.L. Redner, and A.W. Nienhuis. 1988. An oligomer complementary to c-*myc* mRNA inhibits proliferation of HL60 promyelocytic cells and induces differentiation. *Mol. Cell. Biol.* **8:** 963–973.

Holt, J.T., T.V. Gopal, A.D. Moulton, and A.W. Nienhuis. 1986. Inducible production of c-*fos* antisense RNA inhibits 3T3 cell proliferation. *Proc. Natl. Acad. Sci.* **83:** 4794–4798.

Hope, I.A. and K. Struhl. 1985. GCN4 protein, synthesized in vitro, binds HIS3 regulatory sequences: Implications for general control of amino acid biosynthetic genes in yeast. *Cell* **43:** 177–188.

———. 1986. Functional dissection of a eukaryotic transcriptional activator protein, GCN4 of yeast. *Cell* **46:** 885–894.

Hutchison, N. and H. Weintraub. 1985. Localization of DNase I-sensitive sequences to specific regions of interphase nuclei. *Cell* **43:** 471–482.

Ibanez, C.E. and J.S. Lipsick. 1988. Structural and functional domains of the *myb* oncogene: Requirements for nuclear transport, myeloid transformation, and colony formation. *J. Virol.* **62:** 1981–1988.

Iguchi-Ariga, S.M.M., T. Okazaki, T. Itani, M. Ogata, Y. Sato, and H. Ariga. 1988. An initiation site of DNA replication with transcriptional enhancer activity present upstream of the c-*myc* gene. *EMBO J.* **7:** 3135–3142.

Jenkins, J.R., K. Rudge, and G.A. Currie. 1984. Cellular immortalization by a cDNA clone encoding the transformation-associated phosphoprotein p53. *Nature* **312:** 651–653.

Kaddurah-Daouk, R., J.M. Greene, A.S. Baldwin, and R.E. Kingston. 1987. Activation and repression of mammalian gene expression by the c-*myc* protein. *Genes Dev.* **1:** 347–357.

Kahn, P., L. Frykberg, C. Brady, I. Stanley, H. Beug, B. Vennstrom, and T. Graf. 1986. v-*erb*A cooperates with sarcoma oncogenes in leukemic cell transformation. *Cell* **45:** 349–356.

Kelly, K., B.H. Cochran, C.D. Stiles, and P. Leder. 1983. Cell-specific regulation of the c-myc gene by lymphocyte mitogens and platelet-derived growth factor. *Cell* **35:** 603–610.

Klempnauer, K.-H. and A.E. Sippel. 1987. The highly conserved amino-terminal region of the protein encoded by the v-*myb* oncogene functions as a DNA binding domain. *EMBO J.* **6:** 2715–2719.

Klempnauer, K.-H., C. Bonifer, and A. Sippel. 1986. Identification and characterization of the protein encoded by the human c-*myb* proto-oncogene. *EMBO J.* **5:** 1903–1911.

Klempnauer, K., G. Symonds, G. Evan, and J.M. Bishop. 1984. Subcellular localization of proteins encoded by oncogenes of avian myeloblastosis virus and avian leukemia virus E26 and by the chicken c-*myb* gene. *Cell* **37:** 537–547.

Kouzarides, T. and E. Ziff. 1988. The role of the "leucine zipper" in the *fos-jun* interaction. *Nature* **336:** 646–651.

Krystal, G., M. Birrer, J. Way, M. Nau, E. Sausville, C. Thompson, J. Minna, and J. Battey. 1988. Multiple mechanisms for transcriptional regulation of the *myc* gene family in small-cell cancer. *Mol. Cell. Biol.* **8:** 3373–3381.

Lachman, H.M. and A.I. Skoultchi. 1984. Expression of c-*myc* changes during differentiation of mouse erythroleukemia cells. *Nature* **310:** 592–594.

Lamph, W., W. Wamsley, P. Sassone-Corsi, and I.M. Verma. 1988. Induction of proto-oncogene JUN/AP-1 by serum and TPA. *Nature* **332:** 629–631.

Land, H., L.F. Parada, and R.A. Weinberg. 1983. Tumorigenic conversion of primary embryo fibroblasts requires at least two cooperating oncogenes. *Nature* **304:** 596–601.

Landschulz, W.H., P.F. Johnson, and S.L. McKnight. 1988. The "leucine zipper": A hypothetical structure common to a new class of DNA binding proteins. *Science* **240:** 1759–1764.

Lane, D.P. and L. Crawford. 1979. T antigen is bound to a host protein in SV40 transformed cells. *Nature* **278:** 261–263.

Langdon, W.Y., A.W. Harris, S. Cory, and J.M. Adams. 1986. The c-*myc* oncogene perturbs B lymphocyte development in Eu-*myc* transgenic mice. *Cell* **47:** 11–18.

Lech, K., K. Anderson, and R. Brent. 1988. DNA-bound Fos proteins activate transcription in yeast. *Cell* **52:** 179–184.

Lee, W.F., C. Lin, and T. Curran. 1988. Activation of the transforming potential of the human *fos* proto-oncogene requires message stabilization and results in increased amounts of partially modified *fos* protein. *Mol. Cell. Biol.* **8:** 5521–5527.

Lee, W., P. Mitchell, and R. Tjian. 1987. Purified transcription factor AP-1 interacts with TPA-inducible enhancer elements. *Cell* **49:** 741–752.

Li, Y., C.M. Turck, J.K. Teumer, and E. Stavnezer. 1986. Unique sequence, *ski*, in Sloan-Kettering avian retroviruses with properties of a new cell-derived oncogene. *J. Virol.* **57:** 1065–1072.

Linzer, D.I.H. and A.J. Levine. 1979. Characterization of a 54k dalton cellular SV40 tumor antigen present in SV40 transformed cells and uninfected embryonal carcinoma cells. *Cell* **17:** 43–52.

Lipsick, J.S. and W.J. Boyle. 1987. c-*myb* protein expression is a late event during T-lymphocyte activation. *Mol. Cell. Biol.* **7:** 3358–3360.

Lüscher, B. and R.N. Eisenman. 1988. c-*myc* and c-*myb* protein degradation: Effect of metabolic inhibitors and heat shock. *Mol. Cell. Biol.* **8:** 2504–2512.

Lüscher, B., E.A. Kuenzel, E.G. Krebs, and R.N. Eisenman. 1989. Myc oncoproteins are phosphorylated by casein kinase II. *EMBO J.* **8:** 1111–1119.

Maki, Y., T.J. Bos, C. Davis, M. Starbuck, and P.K. Vogt. 1987. Avian sarcoma virus 17 carries the *jun* oncogene. *Proc. Natl. Acad. Sci.* **84:** 2848–2852.

Makino, R., K. Hayashi, and T. Sugimura. 1984. c-*myc* transcript is induced in rat liver at a very early stage of regeneration or by cycloheximide treatment. *Nature* **310:** 697–698.

Mathog, D., M. Hochstrasser, V. Gruenbaum, H. Saumweber, and J. Sedat. 1984. Characteristic folding of polytene chromosomes in *Drosophila* salivary gland nuclei. *Nature* **308:** 414–421.

Mercer, W.E., D. Nelson, A.B. DeLeo, L.J. Old, and R. Baserga. 1982. Microinjection of monoclonal antibody to protein p53 inhibits serum-induced DNA synthesis in 3T3 cells. *Proc. Natl. Acad. Sci.* **79:** 6309–6312.

Miller, A.D., T. Curran, and I.M. Verma. 1984. c-*fos* protein can induce cellular transformation: A novel mechanism of activation of a cellular oncogene. *Cell* **36:** 51–60.

Mohun, T.J., N. Garrett, and R. Treisman. 1987. *Xenopus* cytoskeletal actin and human c-*fos* promoters share a conserved protein binding site. *EMBO J.* **6:** 667–673.

Munoz, A., M. Zenke, U. Gehring, J. Sap, H. Beug, and B. Vennstrom. 1988. Characterization of the hormone binding domain of the chicken c-*erb*A/thyroid hormone receptor protein. *EMBO J.* **7:** 155–159.

Murre, C., P.S. McCaw, and D. Baltimore. 1989. The amphipathic helix-loop-helix: A new apparent DNA-binding and dimerization domain structure in immunoglobulin enhancer binding, *daughterless*, *myo*D, and *myc* proteins. *Cell* **56:** 777–783.

Nakabeppu, Y., K. Ryder, and D. Nathans. 1988. DNA binding activities of three murine Jun proteins: Stimulation by Fos. *Cell* **55:** 907–915.

Nepveu, A., K.B. Marcu, A.I. Skoultchi, and H.M. Lachman. 1987. Contributions of transcriptional and post-transcriptional mechanisms to the regulation of c-*myc* expression in mouse erythroleukemia cells. *Genes Dev.* **1:** 938–945.

Ness, S.A., H. Beug, and T. Graf. 1987. V-*myb* dominance over v-*myc* in doubly transformed chick myelomonocytic cells. *Cell* **51:** 41–50.

Nomura, N., M. Takahashi, M. Matsui, S. Ishii, S. Sasamoto, and R. Ishizaki. 1988. Isolation of human cDNA clones of myb-related genes, A-myb and B-myb. *Nucleic Acids Res.* **16:** 11075–11089.

Norman, C., M. Runswick, R. Pollock, and R. Treisman. 1988. Isolation and properties of cDNA clones encoding SRF, a transcription factor that binds to the c-*fos* serum response element. *Cell* **55:** 989–1003.

Onclercq, R., P. Gilardi, A. Lavenu, and C. Cremisi. 1988. c-*myc* products *trans*-activate the adenovirus E4 promoter in EC stem cells using the same target sequence as E1A products. *J. Virol.* **62:** 4533–4537.

O'Shea, E.K., R.H. Rutkowski, and P.S. Kim. 1989a. Evidence that the leucine zipper is a coiled coil. *Science* **243:** 538–541.

O'Shea, E.K., R.H. Rutkowski, W.S. Stafford III, and P.S. Kim. 1989b. Preferential heterodimer formation by isolated leucine zippers from Fos and Jun. *Science* **245:** 646–648.

Palmieri, S., P. Kahn, and T. Graf. 1983. Quail embryo fibroblasts transformed by four v-*myc*-containing virus isolates show enhanced proliferation but are non-tumorigenic. *EMBO J.* **2:** 2385–2389.

Parada, L.F., H. Land, R.A. Weinberg, D. Wolf, and V. Rotter. 1984. Cooperation between gene encoding p53 tumour antigen and *ras* in cellular transformation. *Nature* **312:** 649–651.

Paz-Ares, J., D. Ghosal, U. Wienand, P.A. Peterson, and H. Saedler. 1987. The regulatory c1 locus of *Zea mays* encodes a protein with homology to *myb* proto-oncogene products and with structural similarities to transcriptional activators. *EMBO J.* **6:** 3553–3558.

Peters, C.W.B., A.E. Sippel, M. Vingron, and K.-H. Klempnauer. 1987. *Drosophila* and vertebrate *myb* proteins share two conserved regions, one of which functions as a DNA binding domain. *EMBO J.* **6:** 3085–3090.

Prendergast, G.C. and M.D. Cole. 1989. Posttranscriptional regulation of cellular gene expression by the c-*myc* oncogene. *Mol. Cell. Biol.* **9:** 124–134.

Pringle, J.R. and L.H. Hartwell. 1981. The *Saccharomyces cerevisiae* cell cycle. In *The molecular biology of the yeast* Saccharomyces (ed. J.N. Strathern et al.), pp. 97–142. Cold Spring Harbor Laboratory, Cold Spring Harbor, New York.

Rauscher, F.J. III, L.C. Sambucetti, T. Curran, R.J. Distel, and B.M. Spiegelman. 1988a. Common DNA binding site for Fos protein complexes and transcription factor AP-1. *Cell* **52:** 471–480.

Rauscher, F.J. III, D.R. Cohen, T. Curran, T.J. Bos, P.K. Vogt, D. Bohmann, R. Tjian, and B.R. Franza, Jr. 1988b. Fos-associated protein p39 is the product of the *jun* proto-oncogene. *Science* **240:** 1010–1016.

Reich, N.C., M. Oren, and A.J. Levine. 1983. Two distinct mechanisms regulate the levels of a cellular tumor antigen, p.53. *Mol. Cell. Biol.* **3:** 2143–2150.

Renz, M., B. Vernier, C. Kurz, and R. Muller. 1987. Chromatin association and DNA binding properties of the c-*fos* proto-oncogene product. *Nucleic Acids Res.* **15:** 277-292.

Rogers, S., R. Wells, and M. Rechsteiner. 1986. Amino acid sequences common to rapidly degraded proteins: The PEST hypothesis. *Science* **234:** 364–368.

Rosson, D. and E.P. Reddy. 1986. Nucleotide sequence of chicken c-*myb* complementary DNA and implications for *myb* oncogene activation. *Nature* **319:** 604–606.

Roussel, M., S. Saule, C. Lagrou, C. Rommens, H. Beug, T. Graf, and D. Staehelin. 1979. Three types of viral oncogene of cellular origin for hematopoietic cell transformation. *Nature* **281:** 452–455.

Ruther, U., C. Garber, D. Komitowski, R. Muller, and E. Wagner. 1987. Deregulated c-*fos* expression interferes with normal bone development in transgenic mice. *Nature* **325:** 412–416.

Ryder, K., L. Lau, and D. Nathans. 1988. A gene activated by growth factor is related to the oncogene v-*jun*. *Proc. Natl. Acad. Sci.* **85:** 1487–1491.

Ryseck, R.-P., S.I. Hirai, M. Yaniv, and R. Bravo. 1988. Transcriptional activation of c-*jun* during the G_0/G_1 transition in mouse fibroblasts. *Nature* **334:** 535–537.

Sakura, H., C. Kanei-Ishii, T. Nagase, H. Nakagoshi, T.J. Gonda, and S. Ishii. 1989. Delineation of three functional domains of the transcriptional activator encoded by the c-myb proto-oncogene. *Proc. Natl. Acad. Sci.* **86:** 5758–5762.

Sap, J., A. Munoz, J. Schmitt, H. Stunnenberg, and B. Vennstrom. 1989. Repression of transcription mediated at a thyroid hormone response element by the v-erb-A oncogene product. *Nature* **340:** 242–244.

Sap, J., A. Munoz, K. Damm, Y. Goldberg, J. Ghysdael, A. Leutz, H. Beug, and B. Vennstrom. 1986. The c-*erb*A protein is a high-affinity receptor for thyroid hormone. *Nature* **324:** 635–640.

Sarnow, P., Y.S. Ho, J. Williams, and A.J. Levine. 1982. Adenovirus E1b-58kd tumor antigen and SV40 large tumor antigen are physically associated with the same 54kd cellular protein in transformed cells. *Cell* **28:** 387–394.

Sassone-Corsi, P., W.W. Lamph, M. Kamps, and I.M. Verma. 1988a. *fos*-associated cellular p39 is related to nuclear transcription factor AP-1. *Cell* **54:** 553–560.

Sassone-Corsi, P., L.J. Ransone, W.W. Lamph, and I.M. Verma. 1988b. Direct interaction between *fos* and *jun* nuclear oncoproteins: Role of the "leucine zipper" domain. *Nature* **336:** 692–695.

Schleif, R. 1988. DNA binding by proteins. *Science* **241:** 1182–1187.

Schonthal, A., P. Herrlich, H.J. Rahmsdorf, and H. Ponta. 1988. Requirement for *fos* gene expression in the transcriptional activation of collagenase by other oncogenes and phorbol esters. *Cell* **54:** 325–334.

Schwab, M., H.E. Varmus, and J.M. Bishop. 1985. The human N-*myc* gene contributes to tumorigenic conversion of mammalian cells in culture. *Nature* **316:** 160–162.

Sejersen, T., J. Sumegi, and N.R. Ringertz. 1985. Density-dependent arrest of DNA replication is accompanied by decreased levels of c-*myc* mRNA in myogenic but not in differentiation-defective myoblasts. *J. Cell. Physiol.* **125:** 465–470.

Sheiness, D. and J.M. Bishop. 1979. DNA and RNA from uninfected vertebrate cells contain nucleotide sequences related to the putative transforming gene of avian myelocytomatosis. *J. Virol.* **31:** 514–521.

Sheiness D. and M. Gardinier. 1984. Expression of a proto-oncogene (proto-*myb*) in hemopoietic tissues of mice. *Mol. Cell. Biol.* **4:** 1206–1212.

Shen-Ong, G.L.C. 1987. Alternative internal splicing of c-*myb* RNAs occurs commonly in normal and tumor cells. *EMBO J.* **6:** 4035–4039.

Shen-Ong, G.L.C., M. Potter, J.F. Mushinski, S. Lavu, and E.P. Reddy. 1984. Activation of the c-*myb* locus by viral insertional mutagenesis in plasmacytoid lymphosarcomas. *Science* **226:** 1077–1080.

Sheng, M., S.T. Dougan, G. McFadden, and M.E. Greenberg. 1988. Calcium and growth factor pathways for c-*fos* transcriptional activation require distinct upstream regulatory sequences. *Mol. Cell. Biol.* **8:** 2787–2796.

Sigler, P.B. 1988. Acid blobs and negative noodles. *Nature* **333:** 210–212.

Simek, S. and N.R. Rice. 1988a. Detection and characterization of the protein encoded by the chicken c-*rel* protooncogene. *Oncogene Res.* **2:** 103–119.

———. 1988b. $p59^{v\text{-}rel}$, the transforming protein of reticuloendotheliosis virus, is complexed with at least four other proteins in transformed chicken lymphoid cells. *J. Virol.* **62:** 4730–4736.

Sinn, E., W. Muller, P. Pattengale, I. Tepler, R. Wallace, and P. Leder. 1987. Coexpression of MMTV/v-Ha-*ras* and MMTV/c-*myc* genes in transgenic mice: Synergistic action of oncogenes *in vivo*. *Cell* **49:** 465–475.

Sorrentino, V., V. Drozdoff, M.D. McKinney, L. Zeitz, and E. Fleissner. 1986. Potentiation of growth factor activity by exogenous c-*myc* expression. *Proc. Acad. Natl. Sci.* **83:** 8167–8171.

Spector, D.L., R.A. Watt, and N.F. Sullivan. 1987. The v- and c-*myc* oncogene proteins colocalize *in situ* with small nuclear ribonucleoprotein particles. *Oncogene* **1:** 5–12.

Stavnezer, E. 1988. "The *SKI* gene." In *The oncogene handbook* (ed. E.P. Reddy et al.), pp. 393–401. Elsevier Science Publishers, The Netherlands.

Stavnezer, E., D.S. Gerhard, R.C. Binari, and I. Balazs. 1981. Generation of transforming viruses in cultures of chicken fibroblasts infected with an avian leukosis virus. *J. Virol.* **39:** 920–934.

Stavnezer, E., A.E. Barkas, L. Brennan, D. Brodeur, and Y. Li. 1986. Transforming Sloan-Kettering viruses generated from the cloned v-*ski* oncogene by *in vitro* and *in vivo* recombinations. *J. Virol.* **57:** 1073–1083.

Stern, D., A. Roberts, N.S. Roche, M.B. Sporn, and R.A. Weinberg. 1986. Differential responsiveness of *myc* and *ras*-transfected cells to growth factors: Selective stimulation of *myc*-transfected cells by epidermal growth factor. *Mol. Cell. Biol.* **6:** 870–877.

Steward, R. 1987. Dorsal, an embryonic polarity gene in *Drosophila*, is homologous to the vertebrate proto-oncogene, c-*rel*. *Science* **238:** 692–694.

Struhl, K. 1987. The DNA-binding domains of the *jun* oncoprotein and the yeast GCN4 transcriptional activator protein are functionally homologous. *Cell* **50:** 841–846.

Thiele, C.J., P.S. Cohen, and M.A. Israel. 1988. Regulation of c-myb expression in human neuroblastoma cell during retinoic acid-induced differentiation. *Mol. Cell. Biol.* **8:** 1677–1683.

Thompson, C.B., P.B. Challoner, P.E. Neiman, and M. Groudine. 1986. Expression of the c-*myb* proto-oncogene during cellular proliferation. *Nature* **319:** 374–380.

Treisman, R. 1985. Transient accumulation of c-*fos* RNA following serum stimulation requires a conserved 5′ element and c-*fos* 3′ sequences. *Cell* **42:** 889–902.

———. 1986. Identification of a protein-binding site that mediates transcriptional response of the c-*fos* gene to serum factors. *Cell* **46:** 567–574.

———. 1987. Identification and purification of a polypeptide that binds to the c-*fos* serum response element. *EMBO J.* **6:** 2711–2717.

Vennstrom, B. and J.M. Bishop. 1982. Isolation and characterization of chicken DNA homologous to the two putative oncogenes of avian erythroblastosis virus. *Cell* **28:** 135–143.

Verma, I.M. 1986. Proto-oncogene *fos*: A multifaceted gene. *Trends Genet.* **2:** 93–96.

Verma, I.M. and P. Sassone-Corsi. 1987. Proto-oncogene *fos*: Complex but versatile regulation. *Cell* **51:** 513–514.

Villares, R. and C.V. Cabrera. 1987. The *achaete-scute* gene complex of *D. melanogaster*: Conserved domains in a subset of genes required for neurogenesis and their homology to *myc*. *Cell* **50:** 415–424.

Vogt, P.K. and R. Tjian. 1988. Jun: A transcriptional regulator turned oncogenic. *Oncogene* **3:** 3–7.

Vogt, P.K., T.J. Bos, and R.F. Doolittle. 1987. Homology between the DNA-binding domain of the GCN4 regulatory protein of yeast and the carboxyl-terminal region of a protein coded for by the oncogene *jun*. *Proc. Natl. Acad. Sci.* **84:** 3316–3319.

Walro, D.S., N.K. Herzog, J. Zhang, M.Y. Lim, and H.R. Bose, Jr. 1987. The transforming protein of reticuloendotheliosis virus is a soluble cytoplasmic protein which is associated with a protein kinase activity. *Virology* **160:** 433–444.

Webster, N.J.G., S. Green, J.R. Jin, and P. Chambon. 1988. The hormone binding domains of the estrogen and glucocorticoid receptors contain an inducible transcription activation function. *Cell* **54:** 199–207.

Weinberger, C., C.C. Thompson, E.S. Ong, R. Lebo, D.J. Gruol, and R.M. Evans. 1986. The c-*erb*A gene encodes a thyroid hormone receptor. *Nature* **324:** 641–646.

Weston, K. and J.M. Bishop. 1989. Transcriptional activation by the v-myb oncogene and its cellular progenitor, c-myb. *Cell* **58:** 85–93.

Westin, E.H., R.C. Gallo, S.K. Arya, A. Eva, L.M. Souza, M.A. Baluda, S.A. Aaronson, and F. Wong-Staal. 1982a. Differential expression of the *amv* gene in human hematopoietic cells. *Proc. Natl. Acad. Sci.* **79:** 2194–2198.

Westin, E.H., F. Wong-Staal, E.P. Gelmann, R. Dalla-Favera, T.S. Papas, J.A. Lautenberger, A. Eva, E.P. Reddy, S.R. Tronik, S.A. Aaronson, and R.C. Gallo. 1982b. Expression of cellular homologues of retroviral *onc* genes in human hematopoietic cells. *Proc. Natl. Acad. Sci.* **79:** 2490–2494.

Wilson, T. and R. Treisman. 1988. Fos C-terminal mutations block down-regulation of c-*fos* transcription during serum stimulation. *EMBO J.* **7:** 4193–4202.

Wingrove, T.G., R. Watt, P. Keng, and I.G. Macara. 1988. Stabilization of myc proto-oncogene proteins during Friend murine erythroleukemia cell differentiation. *J. Biol. Chem.* **263:** 8918–8924.

Wolf, D., N. Harris, and V. Rotter. 1984. Reconstitution of p53 expression in a non-producer Ab-MuLV-transformed cell line by transfection of a functional p53 gene. *Cell* **38:** 119–126.

Yamamoto, K.R. 1985. Steroid receptor regulated transcription of specific genes and gene networks. *Annu. Rev. Genet.* **19:** 209–252.

Zenke, M., P. Kahn, C. Disela, B. Vennstrom, A. Leutz, K. Keegan, M.J. Hayman, H.-Y. Choi, N. Yew, J.D. Engel, and H. Beug. 1988. v-*erb*A specifically suppresses transcription of the avian erythrocyte anion transporter (band 3) gene. *Cell* **52:** 107–119.

Zimmerman, K.A. G.D. Yancopoulos, R.G. Collum, R.K. Smith, N.E. Kohl, K.A. Denis, M.N. Nau, Q.N. Witte, D. Toran-Allerand, C.E. Gee, J.D. Minna, and F.W. Alt. 1986. Differential expression of *myc* family genes during murine development. *Nature* **319:** 780–783.

8

Oncogenes of DNA Tumor Viruses: Papovaviruses

Walter Eckhart
Molecular Biology and Virology Laboratory
The Salk Institute
San Diego, California 92138

I. INTRODUCTION

The papovavirus family includes the polyomaviruses (notably polyoma and SV40) and the papillomaviruses. Polyoma was discovered in 1953 by Ludwik Gross, who noted that extracts from leukemic mice sometimes caused salivary gland tumors. Subsequently, the virus was shown to cause a wide variety of tumors, and the name "polyoma" was proposed by Stewart and Eddy in 1958 to reflect this unusual property.

SV40 was discovered in 1960 by Sweet and Hilleman during a search for contaminants of polio vaccines prepared from monkey cell cultures. The presence of SV40 originally was missed because the virus did not cause pronounced cytopathic effect in cultures of rhesus monkey cells, the most common source for vaccine production.

Papillomas (warts) occur in many species of animals. The first papillomavirus to be well characterized was isolated from cottontail rabbits by Shope in 1933. A variety of papillomaviruses have been isolated from

Oncogenes and the Molecular Origins of Cancer.

human warts, and some of them have been implicated in the progression of benign warts to malignant tumors. Work with these viruses has been hampered by the lack of cell-culture systems in which the viruses will multiply. However, recombinant DNA techniques have allowed much to be learned about the organization and expression of the viral genomes and the functions of the proteins they encode.

Many transforming retroviruses arose because of the incorporation of cellular genetic information into viral genomes. In contrast, the oncogenes of papovaviruses and other DNA tumor viruses seem not to be closely related to cellular genes. Presumably, their transforming potential is incidental to their function in the viral life cycle.

Polyoma and SV40 can produce either of two responses in susceptible cells: The *lytic* response results in virus replication and subsequent death of the host cell; the *abortive* response results in failure of virus replication and survival of the infected cell. Whether the response to infection will be lytic or abortive generally depends on the species of the infected cell. In at least some cases, the presence or absence of factors required for viral DNA replication determines which response will occur.

Occasionally, the viral genome becomes incorporated into the cellular genome after infection, allowing viral genetic information to be inherited by the progeny of the infected cell. The presence and expression of viral oncogenes cause alterations in cell growth control, resulting in cell transformation.

Papovavirus genomes are small: Polyoma and SV40 contain about 5000 bp of DNA, papillomaviruses about 8000 bp. This limited amount of genetic information has evolved to carry out multiple functions. In some cases, the same region of DNA encodes more than one protein. In other cases, a single protein has several functions. This fascinating adaptation complicates the study of the viral oncogenes but makes their characterization especially interesting.

Many excellent reviews of papovaviruses have appeared in recent years. Comprehensive background information can be found in Tooze (1980); Botchan et al. (1986); Salzman (1986); and Salzman and Howley (1987).

II. POLYOMAVIRUS

A. Neoplastic Cell Transformation

Polyoma has the unusual ability to induce neoplasms in a wide variety of cell types in its natural host, the mouse. More than 30 different cell types can be infected in newborn mice inoculated with polyoma, and tumors can arise in more than a dozen of these. The kidney is the major site of virus replication.

Polyoma causes a lytic infection in mouse fibroblasts in culture and an abortive infection in rat and hamster cells. Generally, cell transformation by the intact virus is studied in vitro using rat or hamster cells to avoid the complications caused by cell death from lytic infection. Recombinant DNAs or recombinant retroviruses encoding polyoma transforming proteins do not cause lytic infection and can be used to study transformation of mouse cells.

B. Genome Organization and Expression

The polyoma genome is a double-stranded, covalently closed, circular DNA molecule a little over 5000 bp in size, containing a single origin of replication (ori). DNA synthesis begins at the origin and proceeds bidirectionally, terminating about 180° away. The genome is divided into an early and a late region, about equal in size, on the basis of the time at which genes are expressed during lytic infection. The early region is expressed prior to the onset of viral DNA replication; the late region is expressed predominantly after viral DNA replication begins. Transcription of the early and late regions originates in separate promoter regions near the origin of replication. The early region and the late region are transcribed from opposite strands of the DNA (see Fig. 1). There is a noncoding enhancer region, 100–200 bp in size, on the late side of the origin. The enhancer region interacts with cellular proteins that regulate gene expression and replication.

The early region of the viral genome encodes three proteins, originally called tumor antigens (now generally shortened to T antigens) because they interact with serum from animals bearing polyoma-induced tumors. The T antigens are the oncogenic proteins of polyoma and will be the focus of the discussion of cell transformation. The T antigens are referred to as large T (LT), small T (sT), and middle T (mT), according to their relative sizes. Their sizes, calculated from their deduced amino acid sequences, are 785 amino acids (LT), 195 amino acids (sT), and 421 amino acids (mT).

The T antigens are encoded in overlapping but nonidentical regions of the viral DNA. The coding regions are arranged such that all three proteins share a common amino-terminal region of 79 amino acids. sT and mT share an additional 112 amino acids not found in LT. The carboxy-terminal regions, 4 amino acids for sT, 230 for mT, and 706 for LT, are unique. The unique carboxy-terminal region of mT is encoded by a region of DNA that also encodes part of the carboxy-terminal region of LT but is translated in a different reading frame. This unusual coding arrangement is accomplished by alternative splicing events that produce three unique mRNAs from a single primary transcript (Treisman et al. 1981b). The arrangement of the coding regions is illustrated in Figure 1.

The early region of the polyoma genome is expressed in transformed cells, whereas the late region is not. This observation suggested that the T antigens were important for cell transformation, and stimulated efforts to

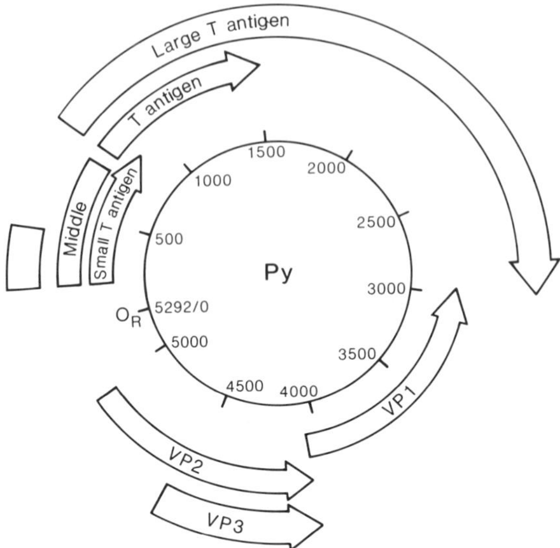

Figure 1 Genome organization of polyomavirus. The early region encodes three T antigens. The late region encodes three capsid proteins. Nucleotide numbers are shown inside the circle. Arrows indicate the direction of transcription.

understand the role of the individual T antigens in lytic infection and transformation.

C. Role of Polyoma T Antigens in Lytic Infection

Infection of a resting cell by polyoma triggers the expression of cellular genes involved in DNA replication and cell cycle control. Presumably, the virus evolved a mechanism for stimulating resting cells in order to provide a favorable environment for the replication of viral DNA. Cellular DNA synthesis begins about 12 hours after infection of resting cells, a time course similar to that produced by growth factor stimulation. Viral DNA synthesis also commences at this time.

Interaction of the viral capsid with a receptor on the cell surface appears to be sufficient to stimulate the transcription of the c-*myc* and c-*fos* genes (Zullo et al. 1987). Increased transcription of these genes also occurs after stimulation of resting cells by growth factors. If no T-antigen synthesis occurs, transcription of c-*myc* and c-*fos* decreases over a period of several hours. However, an elevated level of transcription is maintained if sT is present. These observations raise the intriguing possibility that the polyoma capsid interacts with a receptor that can transmit a mitogenic signal and that sT can maintain an elevated level of c-*myc* and c-*fos* transcription. sT is located primarily in the cytoplasmic fraction of cell extracts but is also present in the nucleus. There is evidence that SV40 sT can regulate transcription from certain promoters (Loeken et al. 1989).

LT is multifunctional. It is involved in transformation, as described below. It also does other, mechanistically unrelated, things in the cell. For example, it binds to viral DNA sequences in the region of the origin and is required for initiation of viral DNA replication. LT is also involved in regulation of transcription of the early region: The levels of early mRNA increase when the amount of LT is reduced. Since early region mRNAs are transcribed from promoters near the origin of replication, the binding of LT in this region may also mediate the effects on transcription.

Mutations affecting sT and mT coordinately (*hr-t* mutations) produce a host range defect: The mutant viruses grow well in some cells but poorly in others (Goldman and Benjamin 1975). The properties of the *hr-t* mutants suggest that some cells provide factors or conditions that render the functions of sT and/or mT dispensable. Cellular factors also influence virus replication in other situations. For example, polyoma fails to replicate in undifferentiated mouse teratocarcinoma cells but replicates in these cells if they are stimulated to differentiate. Mutations in the enhancer region allow the virus to multiply in both kinds of cells (Vasseur et al. 1980; Fujimura et al. 1981).

In summary, LT is absolutely required for viral DNA replication in lytic infection; sT and/or mT are required for efficient growth in some cells but not in others. Cellular factors influence the transcription of viral genes and the replication of viral DNA.

D. Role of Polyoma T Antigens in Transformation

Stable cell transformation generally requires the integration of viral DNA into cellular DNA. The early events in stable transformation require LT because LT is involved in the integration process. Mutations in LT can prevent integration and stable transformation after infection with intact virus, and the presence of functional LT in a permissive cell containing integrated viral DNA results in excision and replication of the viral DNA sequences. Mutations in LT do not block transformation when viral DNA is introduced into a cell by transfection, possibly because recombination events leading to integration take place by a different mechanism after transfection.

Because of the overlapping coding regions of the polyoma T antigens, it was difficult to introduce mutations affecting each of the proteins individually. However, the isolation of cDNA clones of the T antigen mRNAs made it possible to test the role of each of the proteins in transformation. LT alone is not sufficient to transform primary cells or established cell lines. However, LT can act as an oncogenic protein by cooperating with mT. The role of LT appears to be to permit the growth of primary cells at low density and to immortalize primary cells so that they grow as established cell lines (Rassoulzadegan et al. 1982). These changes are necessary for full conversion to tumorigenicity, but are not in themselves sufficient; tumorigenicity also requires actions of mT. (See discussion of collaboration of oncogenes in Chapter 12.)

mT alone is sufficient to transform established cell lines, and under some conditions, it can transform primary cells (Treisman et al. 1981a; Kaplan et al. 1985). The expression of mT allows cells to grow in an anchorage-independent manner, a growth property that is closely correlated with tumorigenic potential (see also Chapter 12).

Little is known about the role of sT in transformation. It seems dispensable for transformation under most conditions, but it can potentiate the transforming effects of mT in some cells. No biochemical function has been assigned to sT; however, its effects on gene expression, mentioned above, suggest that it may be involved in transcriptional regulation.

In summary, mT appears to be primarily responsible for producing the altered growth properties of established cell lines transformed by polyoma, whereas mT and LT cooperate to transform primary cells. Transformation involves interaction of mT with cellular proteins. Characterization of the cellular proteins that interact with mT has led to insights into the mechanisms of cell transformation by polyoma.

E. Interaction of mT with Cellular Proteins: Activation of pp60$^{c\text{-}src}$

Polyoma uses a novel method of oncogene activation as part of its transforming activity. As discussed below, polyoma mT changes the activity of a cellular protein by binding to the protein directly. Immunoprecipitates of polyoma T antigens contain a protein kinase activity that phosphorylates tyrosine residues in mT. The protein kinase activity is due to the presence of pp60$^{c\text{-}src}$, the cellular homolog of the Rous sarcoma virus transforming protein, pp60$^{v\text{-}src}$, which forms a complex with mT (Courtneidge and Smith 1983; see Chapter 6). Only a small fraction of mT and pp60$^{c\text{-}src}$ (5–10%) is found in the complex, but formation of the complex is closely correlated with transformation. All mT mutants that are capable of transformation form the complex, and most mutants that are defective in transformation fail to form the complex (Markland and Smith 1987).

Both mT and pp60$^{c\text{-}src}$ are found in membrane fractions of the cell. mT is anchored in the membrane by a hydrophobic domain near its carboxyl terminus, whereas pp60$^{c\text{-}src}$ is anchored by a myristyl group linked to its amino-terminal glycine residue. Mutations in the amino-terminal region of mT and the carboxy-terminal region of pp60$^{c\text{-}src}$ affect formation of the complex. pp60$^{v\text{-}src}$, which differs from pp60$^{c\text{-}src}$ in its carboxy-terminal region, fails to form a complex with mT. Other cellular protein tyrosine kinases may also be able to associate with mT. For example, pp62$^{c\text{-}yes}$, the cellular homolog of the Y73 virus oncogene product, does so.

The phosphorylation pattern and specific activity of pp60$^{c\text{-}src}$ change as a result of association with mT. Free pp60$^{c\text{-}src}$ is phosphorylated on tyrosine 527; pp60$^{c\text{-}src}$, associated with mT, is phosphorylated on tyrosine 416, as is pp60$^{v\text{-}src}$ (Cartwright et al. 1986). The specific activity of pp60$^{c\text{-}src}$ associated with mT is 10–100-fold higher than that of free pp60$^{c\text{-}src}$ (Bolen et al. 1984). Phosphorylation of tyrosine 527 regulates the protein kinase activity of pp60$^{c\text{-}src}$. Decreased phosphorylation of tyrosine 527 and increased phosphorylation of tyrosine 416 are characteristic of *src* proteins with elevated kinase activity.

The activation of pp60$^{c\text{-}src}$ by association with mT suggested that mT transformation might operate through altered regulation of pp60$^{c\text{-}src}$. In support of this idea, mutations in c-*src* that prevent phosphorylation of tyrosine 527 confer transforming ability on the mutant c-*src* genes (Cartwright et al. 1987; Kmiecik and Shalloway 1987; Piwnica-Worms et al. 1987). However, there are reasons to suspect that mT may have other effects in addition to preventing normal phosphorylation of a small fraction of pp60$^{c\text{-}src}$ in the cell: The phenotypic properties of cells transformed by activated c-*src* are different from those of mT-transformed cells, and some mT mutants that appear to associate with and activate pp60$^{c\text{-}src}$ nevertheless are defective in transformation.

Polyoma mT also binds to other cellular proteins that may affect the properties of transformed cells. For example, there is a phosphatidylinositol (PtdIns) kinase activity associated with mT in immunoprecipitates, and the presence of this activity, like that of pp60$^{c\text{-}src}$, is closely correlated with the transforming activity of mT (Kaplan et al. 1986). It is possible that the PtdIns kinase activity is modulated by mT or pp60$^{c\text{-}src}$. Because PtdIns kinase activity is involved in transduction of signals across cell membranes, it is attractive to think that mT may affect cellular signaling through this mechanism.

Although the magnitude of the contribution of activated pp60$^{c\text{-}src}$ and other associated proteins to transformation by mT is not yet clear, this mechanism suggests that some oncogene products can act at the protein level, causing alterations in cell growth control by binding to other proteins involved in growth regulation.

III. SV40

A. Genome Organization and Expression

SV40 causes a lytic infection of monkey cells and an abortive infection of mouse or rat cells. The organization of the SV40 genome is similar to that of polyoma, with one notable exception: Only two T antigens, sT and LT, are encoded in the early region of SV40; there is no mT. The arrangement of the coding regions is shown in Figure 2. The sT and LT of SV40 are encoded in overlapping regions of the viral DNA in such a way that they

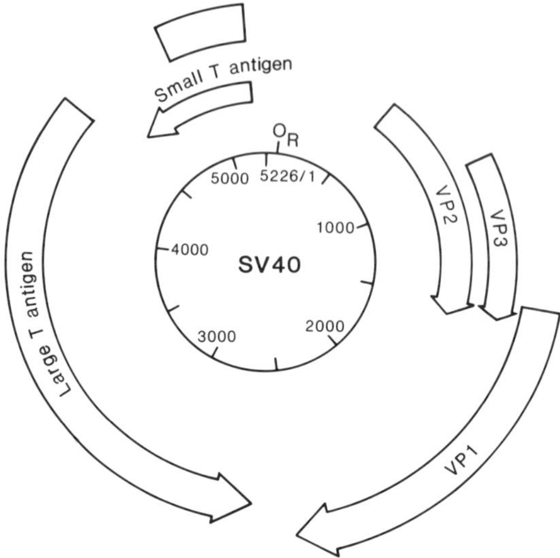

Figure 2 Genome organization of SV40. The early region encodes two T antigens. The late region encodes three capsid proteins. Nucleotide numbers are shown inside the circle. Arrows indicate the direction of transcription.

have identical amino-terminal regions of 82 amino acids but unique carboxy-terminal regions. The size of SV40 sT is 174 amino acids; that of LT is 708 amino acids.

B. Role of SV40 LT in DNA Replication and Transcription

The SV40 LT, like that of polyoma, is located in the nucleus and is required for initiation of viral DNA replication (Tegtmeyer 1972; Li and Kelly 1984). Amino acid sequences including lysine 128 of LT are required for transport of the protein to the nucleus (Kalderon et al. 1984; Lanford and Butel 1984). It may also have a function in events at the growing fork as replication proceeds. SV40 LT binds to regions near the origin of replication in SV40 DNA. Mutations in the region of LT between amino acids 135 and 230 affect this binding and support the conclusion that binding is required for replication (Clark et al. 1983).

Several biochemical activities have been associated with SV40 LT. Prominent among them are nucleotide binding and ATPase activities, which appear to be involved in viral DNA replication. The nucleotide-binding region (amino acids 412–528) includes amino acid sequences homologous to other ATP-binding proteins. The ATPase activity of LT is located in a region including amino acids 371–628. In addition, LT has a helicase activity: It is able to separate duplex DNA in vitro. An attractive model for the initiation of viral DNA replication is that SV40 LT binds to the origin of replication and opens a region of the DNA to allow priming through the synthesis of short initiator RNAs.

Viral DNA replication occurs in cells undergoing a lytic response to infection (permissive cells) but fails to occur in cells undergoing an abortive response (nonpermissive cells), even though LT is present. In vitro DNA replication systems have allowed the identification of cellular components required for replication of viral DNA. These components include a complex of DNA polymerase α and primase. Extracts of nonpermissive mouse cells, supplemented with DNA polymerase α/primase from permissive monkey cells, replicate viral DNA (Murakami et al. 1986). Therefore, the response of a cell to infection appears to be determined, at least in part, by whether its DNA polymerase α/primase complex will interact with LT.

SV40 LT modulates transcription of early mRNAs, presumably by binding to the ori region and affecting the early mRNA promoter sequences, which are located there. SV40 LT also is involved in the activation of late transcription that occurs after DNA replication begins. Before viral DNA replication, transcription occurs predominantly from the early promoter. After viral DNA replication, transcription from the early promoter decreases, and transcription from the late promoter increases, reaching a level 5–10 times higher than transcription from the early promoter. Activation of late transcription requires LT and appears to involve the binding of cellular factors to regulatory sequences on the late side of the viral origin. LT could facilitate binding of cellular transcription factors to the viral DNA, or it could induce new factors or modify existing factors.

C. Role of SV40 LT in Transformation

SV40 LT is mainly responsible for cell transformation by SV40. Under some conditions, sT is also required, but LT alone is sufficient in most cases. Although LT can affect DNA replication and transcription, these effects do not seem to account for its ability to act as an oncogenic protein.

Two observations suggest that direct effects of SV40 LT on cellular DNA replication (e.g., initiation at cellular origins) are not likely to account for transformation. First, mutant LT proteins that are defective in binding to DNA are still capable of transformation (Kalderon and Smith 1984). Second, polyoma LT, which appears to have a similar role in polyoma DNA replication, does not have transforming ability.

Induction or modification of cellular transcription factors is an attractive mechanism for affecting cellular gene expression, and it is possible that this contributes to transformation by SV40. However, there is no direct evidence for a role for such a mechanism.

Recent evidence suggests that interaction of SV40 LT with cellular proteins is important for transformation. LT forms a complex with a cellular protein, p53, in many transformed cells. As a result of this association, the half-life of the p53 protein is extended, and its level is elevated in the transformed cell. Mutation of the cellular p53 gene activates it for cooperation with the *ras* oncogene. The wild-type p53 protein is not transforming; in fact, p53 suppresses transformation when it is cotransfected with *ras* and other oncogenes (Finlay et al. 1989). Several lines of evidence suggest that inactivation of p53 predisposes a normal cell to becoming transformed. Therefore, binding of p53 to SV40 LT may contribute to transformation by sequestering p53 or inactivating its function in growth regulation (see also Chapter 11).

SV40 LT also binds to the protein product of the retinoblastoma susceptibility gene, Rb (the gene whose inactivation triggers retinoblastomas and osteosarcomas) (DeCaprio et al. 1988). Mutations in the domain of LT including amino acids 105–114, which abolish the ability of a fragment of LT to transform established cell lines, also abolish binding to the retinoblastoma protein. The amino acid sequence of the 105–114 region is similar to a domain of the adenovirus E1A gene product that is required for E1A transforming activity (Whyte et al. 1988a). The E1A protein also binds the Rb gene product (Whyte et al. 1988b). Therefore, association with LT or the E1A protein may inactivate or alter the properties of Rb protein, thereby contributing to transformation (see also Chapter 11).

In summary, the overall genetic organization and life cycle of polyoma and SV40 are similar, and the binding of cellular proteins involved in growth control appears to be a common feature of their transforming activities. Because the transforming activities of these viral oncogenes are incidental to their functions in the virus life cycle, it will be interesting to see how the transforming functions arose and what evolutionary pressures encouraged their selection.

IV. PAPILLOMAVIRUSES

A. Genome Organization and Expression

Papillomaviruses cause tumors of the skin and mucosa in many animals. Generally, the tumors are benign and regress. Occasionally, however, benign tumors will progress to malignant carcinomas. The genomes of human papillomavirus (HPV) strains 16 and 18 have been found in more than 70% of human cervical carcinomas examined and, thus, have been implicated as causative agents in these tumors.

Most papillomaviruses are able to replicate only in epithelial cells. However, some are able to induce fibropapillomas, and fibroblasts can be transformed by these viruses in vitro. Infection by papillomaviruses probably begins in the cells of the basal layer, which can be transformed but are nonpermissive for virus replication. As the cells differentiate during their transit to the surface, they become able to support virus growth.

Studies of virus replication have been hampered by the lack of tissue culture systems in which the papillomaviruses can be grown. However, molecular cloning has allowed the genomes of several different papillomaviruses to be characterized extensively. One of the best models is bovine papillomavirus, which has been used to study transformation in vitro and to construct vectors for the introduction of foreign genes into cells (Salzman and Howley 1987).

Figure 3 shows a genetic map of bovine papillomavirus (BPV-1) with the open reading frames (ORFs) indicated outside the circular genome. The

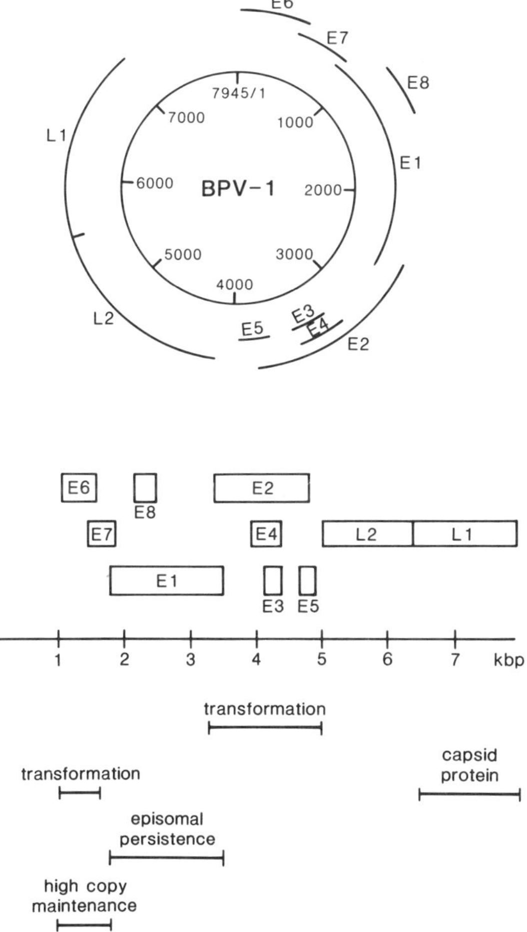

Figure 3 Genome organization of bovine papillomavirus. Nucleotide numbers are shown inside the circle. Open reading frames are shown outside the circle. Regions of the genome involved in various functions are indicated in the linear representation below. (Adapted from Salzman and Howley 1987).

genomic organization of BPV-1 is similar to that of other papillomaviruses. A "consensus" genome based on BPV-1 is shown in linear form in Figure 3. The L1 ORF encodes the major capsid protein of the virion. The L2 ORF encodes a minor capsid protein. The E reading frames encode proteins involved in aspects of virus replication and transformation.

B. Transforming Functions

Much of the information about papillomavirus transformation comes from studies of BPV-1, which can transform fibroblasts in vitro. Integration is not required for transformation by papillomaviruses. The viral DNA in tumors or transformed cells usually is maintained in an extrachromosomal plasmid form. The number of plasmid copies is variable and is affected by viral gene functions.

Genetic studies identified several regions of the viral genome involved in transformation (for review, see Salzman and Howley 1987). Isolation of cDNA clones of the viral mRNAs and cloned ORFs allowed the effects of individual gene products to be tested directly. Two different species of cDNAs are able to transform mouse cells: One encodes the E6 ORF product; the other contains all the 3′ ORFs (E2, E3, E4, E5). The two kinds of cDNAs act synergistically, that is, transfection with both yields more foci than transfection with either alone.

The E6 ORF encodes a 15.5-kD protein that is found in both nuclear and membrane fractions of transformed cells. The predicted amino acid sequence of the E6 protein contains the motif Cys-X-X-Cys repeated four times. The presence of this repeated motif, together with the high lysine and arginine content of the protein, suggests that it may bind to DNA. However, the function of the protein is not known. Generally, E6 proteins are expressed in papilloma-associated carcinomas and cell lines, suggesting that the E6 protein may be important in malignant progression.

The E5 ORF encodes a protein of 44 amino acids that is required for efficient transformation of established mouse cell lines. The protein is very hydrophobic, containing a stretch of 27 hydrophobic amino acids between residues 4 and 30. The carboxy-terminal region of the protein contains several charged and polar amino acids. The hydrophobic region could serve as a membrane-spanning domain, and the protein is located primarily in cellular membranes. Mutations in the hydrophobic region indicate that a stretch of hydrophobic amino acids is required for efficient transformation, but a specific amino acid sequence is not important (Horwitz et al. 1988). The small size and unusual structure of the E5 protein raise intriguing questions about its function and role in transformation. Because the E5 ORF transforms fibroblasts readily and is conserved in papillomaviruses that induce both epidermal and dermal cell growth, the E5 protein may be involved in stimulating the growth of dermal fibroblasts.

The E2 ORF encodes a protein that *trans*-activates the enhancer element in the BPV noncoding region, activating transcription from several viral promoters. A truncated E2 ORF gene product, resulting from initiation of translation at an internal AUG codon, acts as a transcriptional repressor, inhibiting the function of the E2 *trans*-activator. The E2 gene appears to affect transformation by regulating transcription of viral genes involved directly in transformation.

The HPV-16 E2 ORF also encodes a protein that *trans*-activates an enhancer in the HPV-16 genome. The most abundant HPV-16 RNA species in cervical carcinoma tissues and cell lines correspond to the E6 and E7 ORFs, suggesting that expression of these regions may be necessary for maintaining the transformed phenotype.

The E7 ORF encodes a transcriptional *trans*-activation function and a function that can cooperate with an activated *ras* gene to transform primary cells (Phelps et al. 1988). The E7 protein binds to the Rb gene product in vitro (Dyson et al. 1989; Chapter 11) and has amino-terminal amino acid sequences similar to those of the adenovirus E1A gene products that are involved in Rb protein binding and *ras* cooperation for transformation. The carboxy-terminal region of the E7 protein contains the repeated motif Cys-X-X-Cys, which is characteristic of the domain of E1A involved in transcriptional *trans*-activation. Therefore, the E7 protein has biological functions resembling those of the large T antigens of polyoma and SV40, and the E1A proteins of adenovirus (see also Chapter 11).

In summary, transforming functions of BPV-1 are encoded in the E6 and E5 ORFs. The E6 and E5 proteins affect the growth properties of cells in which they are expressed, and cooperate to produce the full transformed phenotype. The E6 protein resembles DNA-binding proteins, whereas the E5 protein appears to be a novel membrane-spanning protein. The E2 ORF encodes proteins that regulate transcription of viral genes and appears to have an indirect effect on transformation. The HPV E7 protein has transcriptional *trans*-activation and transformation functions that resemble those of other DNA tumor viruses.

C. Role in Human Cancer

Three basic types of warts are induced by papillomaviruses in humans: common warts, flat warts, and genital warts. Unlike polyoma and SV40, papillomaviruses are involved in human tumors, both benign and malignant. Warts are benign lesions. Malignant progression of these benign lesions is a relatively rare event. However, papillomaviruses are associated with a variety of squamous cell carcinomas, including cervical and anogenital carcinomas, laryngeal oral carcinomas, and cutaneous carcinomas in patients with epidermodysplasia verruciformis (EV), a disease characterized by disseminated skin lesions resembling flat warts (for review, see

Salzman and Howley 1987). At least 15 types of human papillomaviruses have been associated with EV, but HPV-5 is the type predominantly associated with malignant carcinomas.

EV is influenced by genetic and environmental factors, as well as by HPV. Evidence for the importance of genetic factors includes a high frequency of consanguinity among parents of EV patients and a frequent familial occurrence of the disease. Sunlight appears to be a particularly important environmental factor, because tumors develop primarily in areas of the body that are exposed to the sun.

The most common HPV types associated with human genital cancer are HPV-16 and HPV-18. These viruses are rarely associated with benign genital warts. The viral DNA is often found in an integrated form in cervical cancer cell lines, in contrast to BPV- and other HPV-infected cells, in which the viral genomes are maintained as plasmids.

V. QUESTIONS FOR THE FUTURE

The oncogenes of polyoma, SV40, and papillomaviruses pose a number of intriguing questions. The viruses have multiple oncogenes, which cooperate in transformation and tumorigenesis. How did the oncogenes evolve, and how do they cooperate to exert their effects on cells? In polyoma and SV40, the oncogenes are encoded in overlapping regions of the viral DNA. How did this gene organization come about, and how does it give rise to proteins with diverse functions?

The large T antigens of polyoma and SV40 have multiple biochemical functions. What is the relationship between the functions required in lytic infection (e.g., in DNA replication) and the functions involved in cell transformation?

Finally, how do the oncogenic proteins affect the functions of cellular proteins? The association of T antigens with cellular protein tyrosine kinases, PtdIns kinase, and with the products of cellular "tumor suppressor genes" like the retinoblastoma protein and p53 suggest that modification of cellular proteins is an important mechanism of transformation by the oncogenes of DNA tumor viruses.

REFERENCES

Bolen, J.B., C.J. Thiele, M.A. Israel, W. Yonemoto, L.A. Lipsich, and J.S. Brugge. 1984. Enhancement of cellular *src* gene product associated tyrosyl kinase activity following polyoma virus infection and transformation. *Cell* **38:** 767–777.

Botchan, M., T. Grodzicker, and P.A. Sharp, eds. 1986. *Cancer cells: DNA tumor viruses: Control of gene expression and replication*, volume 4. Cold Spring Harbor Laboratory, Cold Spring Harbor, New York.

Cartwright, C.A., W. Eckhart, S. Simon, and P.L. Kaplan. 1987. Cell transformation by $pp60^{c\text{-}src}$ mutated in the carboxy-terminal regulatory domain. *Cell* **49:** 83–91.

Cartwright, C.A., P.L. Kaplan, J.A. Cooper, T. Hunter, and W. Eckhart. 1986. Altered sites of tyrosine phosphorylation in pp60$^{c\text{-}src}$ associated with polyomavirus middle tumor antigen. *Mol. Cell. Biol.* **6:** 1562–1570.

Clark, R., K. Peden, J.M. Pipas, D. Nathans, and R. Tjian. 1983. Biochemical activities of T-antigen proteins encoded by simian virus 40 A gene deletion mutants. *Mol. Cell. Biol.* **3:** 220–228.

Courtneidge, S.A. and A.E. Smith. 1983. Polyoma virus transforming protein associates with the product of the c-*src* cellular gene. *Nature* **303:** 435–439.

DeCaprio, J.A., J.W. Ludlow, J. Figge, J.-Y. Shew, C.-M. Huang, W.-H. Lee, E. Marsilio, E. Paucha, and D.M. Livingston. 1988. SV40 large tumor antigen forms a specific complex with the product of the retinoblastoma susceptibility gene. *Cell* **54:** 275–283.

Dyson, N., P.M. Howley, K. Münger, and E. Harlow. 1989. The human papilloma virus-16 E7 oncoprotein is able to bind to the retinoblastoma gene product. *Science* **243:** 934–937.

Finlay, C.A., P.W. Hinds, and A.J. Levine. 1989. The p53 proto-oncogene can act as a suppressor of transformation. *Cell* **23:** 809–814.

Fujimura, F.K., P.L. Deininger, T. Friedmann, and E. Linney. 1981. Mutation near the polyoma DNA replication origin permits productive infection of F9 embryonal carcinoma cells. *Cell* **23:** 809–814.

Goldman, E. and T.L. Benjamin. 1975. Analysis of host range of nontransforming polyoma virus mutants. *Virology* **66:** 372–384.

Horwitz, B.H., A.L. Burkhardt, R. Schlegel, and D. DiMaio. 1988. 44-Amino-acid E5 transforming protein of bovine papillomavirus requires a hydrophobic core and specific carboxyl-terminal amino acids. *Mol. Cell. Biol.* **8:** 4071–4078.

Kalderon, D. and A.E. Smith. 1984. *In vitro* mutagenesis of a putative DNA binding domain of SV40 large-T. *Virology* **139:** 109–137.

Kalderon, D., B. Roberts, W.D. Richardson, and A.E. Smith. 1984. A short amino acid sequence able to specify nuclear localization. *Cell* **39:** 499–509.

Kaplan, D.R., M. Whitman, B. Schaffhausen, L. Raptis, R.L. Garcea, D.C. Pallas, T.M. Roberts, and L. Cantley. 1986. Phosphatidylinositol metabolism and polyoma-mediated transformation. *Proc. Natl. Acad. Sci.* **83:** 3624–3628.

Kaplan, P.L., S. Simon, and W. Eckhart. 1985. Polyomavirus middle T protein encoded by a retrovirus transforms nonestablished chicken embryo cells. *J. Virol.* **56:** 1023–1026.

Kmiecik, T.E. and D. Shalloway. 1987. Activation and suppression of pp60$^{c\text{-}src}$ transforming ability by mutation of its primary site of tyrosine phosphorylation. *Cell* **49:** 65–73.

Lanford, R.E. and J.S. Butel. 1984. Construction and characterization of an SV40 mutant defective in nuclear transport of T antigen. *Cell* **37:** 801–813.

Li, J.J. and T.J. Kelly. 1984. Simian virus 40 DNA replication in vitro. *Proc. Natl. Acad. Sci.* **81:** 6973–6977.

Loeken, M., I. Bikel, D.M. Livingston, and J. Brady. 1988. *Trans*-activation of RNA polymerase II and III promoters by SV40 small t antigen. *Cell* **55:** 1171–1177.

Markland, W. and A.E. Smith. 1987. Mutants of polyomavirus middle-T antigen. *Biochim. Biophys. Acta* **907:** 299–321.

Murakami, Y., C.R. Wobbe, L. Weissbach, F.B. Dean, and J. Hurwitz. 1986. Role of DNA polymerase α and DNA primase in simian virus 40 DNA replication *in vitro*. *Proc. Natl. Acad. Sci.* **83:** 2869–2873.

Phelps, W.C., C.L. Yee, K. Münger, and P.M. Howley. 1988. The human papillomavirus type 16 E7 gene encodes transactivation and transformaiton functions similar to those of adenovirus E1A. *Cell* **53:** 539–547.

Piwnica-Worms, H., K.B. Saunders, T.M. Roberts, A.E. Smith, and S.H. Cheng. 1987. Tyrosine phosphorylation regulates the biochemical and biological properties of pp60$^{c\text{-}src}$. *Cell* **49:** 75–82.

Rassoulzadegan, M., A. Cowie, A. Carr, N. Glaichenhaus, R. Kamen, and F. Cuzin. 1982. The roles of individual polyoma virus early proteins in oncogenic transformation. *Nature* **300:** 713–718.

Salzman, N.P. and P.M. Howley, eds. 1987. *The* Papovaviridae, vol. 2. *The Papillomaviruses.* Plenum Press, New York.

Salzman, N.P., V. Natarajan, and G. Selzer. 1986. Transcription of SV40 and polyoma virus and its regulation. In *The* Papovaviridae (ed. N.P. Salzman), vol. 1, pp. 27–98. Plenum Press, New York.

Tegtmeyer, P. 1972. SV40 DNA synthesis: The viral replicon. *J. Virol.* **10:** 591–598.

Tooze, J., ed. 1980. *Molecular biology of Tumor Viruses: DNA tumor viruses, 2nd edition.* Cold Spring Harbor Laboratory, Cold Spring Harbor, New York.

Treisman, R., A. Cowie, J. Favaloro, P. Jat, and R. Kamen. 1981b. The structure of the spliced mRNA's encoding polyoma virus early region proteins. *J. Mol. Appl. Genet.* **1:** 83–92.

Treisman, R., U. Novak, J. Favaloro, and R. Kamen. 1981a. Transformation of rat cells by an altered polyoma virus genome expressing only the middle T protein. *Nature* **292:** 595–600.

Vasseur, M., C. Kress, N. Montreau, and D. Blangy. 1980. Isolation and characterization of polyoma virus mutants able to develop in embryonal carcinoma cells. *Proc. Natl. Acad. Sci.* **77:** 1068–1072.

Whyte, P., H.E. Ruley, and E. Harlow. 1988a. Two regions of the adenovirus early region 1A proteins are required for transformation. *J. Virol.* **62:** 257–265.

Whyte, P., K.J. Buchkovich, J.M. Horowitz, S.H. Friend, M. Raybuck, R.A. Weinberg, and E. Harlow. 1988b. Association between an oncogene and an anti oncogene: The adenovirus E1A proteins bind to the retinoblastoma gene product. *Nature* **334:** 124–129.

Zullo, J., C.D. Stiles, and R.L. Garcea. 1987. Regulation of c-*myc* and c-*fos* mRNA levels by polyomavirus: Distinct roles for the capsid protein VP1 and the viral early proteins. *Proc. Natl. Acad. Sci.* **84:** 1210–1214.

9

Oncogenesis by DNA Viruses: Adenovirus

Thomas Shenk
Department of Molecular Biology
Princeton University
Princeton, New Jersey 08544

I. INTRODUCTION

The adenoviruses are widespread in nature. So far, 31 serotypes have been isolated from humans. They are not important human pathogens. In fact, several adenovirus gene functions suggest they have evolved mechanisms to maintain long-term, inapparent infections of their human hosts.

The adenoviruses contain a 36,000-bp DNA chromosome. Six transcription units are expressed during the early phase of infection, and three late units are activated at the onset of viral DNA replication. Each transcription unit gives rise to a variety of differentially spliced mRNAs. Two of the early units, E1A and E1B, comprise the adenovirus oncogenes (for recent reviews, see Berk 1986; Stillman 1986; Moran and Mathews 1987). All human adenoviruses tested are able to transform cultured rodent fibroblasts, and some serotypes can induce tumors in newborn hamsters and rats.

Like many other DNA tumor virus oncogenes, the adenovirus oncogenes function during normal virus growth. Thus, one of the strengths of the human adenoviruses as an experimental system is that the biochemical functions of their oncogenes can be studied both during viral replication in human cells and within transformed rodent cells.

II. ONCOGENIC POTENTIAL OF ADENOVIRUSES

Human adenoviruses have been divided into five groups, termed A through E, on the basis of DNA homology (Green et al. 1979). These groupings fit well with categorizations based on oncogenicity. Group A adenoviruses (e.g., Ad12, Ad18) are highly oncogenic, inducing tumors in most animals within 4 months; group B members (e.g., Ad3, Ad7) are weakly oncogenic, producing tumors within 4–18 months; and group C, D, and E viruses are nononcogenic. Ad9, a poorly studied group D virus, will, however, induce mammary fibroadenomas in certain strains of female rats (Jonsson and Ankerst 1977).

Both oncogenic and nononcogenic adenoviruses can transform cultured rodent cells. Morphologically, the transformants undergo a change from fibroblastic to an epitheloid, rounded appearance, and they tend to grow as dense, multilayered colonies. These cells can display a variety of the phenotypic hallmarks of transformation, including anchorage-independent growth, growth in reduced serum, and growth to higher saturation densities than normal.

Three main lines of evidence demonstrate that the adenovirus information necessary and sufficient for transformation is contained entirely in the E1A and E1B transcription units, which comprise only 11% of the viral genome. First, virus-transformed cell lines always contain and express the E1A and E1B genes, and some possess only those regions. Second, transfection of rodent cells in vitro with DNA has shown that fragments including only the E1A and E1B genes are sufficient to bring about transformation. Third, mutant viruses with alterations mapping to the E1A or E1B gene are generally unable to induce transformation.

Most of what we know about E1A and E1B function derives from studies of the nononcogenic group C adenoviruses, and, unless otherwise noted, discussion of these genes will focus on the Ad2 and Ad5 (group C) systems. It is likely that differences in the details of E1A and E1B function exist among more distantly related adenoviruses. In fact, such variability is at least in part responsible for the different oncogenic potentials of human adenoviruses.

III. ADENOVIRUS E1A GENE

A. Organization and Protein Products

The E1A transcription unit lies at the left end of the viral chromosome and is apparently the first gene to be expressed subsequent to infection. It encodes at least five mRNAs, which have common 5′ and 3′ ends but differ in their splicing patterns (Fig. 1A). The RNAs are named for their relative sedimentation coefficients: 13S, 12S, 11S, 10S, and 9S. Their corresponding polypeptides are often referred to by the number of amino acids they include. Thus, the 13S, 12S, 11S, 10S, and 9S mRNAs code for 289R, 243R, 217R, 171R, and 55R polypeptides. Nuclear localized products encoded by the four largest mRNAs have been identified in Ad2- or Ad5-infected cells; the 9S-coded 55R polypeptide has not been found within infected cells but can be synthesized in cell-free translation extracts. Perhaps the mRNA is poorly translated in vivo, or the 55R polypeptide turns over rapidly within infected cells. The exons of the four largest mRNAs all utilize the same reading frame. As a result, their protein products are highly related, differing only in the presence or absence of internal domains. The 9S mRNA switches into a second reading frame in its 3′ exon to produce its 55R product.

Comparison of the amino acid sequences of the largest E1A polypeptide from a variety of adenovirus serotypes reveals that the protein contains alternating conserved and nonconserved domains (van Ormondt et al. 1980). The evolutionarily conserved domains have been designated con-

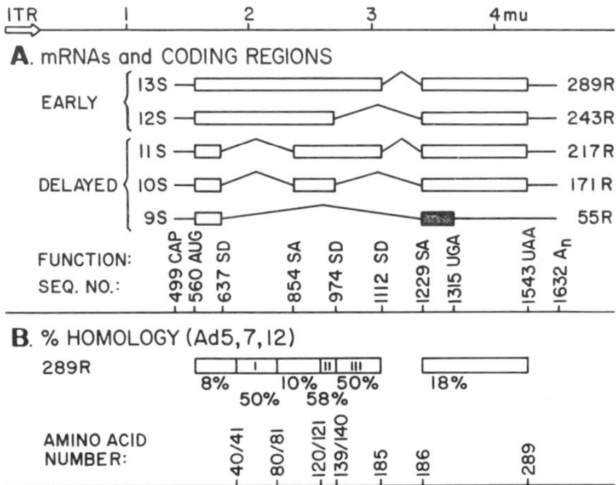

Figure 1 Diagram of the E1A gene and its products. (*A*) E1A mRNAs, coding regions, and polypeptides. mRNAs are indicated by lines, intervening sequences by caret symbols, and polypeptide coding regions by rectangles. Open and shaded rectangles discriminate two translational reading frames. (ITR) Inverted terminal repeat; (mu) map units; (R) amino acid residues; (CAP) mRNA cap site; (AUG) translational start codon; (SD) 5′ splice donor site; (SA) 3′ splice acceptor site; (UGA and UAA) translational termination codons; (A_n) poly(A) addition site. (*B*) Amino acid homology comparison of the 289R E1A polypeptide encoded by Ad5, Ad7, and Ad12 viruses. % Homologies indicate the portion of amino acids in a given domain that are identical among the three viruses. I, II, and III designate the three regions that are highly conserved.

served regions 1–3 (Fig. 1B) (Moran and Mathews 1987), and they are roughly delineated at the mRNA level by splice junctions. The 13S mRNA contains all three regions, the 12S mRNA contains regions 1 and 2 but not 3, the 11S species contains regions 2 and 3 but not 1, and the 10S species carries region 2 but not 1 or 3.

The organization of these four E1A mRNAs raises the question of why the virus produces four different mRNAs and proteins when the largest polypeptide contains all the information present in the other three. The 13S and 12S mRNAs are synthesized very early after infection, whereas the 11S, 10S, and 9S species appear later (Stephens and Harlow 1987; Ulfendahl et al. 1987). If the smaller E1A proteins mediate only a subset of E1A functions, temporal control of their expression could regulate which of the multiple E1A functions predominate at various times during the infectious cycle. It is also possible that the various E1A polypeptides are folded differently to position various domains in optimally functional configurations or locations. If this were true, one of the smaller polypeptides might mediate certain E1A functions more efficiently than the largest member of the set.

Each of the primary translation products of E1A mRNAs undergoes extensive posttranslational modification. By coupling immunoprecipitation with high-resolution, two-dimensional isoelectric focusing polyacrylamide gel electrophoresis, Harlow et al. (1985) resolved the E1A proteins into approximately 60 polypeptide species. The primary translation products of E1A mRNAs migrate faster and at a more basic isoelectric point than the modified forms. E1A proteins are phosphorylated, so many of the E1A forms likely result from differential phosphorylation. Other types of posttranslational modifications might contribute to the variety of E1A products, but, as yet, none have been described.

There is also good evidence that certain E1A proteins form relatively stable complexes with several host-cell proteins in both lytically infected and transformed human cells (Yee and Branton 1985; Harlow et al. 1986). Whyte et al. (1988) have recently shown that the product of the retinoblastoma gene is one of the host-cell proteins bound by the E1A polypeptides (see Chapter 11).

Thus, there are five known primary translation products of the E1A gene, about 60 modified forms arising at least in part from differential phosphorylation, and multiple cellular proteins that complex with subsets of the viral products. This sets the stage for genetic experiments that reveal a variety of functions attributable to the E1A gene.

B. E1A Functions

1. trans-*Activation*

The first insight to E1A function came from the analysis of mutant viruses carrying either point (Berk et al. 1979) or deletion mutations (Jones and

Shenk 1979) within the E1A coding region. These viruses fail to accumulate normal levels of mRNAs from the remaining viral transcription units, indicating than an E1A gene product is required to activate their expression. Subsequent experiments demonstrated that E1A products act at the level of transcription (Nevins 1981). Thus, the E1A gene encodes a transcriptional *trans*-activating activity. Such *trans*-activating genes have also been described for herpesviruses, papovaviruses, and retroviruses.

The *trans*-activation activity of the E1A gene maps to conserved region 3 (Fig. 1B), which is unique to the 13S and 11S mRNA species. Numerous observations support this conclusion. First, point mutations that block the ability of E1A to *trans*-activate map to this region. Second, viruses that carry cDNA copies of the 13S mRNA in place of the normal E1A gene activate early genes with normal efficiency, and products of the 11S mRNA, when expressed subsequent to transfection of cultured cells with a plasmid carrying an 11S cDNA, can activate transcription of other, cotransfected early viral genes. However, viruses carrying cDNA copies of 12S, 10S, or 9S mRNA, which do not encode region 3, fail to efficiently activate their early genes. Third, Lillie et al. (1987) have reported that a 49-amino-acid peptide corresponding to conserved region 3 can activate an E1A-inducible transcriptional control region when the peptide and test gene are simultaneously microinjected into HeLa cells. Apparently, the 49-amino-acid peptide is able to assume an active configuration outside the context of an intact E1A protein. Whereas earlier experiments indicated that conserved region 3 is necessary, this elegant experiment argues that the region is sufficient for *trans*-activation. The assay for activity was not quantitative, so it is not yet clear how the specific activity of the 49-amino-acid peptide compares to that of the intact 289R protein.

E1A gene products have been shown to activate several cellular genes (heat shock: Kao and Nevins 1983; β-tubulin: Stein and Ziff 1984) as well as a variety of cloned cellular genes when they are cotransfected with the E1A gene into a recipient cell. Given the somewhat promiscuous nature of the *trans*-activation activity, it is clear that E1A gene products have the potential to exert profound effects on cellular metabolism.

How do E1A gene products *trans*-activate? Some *trans*-activating proteins bind directly to specific DNA sequences within control regions. This does not appear to be the case for E1A proteins. Although the 289R E1A protein can be photo cross-linked to DNA fragments in vitro (Chatterjee et al. 1988) and contains a Zn^{++} finger motif, characteristic of many DNA-binding proteins (Miller et al. 1985), within conserved region 3, it exhibits no detectable sequence specificity in its binding. Given the lack of sequence-specific binding, the favored hypothesis has been that E1A products act to increase the concentration or activity of a set of essential transcription factors. It could accomplish this directly by interacting with and perhaps modifying a transcription factor, or it could function indirectly by inducing expression of a cellular gene that in turn activates or modifies a transcription factor. Spangler et al. (1987) have reported that the 289R E1A protein produced in *Escherichia coli* can stimulate activity of an E1A-dependent control region when added to a cell-free extract. This would argue for a direct effect of E1A, at least under certain conditions. It could modify the activity of a cellular factor by binding to it and forming a complex. Certain of the complexes of E1A proteins with cellular proteins identified by immunoprecipitation (Yee and Branton 1985; Harlow et al. 1986) are likely candidates for such interactions. Alternatively, E1A products could covalently modify cellular factors. Although no enzymatic activities have been reported for purified E1A proteins, this remains a reasonable hypothesis.

A variety of cellular transcription factors are influenced either directly or indirectly by E1A. The activity of a factor termed E2F that binds DNA sequences within the control regions of the adenovirus E1A and E2 genes is increased within virus-infected cells in an E1A-dependent fashion (Kovesdi et al. 1986). Mutational analysis indicates that another factor, which binds to the TATAA motif, endows E1A-responsiveness on the viral E1B gene (Wu et al. 1987) and the cellular *hsp*70 gene (Simon et al. 1988). E1A products can also enhance polymerase III transcription by increasing the activity of transcription factor IIIC (Hoeffler and Roeder 1985; Yoshinaga et al. 1986). Thus, E1A gene products can activate transcription by both polymerase II and III through several cellular factors. Biochemical characterization of the activated factors should provide clues to the mechanism of activation.

2. trans-*Repression*

Borelli et al. (1984) demonstrated that E1A proteins inhibit transcription of a rabbit β-globin gene linked to the polyomavirus enhancer domain. When HeLa cells were transfected with this recombinant gene, the polyomavirus enhancer element stimulated transcription of the β-globin gene. However, its activity was repressed if the cells were cotransfected with the E1A gene. The SV40 enhancer as well as an immunoglobulin heavy-chain enhancer and insulin enhancer are also inhibited by E1A gene products. The *trans*-repression activity might act at the same target sequence as a cellular repressor present in undifferentiated murine F9 teratocarcinoma cells. This possibility arises from study of a polyomavirus enhancer carrying a point mutation that enables it to function in undifferentiated F9 cells where the wild-type enhancer is inactive. Interestingly, the mutant enhancer also escapes repression by E1A proteins (Hen et al. 1986).

trans-Repression activity has been mapped by analysis of mutations to conserved regions 1 and 2 (Lillie et al. 1986, 1987; Schneider et al. 1987). The fact that two domains on the E1A protein are required for repression raises the possibility that two separate functions cooperate to repress sensitive genes. Alternatively, regions 1 and 2 may be folded together to form a single functional domain.

Both 13S and 12S E1A mRNAs encode proteins with *trans*-repression activities. The 11S and 10S species lack conserved region 1 and would be predicted to encode proteins unable to repress transcription.

There appears to be a difference between the E1A polypeptide domain that mediates *trans*-repression in group B (Ad3) and group C (Ad2 and Ad5) viruses (Larsen and Tibbetts 1987). An Ad3 variant was isolated that contained a sequence duplication within its E1A transcriptional control region and failed to produce detectable E1A mRNA after infection. It could be grown in 293 cells that contain and express the Ad5 E1A and E1B genes. Revertants of the duplication mutant were isolated that could again produce E1A mRNA and grow in normal human cell lines. The revertants contained inframe deletions within the E1A coding region at the junction of conserved regions 2 and 3 (Fig. 1B). Both group B (Ad3) and group A (Ad12) E1A proteins contain as many as 22 additional amino acids at this site as compared to the cognate group C (Ad2 and Ad5) protein. This region is required for efficient repression of the duplicated Ad3 E1A control element, and it might modify or enhance the *trans*-repression capabilities of E1A proteins encoded by the oncogenic group A and B adenoviruses.

As yet, the mechanism by which E1A proteins mediate repression of certain transcription units remains unclear. Since there is no evidence for sequence-specific DNA binding of the E1A proteins, it seems likely that repression, as already discussed for activation, results from interaction of E1A products with specific cellular regulatory proteins.

3. *Cell-cycle Regulation*

The 243R product coded by the 12S mRNA is not required for viral growth in HeLa cells but enhances viral replication in quiescent human cells (Spindler et al. 1985). Therefore, the E1A genes play a role in preparation of the cell for viral DNA replication. These functions are not well understood at the present, but they include stimulation of cellular DNA synthesis, induction of cell-cycle-specific gene products, and secretion of one or more growth factors. They appear to map to conserved regions 1 and 2 (Fig. 1B).

4. *Transformation*

Houweling et al. (1980) demonstrated that a DNA fragment carrying the Ad5 E1A gene could "immortalize" but not fully transform primary rodent cells. E1A-immortalized cells can be passaged indefinitely in culture without undergoing senescence. However, unlike cells transformed by the intact virus, they exhibit fibroblastic rather than epitheloid morphology, they are unable to grow to high cell densities, and they are not tumorigenic in nude mice. The E1A gene alone has little effect on the growth characteristics of established rodent cells (cells that are already immortalized) such as NIH-3T3 cells. However, if expressed at higher levels using a heterologous transcriptional control region, the E1A gene is indeed able to transform NIH-3T3 cells (Senear and Lewis 1986). The E1A gene, under control of its own regulatory elements, can cooperate with the E1B gene to fully transform both primary and established rodent cells. This implies that the two adenovirus oncogenes have distinct and complementary effects on the growth phenotype of transformed cells. The E1A gene can also cooperate with the activated Ha-*ras* oncogene to produce a fully transformed phenotype in primary rat cells (Ruley 1983; see also Chapter 12).

The 243R product of the 12S mRNA is as efficient as the 13S-coded 289R product in inducing immortalization of rodent cells, and both E1A proteins produce a fully transformed phenotype when cooperating with the Ha-*ras* oncogene. However, the products of the 11S and 10S E1A mRNAs fail to cooperate with Ha-*ras* in transformation of primary cells (Stephens and Harlow 1987; Ulfendahl et al. 1987), suggesting that conserved region 1, which they lack, is important for oncogene cooperation. Consistent with the results for cDNAs, mutational analysis indicates that conserved regions 1 and 2 but not 3 are required for E1A transforming ability (Lillie et al. 1986, 1987; Moran et al. 1986; Schneider et al. 1987). Thus, the two conserved domains required for *trans*-repression, but not the domain that mediates *trans*-activation, are required for transformation. The coincidence of domains required for *trans*-repression and transformation raises the intriguing possibility that E1A proteins exert their immortalization and transformation effects at least in part by repressing expression of one or more cellular genes.

A second model for the role of conserved regions 1 and 2 in transformation arises from the recent demonstration that binding of E1A proteins to the retinoblastoma susceptibility gene product is inhibited by deletions within these conserved E1A domains (P. Whyte et al., pers. comm.). Loss of retinoblastoma susceptibility gene function (e.g., by mutation) is strongly associated with the appearance of retinoblastomas or other tumors. Perhaps function of the retinoblastoma susceptibility gene product is inhibited by the binding of the E1A proteins. E1A proteins could exhibit their oncogenic activity, at least in part, by interfering with the normal function of a cellular "tumor suppressor" or "anti-oncogene."

IV. ADENOVIRUS E1B GENE

A. Organization and Protein Products

The E1B transcription unit lies immediately to the right of the E1A unit on the conventional adenovirus map. In fact, the E1A poly(A) addition site is only 67 bp upstream of the E1B 5′ cap site. The E1B unit encodes at least five mRNAs. As was the case for E1A, all E1B mRNAs share common 5′ and 3′ ends but differ in their splicing patterns (Fig. 2A). The two major E1B mRNAs have sedimentation coefficients of 22S and 13S, and there are also minor 14.5S, 14S, and 11S species (Pettersson et al. 1983; Lewis and Anderson 1987). All mRNAs except the 11S species encode a 175R polypeptide. The 22S, 14.5S, 14S, 13S, and 11S mRNAs encode 495R, 92R, 155R, 82R, and 168R polypeptides, respectively, that are translated from a different reading frame than the 175R moiety. All of the polypeptides have been identified within Ad2-infected human cells with the exception of the 92R species. Its existence is inferred from the structure of the 14.5S mRNA.

A sixth mRNA is encoded within the E1B region. It is derived from an independent, late transcription unit, and it encodes a minor structural component of the adenovirus virion called pIX. As such, it is unlikely that this mRNA and encoded protein are involved in the oncogenic activities of

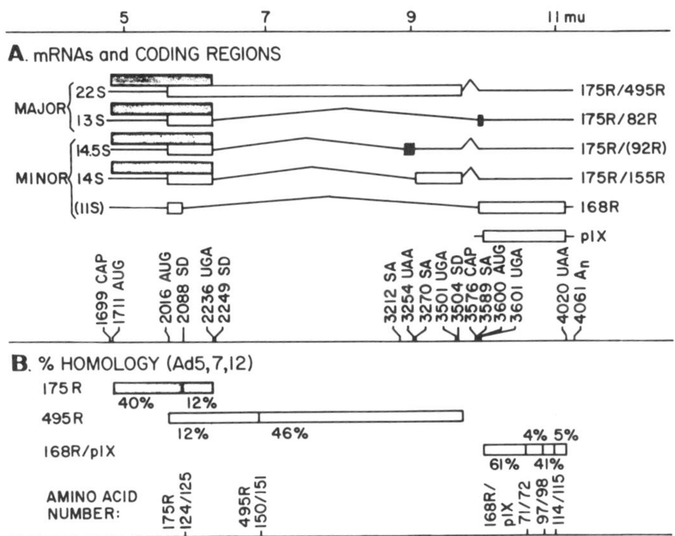

Figure 2 Diagram of the E1B gene and its products. (*A*) E1B mRNAs, coding regions, and polypeptides. mRNAs are indicated by lines, intervening sequences by caret symbols, and polypeptide coding regions by rectangles. Open, shaded, and solid rectangles discriminate the three translational reading frames. (mu) Map units; (R) amino acid residues; (CAP) mRNA cap site; (AUG) translational start codon; (SD) 5′ splice donor site; (SA) 3′ splice acceptor site; (UGA and UAA) translational termination codons; (A_n) poly(A) addition site. (*B*) Amino acid homology comparisons of E1B polypeptides encoded by Ad5, Ad7, and Ad12 viruses. % Homologies indicate the portion of amino acids in a given domain that are identical among the three viruses.

the E1B region. Interestingly, pIX is highly related in its sequence to the E1B-168R polypeptide (Fig. 2A).

Comparison of the amino acid sequence for the major 495R and 175R polypeptides among a variety of adenovirus serotypes indicates that each protein contains one evolutionarily conserved and one variable domain (van Ormondt and Hesper 1983). The variable domains roughly correspond to the portions of the two polypeptides whose coding regions overlap in different reading frames (Fig. 2B). This suggests, by analogy with the better-studied E1A polypeptides, that the key functional domains of the 495R and 175R polypeptides are those coded outside the region of overlap.

Immunofluorescence and fractionation studies indicate the E1B-495R polypeptide is localized predominantly in the nucleus of infected human cells, but it can also be detected outside the nucleus. The 495R protein is phosphorylated, and a portion of it is complexed with an adenovirus protein encoded by early region 4 (E4-34K polypeptide) within infected human cells (Sarnow et al. 1984). Generally, the E4-34K polypeptide is not produced within adenovirus-transformed cells. In fact, the E4 gene is often lost from Ad2 or Ad5 transformants. Thus, it is unlikely that the complex of E1B and E4 proteins plays a role in transformation.

Sarnow et al. (1982) have shown that a portion of the E1B-495R protein is complexed with the cellular p53 tumor antigen in transformed cells. The p53 polypeptide was first identified in a complex with SV40 large T antigen and can function as an oncogene in its own right. Curiously, the complex of Ad5 E1B-495R polypeptide and p53 is found in a cluster of 8-nm filaments adjacent to the nucleus within the cytoplasm (Zantema et al. 1985).

The 175R species is initially produced in small quantities and is then synthesized at higher levels after the onset of viral DNA replication. It is not detectably phosphorylated or glycosylated; it is present in both the nuclear envelope and cytoplasmic membranes early after infection, but accumulates exclusively in the nuclear envelope after the onset of DNA replication. The protein is present in both locations within transformed cells.

B. E1B Functions

1. E1B-495R: Control of mRNA Accumulation

Analysis of mutant viruses suggests that the E1B-495R polypeptide mediates shutoff of host-cell mRNA accumulation and enhances cytoplasmic accumulation of late viral mRNAs (Babiss et al. 1985; Pilder et al. 1986; Williams et al. 1986). Whereas host-cell mRNAs fail to be transported from nucleus to cytoplasm late after infection with wild-type virus, E1B-495R mutants fail to induce host-cell shutoff. In addition, these mutants display a reduced cytoplasmic accumulation of late viral mRNAs.

This reduction can be observed at a time when transcription rates are very nearly normal, suggesting the defect is primarily posttranscriptional. Viral RNAs present in the nucleus appear to be processed normally in mutant-infected cells, placing the defect after mRNA maturation and before its appearance in the cytoplasm. It seems likely that the E1B-495R polypeptide mediates two related reactions: inhibition of host-cell mRNA transport and enhancement of late viral mRNA transport from nucleus to the cytoplasm.

Two alternative models could explain how the E1B-495R polypeptide might control mRNA transport in virus-infected cells. The first postulates a signal in the sequence or structure of viral mRNA molecules, enabling them to be distinguished by the E1B-495R polypeptide from host mRNAs. However, since cellular mRNAs expressed from genes on the viral chromosome accumulate in the cytoplasm late after infection, it seems unlikely that a discrimination signal is built into viral mRNAs. The second model proposes that the E1B-495R polypeptide functions to localize the viral chromosome within the nucleus such that it can dominate transport of mRNAs to the cytoplasm at its local nuclear pore or so host-cell transcription units are displaced from sites at which efficient transport can occur. A localization model fits a variety of observations. (1) It predicts transport of nonviral mRNAs encoded by genes on the adenovirus chromosome. (2) Host-cell shutoff cannot occur if viral DNA replication is inhibited, and this is also consistent with the model. It could be necessary for the viral chromosome to colonize and dominate most, if not all, nuclear mRNA transport sites to achieve host shutoff. (3) A localization model can accommodate the recent demonstration that mRNAs of induced cellular genes can be transported late after adenovirus infection (Moore et al. 1987). Induction could localize a cellular gene so it can effectively compete with a viral chromosome that is attempting to dominate transport. Indeed, Blobel (1985) has hypothesized that transcriptionally active genes might be positioned near nuclear pore complexes.

A portion of the E1B-495R polypeptide is present in a complex with a 34-kD polypeptide encoded by adenovirus early region 4 (Sarnow et al. 1984). A mutant lacking the E4-34-kD coding region exhibits a phenotype similar to that displayed by E1B-495R mutants (Halbert et al. 1985), arguing that mRNA accumulation is controlled by the complex.

Some E1B-495R mutants (Stillman 1983), as well as the E4-34-kD mutant, exhibit delays in the onset of viral DNA replication subsequent to infection. The role of these proteins in DNA replication is almost certainly indirect, since neither is required in cell-free replication systems.

2. *E1B-175R: Down-regulation of Viral Replication*

Mutants containing lesions in the E1B-175R coding region exhibit pleiotropic phenotypes. The onset of cytopathic effect is dramatically accelerated, and both host-cell and viral DNAs are extensively degraded late after infection (Lai Fatt and Mak 1982; Pilder et al. 1984; Subramanian et al. 1984; White et al. 1984). E1A gene function is required for expression of the cytolytic phenotype (White and Stillman 1987). The E1A requirement is not merely to *trans*-activate another early viral gene, since infection of cells with a double E1A/E1B-175R mutant at high multiplicity activates viral gene expression and leads to viral replication without enhanced cytopathogenicity or DNA degradation. Therefore, E1A proteins play either a direct role in the phenotype, or, more likely, an indirect role, perhaps inducing or repressing cellular genes.

Viruses with mutations in the E1B-175R coding region also display a curious host-range effect (White et al. 1986). Whereas the mutants produce near-wild-type yields in HeLa cells, they grow considerably better than the wild-type virus in WI38 cells, a human diploid fibroblast line. The enhanced yield correlates with increased expression of early viral genes, suggesting the E1B gene product inhibits E1A function in WI38 cells.

It appears, then, that the E1B-175R polypeptide regulates the activity of E1A proteins. Normally, the protein serves to down-regulate the ability of E1A products to activate other viral genes (at least in WI38 cells) and to inhibit an E1A function that leads to enhanced cytopathogenicity and DNA degradation. The E1B product may enforce correct temporal control of the viral replication cycle or simply slow it down. A slow-down function could be very useful to the virus in its natural setting, allowing it to replicate and spread within its host at a moderate pace. This could prevent undue injury to the human host, facilitating a long-term inapparent infection.

3. *Additional E1B-coded Polypeptides*

The common 5′ splice site in 145S, 14S, 13S, and 11S mRNAs, as well as the unique 3′ splice site in the 14S mRNA, have been rendered nonfunctional by mutations, and these mutant viruses grow normally in HeLa cells and transform rat fibroblasts. Therefore, the minor E1B-coded polypeptides do not play an essential role during viral infection of cultured cells. Possibly they result from spurious splicing or translational initiation events, and they never play a meaningful role in adenovirus growth. Alternatively, the minor polypeptides could perform functions during viral growth in their normal human host that are not required during viral propagation in the laboratory.

4. *Transformation*

In the absence of E1A, the E1B gene does not exhibit detectable transforming activity. Cells are not transformed by an E1B gene whose expression is controlled by a constitutively active promoter (van den Elsen et al. 1983). The E1B gene very clearly contributes to the transformed phenotype when cooperating with E1A functions. The E1A region alone can immortalize primary rat cells at low frequency; when the E1 region is included, the frequency is substantially increased and a fully transformed phenotype results. There appear to be three components to the E1B contribution to transformation: a *cis*-acting activity that enhances E1A expression, the E1B-495R polypeptide, and the E1B-175R moiety.

E1A-immortalized cells express E1A mRNAs at substantially reduced levels as compared to transformants that contain both E1A and E1B genes. Jochemsen et al. (1987) have shown that presence of the E1B gene leads to enhanced transcription of the E1A gene and that the transcriptional activation is dependent to a large extent on a physical linkage between the E1A and E1B units. This suggests that a *cis*-acting element is present within the E1B coding region that enhances E1A transcription, possibly a 3′ enhancer element. Since a DNA segment that contains the entire E1A gene but only the 5′ half of the E1B gene can elicit complete transformation, it seems likely the element resides in the 5′ half of the E1B unit.

Barker and Berk (1987) have constructed an Ad2 variant carrying two mutations within the E1B-495R gene: an amino-terminal nonsense mutation and a deletion within the region coding the carboxy-terminal half of the molecule. Both the virus and its DNA are extremely defective for transformation, demonstrating that the E1B-495R polypeptide is required for transformation by adenovirus. Evidently, very low levels of the amino-terminal half of the molecule are sufficient for E1B-495R transforming activity. Rowe et al. (1984) have described Ad5 transformed hamster cell lines that contain only the amino-terminal half of the 495R coding region. It was not possible to detect a fragment of the 495R polypeptide within these cells by immunoprecipitation, yet, when these cells were injected into hamsters, they elicited production of antitumor serum able to precipitate the normal 495R protein. Therefore, a truncated form of the 495R polypeptide must have been expressed within the transformed hamster cells at undetectable levels.

The role played by the E1B-495R polypeptide in transformation is not at all clear. There is no reason to assume its transforming role is related to its ability to regulate viral and cellular mRNA transport during productive infection, since the E4-34-kD polypeptide, which is also required for this lytic function (Halbert et al. 1985), is not usually present in transformed cells. As mentioned above, the 495R polypeptide is complexed with the product of the cellular p53 oncogene in rodent cells (Sarnow et al. 1982). The association stabilizes the cellular transforming protein. Perhaps the 495R polypeptide contributes to transformation through its interaction with the p53 protein.

Although it is clear from mutant studies that the 175R polypeptide is required for adenovirus transformation, its role is, again, uncertain. Perhaps, in this case, the role of the protein in viral replication is identical to its role in transformation, and it regulates one or more E1A activities. An

E1A-regulatory role predicts the 175R polypeptide probably would not cooperate with other nuclear oncogenes such as polyomavirus large T antigen or the cellular p53 tumor antigen to transform cells. Work of Subramanian et al. (1985) demonstrates that the 175R polypeptide is responsible for the ability of adenovirus transformants to grow in medium containing low concentrations of Ca^{++} ions. Perhaps the E1B-175R polypeptide contributes to transformation by modulating intracellular Ca^{++} storage and release, an important growth process.

V. ADENOVIRUS TUMOR INDUCTION AND THE HOST IMMUNE SYSTEM

Rat cells transformed by the highly oncogenic Ad12 are invariably tumorigenic in newborn syngeneic rats, whereas cells transformed by the nononcogenic Ad2 or Ad5 generally are not able to produce tumors. A portion of Ad2-transformed rat cells become tumorigenic in immunosuppressed rats (Gallimore 1972), suggesting that cells transformed by nononcogenic adenoviruses are rejected by the host's immune system. The thymus-dependent cellular immune system plays a key role in this rejection. Newborn hamsters, which have not yet developed a thymus-dependent immune response, are susceptible to tumor formation by Ad2 transformants. Thymectomized hamsters remain susceptible, but normal animals become resistant to challenge at the age of 3 weeks when their thymic response has developed (Cook and Lewis 1979).

The thymus-dependent, cytotoxic T lymphocyte (CTL) response that prevents tumor formation by cells transformed with nononcogenic adenoviruses is inhibited by an Ad12 E1A gene product (Bernards et al. 1983). Schrier et al. (1983) demonstrated that Ad12-transformed rat cells express reduced quantities of class I major histocompatibility (MHC) antigen on their cell surface. CTLs can recognize foreign antigens at the cell surface only in the context of class I MHC molecules. It follows, then, that tumor cells expressing reduced quantities of class I antigens might well evade CTL-mediated lysis. Consistent with this interpretation, tumorigenicity of Ad12-transformed mouse cells was inhibited after introduction by transfection of a functional class I MHC gene that could not be down-modulated by the Ad12 E1A proteins (Tanaka et al. 1985). These observations can nicely explain the resistance of Ad12 transformants to a CTL response. The Ad12 E1A gene represses expression of the class I antigen which, in turn, prevents recognition of the transformed cell by CTLs. Given the ability of the E1A gene to repress transcription of certain genes, it seems probable that expression of class I antigen might be repressed at the level of transcription, but this has not been clearly established as yet. Furthermore, not all Ad12 transformants have proven resistant to CTL lysis (Mellow et al. 1984).

It is clear that thymus-mediated immune surveillance plays a key role in preventing tumor formation by cells transformed with nononcogenic adenoviruses. However, additional factors must play a role, since Ad2 transformed cells are markedly less efficient than their Ad12 counterparts in their ability to form tumors in athymic nude mice that are unable to mount a CTL response. This effect is likely mediated by a class of immunologically nonspecific cytotoxic lymphocytes termed natural killer (NK) cells. Nude mice contain functional NK cells, and Ad2 transformants are much more susceptible to NK cell-mediated lysis than their Ad12 counterparts (Cook et al. 1982; Raska and Gallimore 1982). Analysis of cells transformed by either mutant viruses or chimeric Ad5/Ad12 viruses indicates that susceptibility or resistance to NK killing is governed by the E1A gene (Sawada et al. 1985; Cook et al. 1987). Expression of the Ad5 E1A gene leads to cytolysis, whereas expression of the Ad12 homolog does so at greatly reduced efficiency. It is not yet known if an E1A polypeptide serves directly as a target on the cell surface, or whether E1A gene products indirectly mediate susceptibility by influencing expression of cellular genes.

Recent experiments have shown that the E1A genes of Ad2, Ad5, and Ad12 induce susceptibility of transformants to lysis by tumor necrosis factor (Chen et al. 1987), and a 14.7-kD polypeptide encoded by early region 3 of the adenovirus genome protects against cytolysis (Gooding et al. 1988). Thus, adenovirus gene products encoded outside the E1A and E1B regions might play roles in the complex interactions that take place during virus-mediated tumor formation. Roles for additional genes fit well with the observation that recombinant Ad5 viruses carrying an Ad12 E1A and E1B region in place of the corresponding Ad5 domain fail to induce tumors in newborn rats or hamsters (Bernards et al. 1984).

VI. SUMMARY

The human adenoviruses encode two oncogenes, E1A and E1B, that cooperate to oncogenically transform rodent cells. A variety of functions have been described for the E1A gene, including transcriptional *trans*-activation and *trans*-repression. Mutational analyses suggest the transforming capacity of the E1A gene coincides with its ability to bind to the cellular retinoblastoma protein. The E1B gene encodes two products that play roles in transformation, but neither of their biochemical functions in oncogenesis is well delineated. Available evidence suggests the E1B-495R polypeptide might contribute to transformation by binding the product of the cellular p53 oncogene, and the E1B-175R protein appears to regulate one or more activities of the E1A gene. The E1A gene can transform cells in the absence of E1B when expressed at high levels or in cooperation with the *ras* oncogene. The E1B unit has not been shown to have oncogenic activity in the absence of the E1A gene.

Although all adenoviruses can transform cells in culture, only certain serotypes are oncogenic. Some, but not all, cells transformed by oncogenic adenoviruses are resistant to lysis by cytotoxic T lymphocytes. Resistance appears to result from an E1A-mediated reduction in cell-surface levels of class I major histocompatability antigen. In contrast, cells transformed by nononcogenic adenoviruses contain normal levels of class I antigen, and, as a result, are lysed by cytotoxic T lymphocytes. Furthermore, the E1A gene of nononcogenic adenoviruses somehow makes transformed cells susceptible to NK cell-mediated cytolysis. Thus, oncogenicity of adenovirus-transformed cells appears to be controlled primarily through interactions with the host's cellular immune defenses.

ACKNOWLEDGMENTS

I thank my colleagues who kindly communicated unpublished results and who read and commented on this manuscript. The author is an American Cancer Society Research Professor.

REFERENCES

Babiss, L.E., H.S. Ginsberg, and J.E. Darnell. 1985. Adenovirus E1B proteins are required for accumulation of late viral mRNA and for effects on cellular mRNA translation and transport. *Mol. Cell. Biol.* **5:** 2552–2558.

Barker, D.D. and A.J. Berk. 1987. Adenovirus proteins from both E1B reading frames are required for transformation of rodent cells by viral infection and DNA transfection. *Virology* **156:** 107–121.

Berk, A.J. 1986. Functions of adenovirus E1A. *Cancer Surv.* **5:** 367–387.

Berk, A.J., F. Lee, T. Harrison, J. Williams, and P.A. Sharp. 1979. Pre-early adenovirus 5 gene product regulates synthesis of early viral gene mRNAs. *Cell* **17:** 935–944.

Bernards, R., M.G.W. deLeeuw, M. Vaessen, A. Houweling, and A.J. van der Eb. 1984. Oncogenicity by adenovirus is not determined by the transforming region only. *J. Virol.* **50:** 847–853.

Bernards, R., P.I. Schrier, A. Houweling, J.V. Bos, A.J. van der Eb, M. Zijlstra, and C.J.M. Melief. 1983. Tumorigenicity of cells transformed by adenovirus type 12 by evasion of T-cell immunity. *Nature* **305:** 776–779.

Blobel, G. 1985. Gene gating: A hypothesis. *Proc. Natl. Acad. Sci.* **82:** 8527–8529.

Borrelli, E., R. Hen, and P. Chambon. 1984. Adenovirus-2 E1A products repress enhancer-induced stimulation of transcription. *Nature* **312:** 608–612.

Chatterjee, P.K., M. Bruner, S.J. Flint, and M.L. Harter. 1988. DNA-binding properties of an adenovirus 289R E1A protein. *EMBO J.* **7:** 835–841.

Chen, M.-J., B. Hoskin, J. Strickler, J. Gorniak, M.A. Clark, P.J. Johnson, M. Mitcho, and D. Shalloway. 1987. Induction by E1A oncogene expression of cellular susceptibility to lysis by TNF. *Nature* **330:** 581–583.

Cook, J.L. and A.M. Lewis. 1979. Host response to adenovirus 2-transformed hamster embryo cells. *Cancer Res.* **39:** 1455–1461.

Cook, J.L., J.B. Hibbs, and A.M. Lewis, Jr. 1982. DNA virus transformed hamster cell-host effector cell interactions: Level of resistance to cytolysis is correlated with tumorigenicity. *Int. J. Cancer* **30:** 795–803.

Cook, J.L., D.L. May, A.M. Lewis, Jr., and T.A. Walker. 1987. Adenovirus E1A gene induction of susceptibility to lysis by natural killer cells and activated macrophages in infected rodent cells. *J. Virol.* **61:** 3510–3520.

Gallimore, P.H. 1972. Tumor production in immunosuppressed rats with cells transformed *in vitro* by Ad2. *J. Gen. Virol.* **62:** 99–102.

Gooding, L.R., L.W. Elmore, A.E. Tollefson, H.A. Brady, and W.S.M. Wold. 1988. A 14,700 MW protein from the E3 region of adenovirus inhibits cytolysis by tumor necrosis factor. *Cell* **53:** 341–346.

Green, M., J.K. MacKay, W.S.M. Wold, and P. Rigden. 1979. Thirty-one human adenovirus serotypes (Ad1-31) form five groups (A–E) based upon DNA genome homologies. *Virology* **93:** 481–492.

Halbert, D.N., J.R. Cutt, and T. Shenk. 1985. Adenovirus early region 4 encodes functions required for efficient DNA replication, late gene expression and host cell shutoff. *J. Virol.* **56:** 250–257.

Harlow, E., B.R. Franza, and C. Schley. 1985. Monoclonal antibodies specific for adenovirus early region 1A proteins: Extensive heterogeneity in early region 1A products. *J. Virol.* **55:** 533–546.

Harlow, E., P. Whyte, B.R. Franza, and C. Schley. 1986. Association of adenovirus early region 1A proteins with cellular polypeptides. *Mol. Cell. Biol.* **6:** 1579–1589.

Hen, R., E. Borrelli, C. Fromental, P. Sassone-Corsi, and P. Chambon. 1986. A mutated polyoma virus enhancer which is active in undifferentiated embryonal carcinoma cells is not repressed by adenovirus-2 E1A products. *Nature* **321:** 249–251.

Hoeffler, W.K. and R.G. Roeder. 1985. Enhancement of RNA polymerase III transcription by the E1A gene product of adenovirus. *Cell* **41:** 955–963.

Houweling, A., P.J. van den Elsen, and A.J. van der Eb. 1980. Partial transformation of primary rat cells by the left most 4.5% fragment of adenovirus 5 DNA. *Virology* **105:** 537–550.

Jochemsen, A.G., L.T.C. Peltenburg, M.F.W. tePas, C.M. deWit, J.L. Bos, and A.J. van der Eb. 1987. Activation of adenovirus 5 E1A transcription by region E1B in transformed primary rat cells. *EMBO J.* **6:** 3399–3405.

Jones, N. and T. Shenk. 1979. An adenovirus type 5 early gene function regulates expression of other early viral genes. *Proc. Natl. Acad. Sci.* **76:** 3665–3669.

Jonsson, N. and J. Ankerst. 1977. Studies on adenovirus 9-induced mammary fibroadenomas in rats and their malignant transformation. *Cancer* **39:** 2513–2519.

Kao, H.-T. and J.R. Nevins. 1983. Transcriptional activation and subsequent control of the human heat shock gene during adenovirus infection. *Mol. Cell. Biol.* **3:** 2058–2065.

Kovesdi, I., R. Reichel, and J.R. Nevins. 1986. Identification of a cellular transcription factor involved in E1A *trans*-activation. *Cell* **45:** 219–228.

Lai Fatt, R.B. and S. Mak. 1982. Mapping of an adenovirus function involved in the inhibition of DNA degradation. *J. Virol.* **42:** 969–977.

Larsen, P.L. and C. Tibbetts. 1987. Adenovirus E1A gene products have a functional domain associated with enhancer-targeted autorepression. *Proc. Natl. Acad. Sci.* **84:** 8185–8189.

Lewis, J.B. and C.W. Anderson. 1987. Identification of adenovirus type 2 early region 1B proteins that share the same amino terminus as do the 495R and 155R proteins. *J. Virol.* **61:** 3879–3888.

Lillie, J.W., M. Green, and M.R. Green. 1986. An adenovirus E1A protein region required for transformation and transcriptional repression. *Cell* **46:** 1043–1051.

Lillie, J.W., P.M. Loewenstein, M.R. Green, and M. Green. 1987. Functional domains of adenovirus type 5 E1A proteins. *Cell* **50:** 1091–1100.

Mellow, G.H., B. Fohring, J. Dougherty, P.H. Gallimore, and K. Raska, Jr. 1984.

Tumorigenicity of adenovirus transformed rat cells and expression of class I major histocompatibility antigen. *Virology* **134:** 460–465.

Miller, J., A.D. McLachlan, and A. Klug. 1985. Repetitive zinc-binding domains in the protein transcription factor IIIA from *Xenopus* oocytes. *EMBO J.* **4:** 1609–1614.

Moore, M., J. Schaack, S.B. Baim, R.I. Morimoto, and T. Shenk. 1987. Induced heat shock mRNAs escape the nucleocytoplasmic transport block in adenovirus-infected HeLa cells. *Mol. Cell. Biol.* **7:** 4505–4512.

Moran, E. and M.B. Mathews. 1987. Multiple functional domains in the adenovirus E1A gene. *Cell* **48:** 177–178.

Moran, E., B. Zerler, T.M. Harrison, and M.B. Mathews. 1986. Identification of separate domains in the adenovirus E1A gene for immortalization activity and the activation of virus early genes. *Mol. Cell. Biol.* **6:** 3470–3480.

Nevins, J.R. 1981. Mechanism of activation of early viral transcription by the adenovirus E1A gene product. *Cell* **26:** 213–220.

Pettersson, U., A. Virtanen, M. Perricaudet, and G. Akusjarvi. 1983. The messenger RNAs from the transforming region of human adenoviruses. *Curr. Top. Microbiol. Immunol.* **109:** 107–123.

Pilder, S., J. Logan, and T. Shenk. 1984. Deletion of the gene encoding the adenovirus type 5 E1B-21K polypeptide leads to degradation of viral and host cell DNA. *J. Virol.* **52:** 664–671.

Pilder, S., M. Moore, J. Logan, and T. Shenk. 1986. The adenovirus E1B-55K transforming polypeptide modulates transport or cytoplasmic stabilization of viral and host cell mRNAs. *Mol. Cell. Biol.* **6:** 470–476.

Raska, K., Jr. and P.H. Gallimore. 1982. An inverse relation of the oncogenic potential of adenovirus-transformed cells and their sensitivity to killing by syngeneic natural killer cells. *Virology* **123:** 8–18.

Rowe, D.T., P.E. Branton, S. Yee, S. Bacchetti, and F.L. Graham. 1984. Establishment and characterization of hamster cell lines transformed by restriction endonuclease fragments of adenovirus 5. *J. Virol.* **49:** 162–170.

Ruley, H.E. 1983. Adenovirus early region 1A enables viral and cellular transforming genes to transform primary cells in culture. *Nature* **304:** 602–606.

Sarnow, P., Y.S. Ho, J. Williams, and A.J. Levine. 1982. Adenovirus E1b-58kd tumor antigen and SV40 large tumor antigen are physically associated with the same 54kd cellular protein in transformed cells. *Cell* **28:** 387–394.

Sarnow, P., P. Hearing, C.W. Anderson, D.N. Halbert, T. Shenk, and A.J. Levine. 1984. Adenovirus E1B-55K tumor antigen is physically associated with an E4-25K protein in productively infected cells. *J. Virol.* **49:** 692–700.

Sawada, Y., B. Fohring, T. Shenk, and K. Raska. 1985. Tumorigenicity of adenovirus-transformed cells: Region E1A of adenovirus 12 confers resistance to natural killer cells. *Virology* **147:** 413–421.

Schneider, J.F., F. Fisher, C.R. Coding, and N.C. Jones. 1987. Mutational analysis of the adenovirus E1A gene: The role of transcriptional regulation in transformation. *EMBO J.* **6:** 2053–2060.

Schrier, P.I., R. Bernards, T.J. Vaessen, A. Houweling, and A.J. van der Eb. 1983. Expression of class I major histocompatibility antigens switched off by highly oncogenic adenovirus 12 in transformed rat cells. *Nature* **305:** 771–775.

Senear, A.W. and J.B. Lewis. 1986. Morphological transformation of established rodent cell lines by high-level expression of the adenovirus type 2 E1A gene. *Mol. Cell. Biol.* **6:** 1253–1260.

Simon, M.C., T.M. Fisch, B.J. Benecke, J.R. Nevins, and N. Heintz. 1988. Definition of multiple, functionally distinct TATA elements, one of which is a target in the *hsp*70 promoter for E1A regulation. *Cell* **52:** 723–729.

Spangler, R., M. Bruner, B. Dalie, and M.L. Harter. 1987. Activation of adenovirus promoters by the adenovirus E1A protein in cell-free extracts. *Science* **237:** 1044–1046.

Spindler, K.R., C.Y. Eng, and A.J. Berk. 1985. An adenovirus early region 1A protein is required for maximal viral DNA replication in growth-arrested human cells. *J. Virol.* **53:** 742–750.

Stein, R.W. and E.B. Ziff. 1984. HeLa cell β-tubulin gene transcription is stimulated by adenovirus 5 in parallel with viral early genes by an E1A-dependent mechanism. *Mol. Cell. Biol.* **4:** 2792–2801.

Stephens, C. and E. Harlow. 1987. Differential splicing yields novel adenovirus 5 E1A mRNAs that encode 30kd and 35kd proteins. *EMBO J.* **6:** 2027–2035.

Stillman, B.W. 1983. The replication of adenovirus DNA. *UCLA Symp. Mol. Cell. Biol.* **10:** 381–393.

———. 1986. Functions of the adenovirus E1B tumor antigens. *Cancer Surv.* **5:** 389–404.

Subramanian, T., M. Kuppuswamy, and G. Chinnadurai. 1985. An adenovirus 2-coded tumor antigen located on the endoplasmic reticulum and nuclear envelope is required for growth of transformed cells in Ca^{2+}-deficient medium. *Mol. Cell. Biol.* **5:** 3297–3300.

Subramanian, T., M. Kuppuswamy, S. Mak, and G. Chinnadurai. 1984. Adenovirus *cyt*$^+$ locus, which controls cell transformation and tumorigenicity, is an allele of lp$^+$ locus, which codes for a 19 kilodalton tumor antigen. *J. Virol.* **52:** 336–343.

Tanaka, K., K.J. Isselbacher, G. Khoury, and G. Jay. 1985. Reversal of tumorigenicity by expression of a major histocompatibility complex class I gene. *Science* **228:** 226–230.

Ulfendahl, P.J., S. Linder, J.-P. Kreivi, K. Nordquist, C. Sevensson, H. Hultberg, and G. Akusjarvi. 1987. A novel adenovirus-2 E1A mRNA encoding a protein with transcription activation properties. *EMBO J.* **6:** 2037–2044.

van den Elsen, P., A. Houweling, and A. van der Eb. 1983. Expression of region E1b of human adenovirus in the absence of E1A is not sufficient for complete transformation. *Virology* **128:** 377–390.

van Ormondt, H. and B. Hesper. 1983. Comparison of the nucleotide sequences of early region E1B DNA of human adenoviruses types 12, 7 and 5 (subgroups A, B and C). *Gene* **21:** 217–226.

van Ormondt, H.J. Maat, and R. Dijkema. 1980. Comparison of nucleotide sequences of the early E1a regions for subgroups A, B and C of human adenoviruses. *Gene* **12:** 63–76.

White, E. and B. Stillman. 1987. Expression of adenovirus E1B mutant phenotypes is dependent on the host cell and on synthesis of E1A proteins. *J. Virol.* **61:** 426–435.

White, E., B. Faha, and B. Stillman. 1986. Regulation of adenovirus gene expression in human W138 cells by an E1B-encoded tumor antigen. *Mol. Cell. Biol.* **6:** 3763–3773.

White, E., T. Grodzicker, and B.W. Stillman. 1984. Mutations in the gene encoding the adenovirus early region 1B 19,000 molecular weight tumor antigen cause the degradation of chromosomal DNA. *J. Virol.* **42:** 410–419.

Whyte, P., K.J. Buchkovich, J.M. Horowitz, S.H. Friend, M. Raybuck, R.A. Weinberg, and E. Harlow. 1988. Association between an oncogene and an anti-oncogene: The adenovirus E1A proteins bind to the retinoblastoma gene product. *Nature* **334:** 124–129.

Williams, J., B.D. Karger, Y.D. Ho, C.L. Castiglia, T. Mann, and S.J. Flint. 1986. The adenovirus E1B 495R protein plays a role in regulating the transport and stability of the viral late messages. *Cancer Cells* **4:** 275–284.

Wu, L., D.S. Rosser, M.C. Schmidt, and A. Berk. 1987. A TATA box implicated in E1A transcriptional activation of a simple adenovirus 2 promoter. *Nature* **326:** 512–515.

Yee, S. and P. Branton. 1985. Detection of cellular proteins associated with human adenovirus type 5 early region 1A polypeptides. *Virology* **147:** 142–153.

Yoshinaga, S., N. Dean, M. Han, and A.J. Berk. 1986. Adenovirus stimulation of transcription by RNA polymerase III: Evidence for an E1A dependent increase in transcription factor III C concentration. *EMBO J.* **5:** 343–354.

Zantema, A., P.I. Schrier, A. Davis-Oliver, T. van Laar, R.T.M.J. Vaessen, and A.J. van der Eb. 1985. Adenovirus serotype determines association and localization of the large E1B tumor antigen and cellular tumor antigen p53 in transformed cells. *Mol. Cell. Biol.* **5:** 3084–3091.

10
Oncogenesis by Herpesviruses

Elliott Kieff and David Liebowitz
Departments of Medicine and Microbiology
and Molecular Genetics
Harvard Medical School
Boston, Massachusetts 02115

I. INTRODUCTION

The herpesviruses are a diverse group of animal viruses that share common structural features and common intracellular replication schemes (for review, see Roizman and Batterson 1985). Herpesviruses have a complex core consisting of linear, double-strand DNA (100–250 kbp) wrapped around a protein toroid, a proteinaceous nucleocapsid shell, and an outer

Oncogenes and the Molecular Origins of Cancer.

protein phospholipid bilayer membrane with glycoprotein spikes. Almost every animal species has at least one herpesvirus that is highly prevalent in that species and rarely, if ever, infects heterologous species. Herpesviruses vary widely in oncogenicity. Epstein-Barr virus (EBV), a human herpesvirus, and Marek's disease virus (MDV), a chicken herpesvirus, are important causes of natural malignancies. EBV has been the dominant focus of oncogenic herpesvirus research and is therefore considered in greatest depth throughout this review. Another herpesvirus, herpesvirus saimiri (HVS), does not cause naturally occurring malignancies but efficiently induces tumors in heterologous species and transforms cells in vitro. Most herpesviruses, however, have little obvious direct oncogenic activity.

A. Properties of Herpesviruses Relevant to Their Oncogenicity

Despite the wide variation in oncogenicity among herpesviruses, there are themes in herpesvirus oncogenicity that derive from the common properties of the herpesvirus class. Herpesviruses have more than 50 genes. They replicate their DNA within the cell nucleus and assemble into nucleocapsids at the nuclear periphery. The cell nucleus is profoundly altered by virus replication. Nucleoli are disaggregated. Chromatin becomes marginated to the nuclear periphery. Cell DNA transcription and replication cease as virus DNA transcription and replication proceed. Nucleocapsids are initially enveloped by budding through the inner lamella of the nuclear membrane. Herpesvirus replication also produces profound changes in the cell cytoplasm. Translation of cell RNAs is inhibited and replaced by translation of viral RNAs. Cytoplasmic membranes are extensively modified by insertion of virus-encoded proteins, including several prominent glycoproteins. The extensively modified endoplasmic reticulum appears to be a conduit for virus egress. Because herpesvirus replication so extensively alters the infected cell, cell death always accompanies virus replication. Consequently, oncogenic transformation cannot occur unless a herpesvirus has infected a cell in which the virus does not replicate.

In fact, virus replication is not an invariant outcome of infection. In complex multicellular organisms, cells fixed in different stages of growth or differentiation differ in their permissivity for herpesvirus replication. During primary virus infection, herpesviruses disseminate widely through many tissues and infect some cells in which the virus can persist without replicating. This state of nonreplicative virus infection is termed latency. For most herpesviruses, little is known about the virus or cell genes involved in initiating and maintaining latent infection. Latency has been studied most extensively in the case of EBV infection of B lymphocytes, because in this instance, the latently infected cell is transformed by the infection and consequently can be grown in vitro as an "immortalized," latently infected, cell line (Pope et al. 1968).

The EBV genome usually persists in latently infected cells as a covalently closed circular episome (Lindahl et al. 1976). Herpesvirus DNAs have a repeat DNA sequence at both termini that is recognized by a virus enzyme(s) that cleaves and packages unit length linear viral DNA from newly replicated concatenates. Following the infection, the viral DNA usually circularizes through end ligation of the terminal repeat DNA. EBV encodes a nuclear protein in latently infected cells (EBNA-1) that binds to a specific DNA sequence (ori-P) and facilitates persistence of the newly circularized DNA as an episome (Rawlins et al. 1985; Reisman et al. 1985). Less commonly, the entire EBV genome can persist in cells by integration of the EBV terminal repeat DNA into nonhomologous chromosomal DNA (Matsuo et al. 1984). Episomal and linear integrated EBV DNA may coexist in the same cell. In latently infected cells, EBV episomes are replicated by cell DNA polymerase early in S phase (Hampar et al. 1974).

Latent persistence is important for herpesviruses because changes in the latently infected cell can render it permissive for herpesvirus replication. The virus can then replicate and infect other cells of the same host or other hosts. Herpesvirus infections are usually acquired early in life, and almost all individuals become infected and thereafter are immune. Since most people are immune, herpesviruses cannot sustain themselves in a population by spreading from one acutely infected person to nonimmune, susceptible people. Reactivation of virus from latency is therefore important in herpesvirus epidemiology, since reactivation provides a necessary long-term source of virus that can infect the next generation of immunologically naive individuals.

The fact that herpesviruses can infect some cells and persist in a latent state makes it possible for herpesviruses to persistently alter cells. With regard to oncogenesis, it is important to note that there would be positive selection for genes that would increase the number of latently infected cells by causing cell proliferation. In this light, the oncogenic properties of herpesviruses can be seen as a manifestation of the significance of latent infection to the herpesvirus life cycle.

The specter of cells transformed by herpesvirus infection having been raised, it should be pointed out from the start that there are important characteristics of such cells that distinguish them from uninfected tumor cells transformed through overexpression or mutation of a cellular oncogene. First, since transformation is dependent on virus gene products that differ from cell gene products, the viral proteins are potential targets for natural immunity, for immunotherapy against the transformed cells, or for chemotherapy. Second, since the virus genome is resident within the cell, induction of virus replication would destroy the transformed cell from within.

B. General Strategies in Oncogenic Transformation

Given their ability to persist within some cells in a latent state, there are several mechanisms by which herpesviruses could cause oncogenic transformation. First, herpesvirus DNA can integrate into cell DNA (Matsuo et al. 1984) and thereby alter expression or function of a crucial cell gene. Since herpesviruses can undergo many cycles of reactivated infection in a single host, there is ample opportunity for a rare, untoward integration to occur. Integration of herpesvirus DNA into cell DNA has so far not been demonstrated to have caused malignant transformation. Second, following the model of papovaviruses or adenoviruses (reviewed in Chapters 8 and 9), herpesviruses could transform cells through expression of protein(s) that alters expression or function of a putative key cell growth regulatory gene. Herpesviruses encode for a number of proteins that regulate their gene expression and could affect cell gene expression as well. In herpesvirus replication, virion protein(s) up-regulates herpesvirus immediate early genes. Immediate early genes turn on early genes, which then turn on late genes. Gene expression is also negatively affected by high-level accumulation of proteins of the same class or through expression of proteins encoded by a later viral gene class. Genes of various classes are interspersed through herpesvirus genomes. Thus, *trans*-regulation of gene expression and *cis*-acting, DNA regulatory elements recognized by these factors are important features of virus replication that could incidentally alter expression of cell genes, and in the absence of cytocidal virus replication, cause malignancy. Third, despite the conservation of some genes among herpesviruses, herpesvirus genomes vary in size from 100 to 250 kb. Given this genome variability and an identical virion structure, most herpesviruses should have room for incorporating additional DNA. Moreover, recombination is remarkably efficient in cells in which herpesviruses are replicating. Therefore, it is not surprising that DNA with extensive homology to cell DNA has been identified in some herpesvirus genomes (Heller et al. 1985; Trimble et al. 1988). In fact, EBV or HVS genes associated with cell transformation are not found in other herpesviruses and may have arisen from cell DNA.

II. HERPESVIRUS ONCOGENESIS

Herpesviruses cause some malignancies in humans, nonhuman primates, frogs, fish, and birds. Some of these oncogenic herpesviruses and other herpesviruses not as yet demonstrated to be naturally oncogenic can induce tumors in experimental animals or can oncogenically transform cells in culture. The oncogenic activity of the viruses is a necessary context for evaluating the oncogenic properties of specific virus genes.

A. Epstein-Barr Virus, B Lymphomas, and Nasopharyngeal Carcinoma

Almost everyone becomes infected with EBV before age 25 (Fig. 1) (for reviews, see Henle and Henle 1979; Klein 1979; Tosato and Blaese 1985; Dambaugh et al. 1986a; de The and Zeng 1986). Primary EBV infection begins in the pharyngeal epithelium, which is permissive for virus replication. Virus soon spreads to subepithelial B lymphocytes where it establishes latent infection. Primary EBV infection is the usual cause of infectious mononucleosis. In people with normal immune function, acute infectious mononucleosis is a self-limited, EBV-infected, B-lymphocyte proliferative disease.

1. *Effects of EBV on B-lymphocyte Growth*

Latently infected B lymphocytes circulate at a high frequency (1 in 10^2–10^3 B lymphocytes) in acute infectious mononucleosis and at a low frequency (1 in 10^6) in the peripheral blood of latently infected humans after primary infection. EBV-infected B lymphocytes constitutively express cell activation markers, secrete growth factors, and respond to T-cell-derived or B-cell-derived growth factors in the same way as B lymphocytes transiently activated by antigen or mitogen (Gordon et al. 1985; Calender et al. 1987; Swendeman and Thorley-Lawson 1987; Cairns et al. 1988; Tosato et al. 1988; for review, see Kishimoto and Hirano 1988). Some of these growth factors or growth factor receptors are B-lymphocyte-specific. Latently infected human B lymphocytes, in vivo, or normal human B lymphocytes infected by EBV, in vitro, differ fundamentally from normal B lymphocytes because they are able to proliferate indefinitely when maintained in vitro. Uninfected B lymphocytes can only be maintained in vitro for a limited number of cell divisions, even in the presence of mitogens, helper cells, or growth factors. EBV-infected lymphocytes are also tumorigenic on inoculation into nude mouse brains but not in nude mouse skin or subcutaneous tissue. Moreover, experimental primary EBV infection uniformly induces acute, malignant, fatal, polyclonal, EBV-infected cell lymphoproliferation in some species of new world primates, particularly cottontop tamarins (Shope et al. 1973). The fact that EBV infection acutely and efficiently enables lymphocytes to proliferate in vitro and to form tumors in nude mouse brain or in cottontop tamarins indicates that EBV must express an oncogene(s) in primate B lymphocytes. Consistent with the oncogenic activity of EBV in experimental infection of primate B lymphocytes, latently infected proliferating B lymphocytes can be tumorigenic in

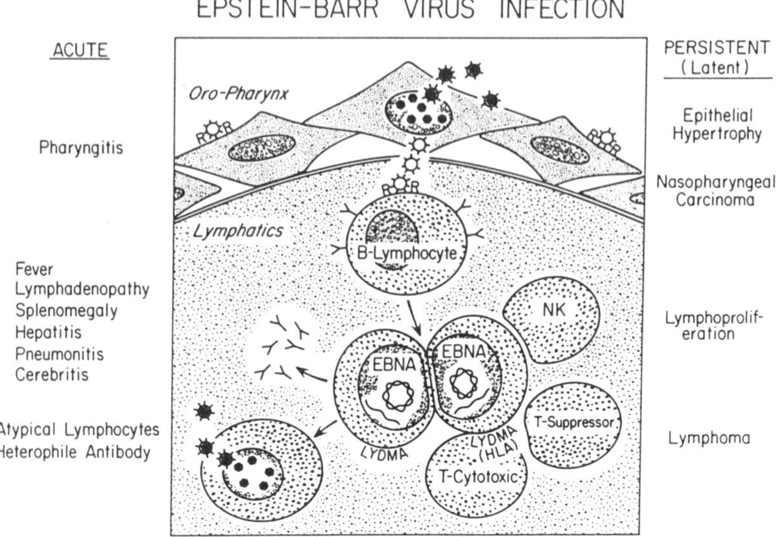

Figure 1 Pathogenesis of EBV infection. Virus is spread in saliva and attaches to a CR2-related receptor on oropharyngeal epithelial cells. EBV replicates epithelial cells, kills the infected cell, and invades adjacent epithelial cells and B lymphocytes. Infection of epithelial cells remains persistent (low-level replication), whereas infection in B lymphocytes is largely latent. Latently infected B lymphocytes contain EBV episomes or integrated EBV genomes and are driven to proliferate and secrete Ig. In B lymphocytes, EBV gene expression is restricted to six nuclear protein genes (EBNAs) and an integral membrane protein (LMP). EBNA-1 is necessary for episome persistence. EBNA-2 specifically *trans*-activates CD23, a putative B cell growth factor or growth factor receptor, and LMP is a transforming oncogene. The proliferation of EBV-infected B lymphocytes is initially contained by NK and B-cell specific suppressor cells. Late in acute infection, an HLA and antigen-specific cytotoxic T-cell response develops. Antigens recognized by cytotoxic T cells, initially given the acronym LYDMA, include LMP and EBNA proteins. In immune-suppressed people or in experimental marmoset infection, polyclonal EBV-infected B-cell lymphoproliferation can be malignant. EBV-infected B lymphocytes can become progressively more malignant. Increased c-*myc* expression is an important event in the evolution of uniclonal malignant lymphomas. EBV can also cause benign epithelial proliferation in patients with AIDS and is an etiologic agent in most nasopharyngeal cancer.

humans with markedly abnormal immune responses (Robinson et al. 1980; Pelicci et al. 1986; Weisenberger and Purtillo 1986; for review, see Cleary et al. 1986). EBV causes malignant B-lymphocyte proliferation in children with X-linked immunodeficiency, rare children of either sex without known genetic predisposition, patients with acquired immunodeficiency syndrome (AIDS), or patients undergoing high-level immunosuppression for organ transplantation. However, EBV-infected B lymphocytes are found regularly in normal humans, and EBV is not a common cause of B lymphomas in normal people. This is because natural killer (NK) cells, T-suppressor cells, and HLA and antigen-restricted T-cytotoxic and T-suppressor cells restrict virus-infected B-lymphocyte proliferation at different stages of human EBV infection (for reviews, see Tosato and Blaese 1985; Rickinson 1986).

2. *Interaction between EBV and c*-myc

Some immune-deficient patients at risk for fatal EBV-infected cell lymphoproliferative disease recover and succumb later to proliferation of a clone of EBV-infected cells carrying an 8:14, 8:2, or 8:22 reciprocal translocation (Weisenberger and Purtillo 1986; for review, see Cleary et al. 1986). The translocations result in constitutively high c-*myc* expression (for review, see Showe and Croce 1987). In vitro, induction of constitutive c-*myc* expression in EBV-infected lymphocytes by gene transfer enhances their anchorage-independent growth (Lombardi et al. 1987). c-*myc* is an oncogene that can immortalize primary rat embryo fibroblasts in vitro (Land et al. 1983). In transgenic animals, c-*myc* expression in B lymphocytes or breast cells under control of tissue-specific regulators results in uniclonal malignancies (Adams et al. 1985; Leder et al. 1986). The fact that in transgenic mice only a rare B lymphocyte or breast cell with altered c-*myc* expression becomes malignant indicates that malignancy in vivo is a multistep process in which constitutive c-*myc* expression is a significant step. The role of continued EBV gene expression in a malignant human B lymphocyte that has progressed beyond constitutive c-*myc* activation is uncertain. Other malignant immature B lymphocytes that have c-*myc* translocation without EBV infection have additional abnormalities on chromosome 1, providing in vivo evidence for accessory functions in c-*myc*-associated malignancies (Berger and Bernheim 1985).

Almost all Burkitt's lymphomas in equatorial Africa are uniclonal malignancies characterized by both latent EBV infection and c-*myc* translocation (zur Hausen et al. 1970; for review, see Berger and Bernheim 1985). These tumors occur several years after primary EBV infection, preferentially among individuals with abnormally high antibody responses to EBV, presumably indicative of more severe primary or persistent EBV infection. Immunosuppressive effects of malaria and malnutrition appear to facilitate oncogenicity. In Burkitt's tumors, EBV infection of each tumor cell is uniclonal with regard to virus repeat DNA sequences that otherwise vary among different cells infected with a single virus isolate (Raab-Traub and Flynn 1986; Brown et al. 1988). This indicates that EBV contributes quite specifically to an early stage of lymphomagenesis. A unifying hypothesis is that EBV increases the pool of proliferating lymphocytes, that immunosuppression allows a further expansion of the number of EBV-infected B lymphocytes, and that c-*myc* translocation is an important subsequent step that creates a more malignant cell. Beyond a general increase in B-lymphocyte proliferation, EBV has a specific proliferative effect on the immature B lymphocyte that is rearranging its immunoglobulin genes, and in this way, may specifically predispose to c-*myc* recombination.

3. Other EBV-associated Malignancies

Similar data to those linking EBV to African Burkitt's lymphoma indicate that EBV is a significant etiologic factor in human anaplastic nasopharyngeal carcinoma (NPC), a common tumor among some Mongoloid populations, and in papillomatous proliferation of epithelial cells ("hairy leukoplakia") in AIDS patients. NPC occurs with a high incidence in genetically susceptible Chinese, long after primary EBV infection. High EBV antibody titers correlate with subsequent NPC (Zeng and de The 1985). NPC tumors are monoclonal in latent EBV infection (Klein 1979; Raab-Traub and Flynn 1986).

B. MDV and T-cell Lymphomas

MDV is the major cause of domestic chicken and turkey lymphomas (for reviews, see Kato and Hirai 1985; Calnek 1986). Cell-free transmission of virus to uninfected birds rapidly produces fatal T-cell lymphoma. Tumor cells contain the MDV genome, and virus replication in tumor tissue is not unusual. T-cell immune surveillance is believed to determine whether the outcome of MDV infection is malignant or benign. Initial experiments indicate that MDV can transform T lymphocytes in vitro (Nakajima et al. 1987). Early identification of MDV led to the development and widespread use of live attenuated MDV vaccines. These vaccines have been remarkably effective in preventing Marek's-disease-associated lymphomas in domestic flocks.

C. Lucke Herpesvirus

Lucke herpesvirus was discovered in microscopic sections of frog "Lucke type" renal adenocarcinomas (for review, see Mizell 1985). These malignant renal tumors occur with a high frequency in frogs from northern United States and southern Canada, where the frog population is particularly dense. The virus emerges from a latent state within tumor cells when frogs are held at 5°C. Injection of virus into embryos obtained from frogs that otherwise have a low tumor incidence results in a high rate of tumor induction. In fact, the stage and site of embryo injection is predictive of the site of renal tumor development.

D. Herpes Simplex Virus and Cervical Cancer

Considerable attention has been given over the years to the epidemiologic association between herpes simplex virus type 2 (HSV-2) and cervical cancer. Although studies of HSV-2 antibody prevalence in various human populations have shown a good correlation with cervical cancer incidence, there has been little evidence of herpesvirus DNA, RNA, or proteins in tumor tissue.

E. Herpesvirus Saimiri or Aeteles and Experimental Induction of T-cell Lymphoma

HVS and herpesvirus aeteles are examples (as yet enigmatic) of herpesviruses that are not associated with malignant disease of their natural host species (squirrel monkeys) but are highly oncogenic in experimental infection of other primate species. In owl monkeys, cottontop or common marmosets, or in New Zealand white rabbits, HVS rapidly induces malignant T-cell lymphomas. Susceptible animals die of virus-induced leukemic lymphoma in 30–40 days. The virus genome is found in a latent state in the lymphoma cells. In vitro, HVS immortalizes owl monkey, cottontop marmoset, or common marmoset T lymphocytes, albeit with a low efficiency (Desrosiers et al. 1986).

III. MECHANISMS OF HERPESVIRUS ONCOGENESIS

A. Herpesvirus Oncogenes

EBV infection in vitro immediately and efficiently transforms normal resting human B lymphocytes into perpetually proliferating lymphoblasts. In addition, EBV induces acute, uniformly fatal, malignant lymphoma in vivo in cottontop marmosets. Therefore, EBV is an acute, efficiently transforming herpesvirus. It is therefore likely to carry one or more genes that are necessary and sufficient for malignant B-lymphocyte growth transformation. These EBV genes (and those necessary for latent persistence but not other genes necessary for virus replication) would be expected to be expressed in latently infected, growth-transformed lymphocytes.

1. EBV Gene Expression in Transformed Lymphocytes

A schematic diagram of the RNAs expressed from the EBV episome in latently infected growth-transformed lymphocytes is shown in Figure 2 (for review, see Dambaugh et al. 1986a). The most significant aspects of latent-cycle EBV gene expression are: (1) Two small, non-polyadenylated, largely self-complementary RNAs are transcribed by cellular RNA polymerase III. These RNAs (designated EBERs) are the most abundant EBV

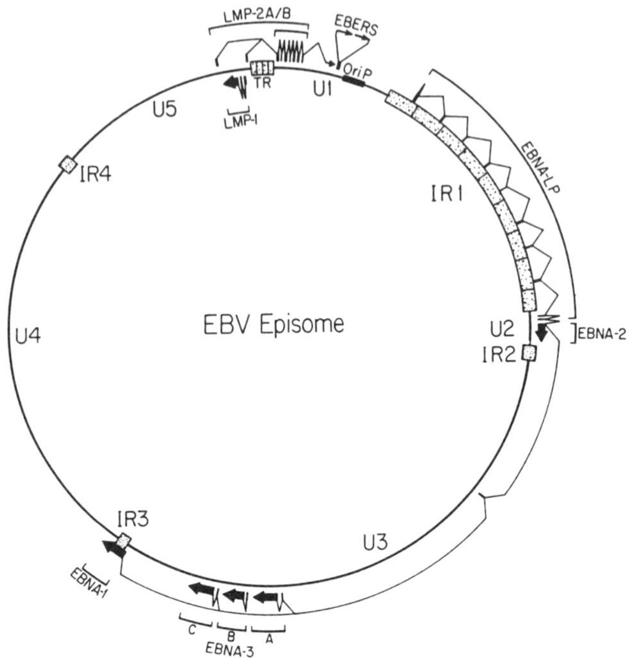

Figure 2 EBV episome, transcripts, and mRNAs in latent B-lymphocyte infection. Largely unique (U1–U5) and highly repetitive internal (IR1–4) or terminal (TR) repeat DNA domains, the episomal replicon (ori-P) and the location of exons encoding EBV nuclear proteins (EBNA-1, -2, -3A, -3B, -3C, -LP) or LMP genes are indicated by dark boxes. The five EBNA protein mRNAs are spliced from a single transcript. EBNA-LP is encoded by an open reading frame at the beginning of the mRNAs, whereas EBNA-1, -2, -3A, -3B, or -3C are encoded by open reading frames at the ends of their respective mRNAs. The EBERs are two small, nonpolyadenylated, palindromic RNAs transcribed in latent or productive infection. LMP-2A/B are predicted proteins based on cDNA clone sequence. Unlike the other latent infection proteins, LMP-2A/B have not been directly demonstrated to be expressed in each latently infected cell.

RNAs in latent infection and increase in abundance as EBV DNA replicates late in productive infection. These small RNAs are largely confined to the nucleus and may function in mRNA processing (Glickman et al. 1988). A second possibility (based on their similarity to adenovirus viral-associated RNAs) is that the EBERs affect mRNA translation. (2) An RNA polymerase II promoter in the large internal EBV DNA repeat element (IR1) initiates transcription of at least 130 kb of the R strand of EBV DNA. The transcript initiated by the IR1 promoter gives rise to five different mRNAs. The five mRNAs have a common 1.5-kb leader largely derived from IR1 that contains a long open reading frame encoding a

35-kD nuclear protein (EBNA-LP, for EBNA mRNA leader protein) that is expressed in all latently infected cells (Bodescot and Perricaudet 1986; Sample et al. 1986; Wang et al. 1987a). EBNA-LP is associated with subnuclear, nonnucleolar particles. After the EBNA-LP termination codon, the five mRNAs have short, untranslated domains and a second long open reading frame. The second long open reading frames encode five different nuclear proteins. Three of these (EBNA-3A, -3B, and -3C) are nonnucleolar, nucleoplasmic proteins that are encoded by three distantly homologous, tandemly placed, EBV DNA segments (Petti and Kieff 1988; Petti et al. 1988). The two other 3′ open reading frames are single exons that encode EBNA-1 or EBNA-2. EBNA-1 is pan-nuclear in localization, whereas EBNA-2 localizes to large, extranucleolar nuclear aggregates. (3) A second polymerase II promoter (near the right end of the linear virion EBV genome map) initiates transcription of the L strand of episomal EBV DNA. This transcript encodes an integral membrane protein, designated LMP for latent infection membrane protein (Hennessy et al. 1984). (4) Two other mRNAs have been detected in latently infected lymphocytes (Laux et al. 1988; Sample et al. 1989). On the basis of cDNA sequence and the properties of the in vitro translation product, these two mRNAs encode integral membrane proteins that differ only in the presence or absence of an amino-terminal domain. Although the proteins have not as yet been demonstrated to exist in latently infected cells, they are tentatively designated LMP-2A and LMP-2B. In summary, a complex repertoire of two short nonpolyadenylated RNAs and at least six and possibly as many as eight mRNAs encode six nuclear proteins and at least one and possibly as many as three integral membrane proteins in EBV-transformed cells.

2. *Activity of EBV Genes in Transformation*

The potential activity of these EBV genes in maintaining EBV latency and cell growth transformation has been assayed by gene transfer into a variety of cells, including primary or early passage continuous rodent fibroblast or human B-lymphoma cell lines. Human B lymphocytes are a necessary assay for EBV transforming gene(s), since EBV latent infection turns on specific B-lymphocyte activation markers, growth factors, or growth factor receptors that are unlikely to be turned on in other cells (Gordon et al. 1985; Amen et al. 1986; Calendar et al. 1987; Swendeman and Thorley-Lawson 1987; Wang et al. 1987b; Cairns et al. 1988; for review, see Kishimoto and Hirano 1988). Fortunately, immature B lymphomas that occur outside of Africa frequently lack EBV, still grow in vitro, and are at a similar stage of differentiation as EBV-infected African Burkitt's tumors. These non-EBV-infected Burkitt's-type lymphoma cell lines are useful for assaying EBV effects on some human B-lymphocyte-specific genes. Despite transformation by altered c-*myc* expression and possibly by activation of other oncogenes (duplications and rearrangements of chromosome 1 are common), these cells frequently grow as single cells to a low cell density and express some B-cell activation markers, growth factors, or growth factor receptors and not others. EBV infection in vitro causes these cells to grow in tight clumps to a higher cell density and turns on many of the cell activation markers expressed in EBV growth-transformed lymphoblastoid cell lines (LCLs). In a third type of assay, latently infected B lymphocytes are useful for analyzing EBV DNA *cis*-acting elements in latent infection or transformation, because they already express EBV *trans*-acting elements (Reisman et al. 1985).

a. EBNA-1. EBNA-1 was the first EBV latent infection-associated protein demonstrated to have a specific function. An EBV repetitive DNA element, ori-P, was defined as being important in episome maintenance because its presence on a plasmid enables the plasmid to persist as an episome in latently infected cells (Reisman et al. 1985). EBNA-1 expression is sufficient for stable maintenance of ori-P-containing plasmids in some human cell lines. EBNA-1 is highly sequence-specific and binds directly to ori-P (Rawlins et al. 1985). In binding to ori-P, EBNA-1 also *trans*-activates an ori-P-associated enhancer activity. EBNA-1 has no apparent direct effect on primary or continuous rodent fibroblast growth alone or in cotransfection with *myc* or *ras* and has no effect on human B-lymphoma cell growth (Dambaugh et al. 1986b; Wang et al. 1987b).

b. EBNA-2. Several lines of evidence indicate that EBNA-2 is directly involved in B-lymphocyte transformation. First, there is a correlation between EBV strain EBNA-2 genotype and cell transformation. EBV strains carrying one EBNA-2 allele transform cells inefficiently, and the transformed cells initially grow poorly in vitro (Dambaugh et al. 1986a; Rickinson et al. 1987). Second, in two instances, EBV strains have been identified that are deleted for EBNA-2. The resultant viruses are unable to initiate growth transformation (Miller et al. 1974). These viruses can infect and persist in cells that are already immortalized. Thus, the defect is more likely to be due to lack of a transforming function than to lack of a genome maintenance or virus replication repressor function. Recombinants between an EBNA-2-deleted virus and another defective EBV genome were selected by their ability to initiate growth transformation. All of the transforming recombinants had a reconstituted EBNA-2 gene (Skare et al. 1985). (All of the recombinants also had a reconstituted EBNA-LP gene, complicating the interpretation of the experiment.) Third, in Rat-1, a continuous fibroblast cell line, EBNA-2 expression following gene transfer enabled the cells to grow, albeit at a reduced rate, in medium supplemented with less serum than is required for similar growth of Rat-1 control cells (Dambaugh et al. 1986b). Fourth, liposome-mediated EBNA-2 gene transfer into normal human lymphocytes caused a transient increase in DNA synthesis (Volsky et al. 1984). Fifth, in Burkitt's lymphoma cells, EBNA-2 caused the cells to grow in tight clumps and activated high-level expression of the B-cell activation marker, CD23 (Wang et al. 1987a). CD23 mRNA level is increased in those cells in which EBNA-2 is expressed. Other B-lymphocyte activation markers are not affected by EBNA-2 expression. CD23 is an unusual plasma membrane glycoprotein first identified as a prominent B-cell surface antigen induced by EBV infection (Sugden and Metzenberg 1982). Its expression is also induced by mitogen stimulation or by interleukin-4. Some monoclonal antibodies to CD23 block low-molecular-weight B-cell growth factor adsorption to B lymphocytes, whereas other CD23-specific monoclonal antibodies mimic the effects of B-cell growth factor, suggesting that CD23 is a receptor for this growth factor. A soluble CD23 component, cleaved from CD23 by proteases, also has B-cell growth factor activity (Swendeman and Thorley-Lawson 1987; Cairns et al. 1988). Thus, CD23 has at least two roles in B-cell growth regulation. Interestingly, EBNA-2 has no transforming or immortalizing activity in primary rodent fibroblast cells alone or in combination with *myc* or *ras* (F. Wang et al., unpubl.).

c. LMP. Following gene transfer, LMP has transforming effects in continuous rodent fibroblast cell lines, but not in primary rodent fibroblasts, alone or in combination with *myc* or *ras* (Wang et al. 1985, 1988a). In Rat-1 or NIH-3T3 cells, LMP alters cell morphology and enables cells to grow in medium supplemented with low serum. In Rat-1 cells, LMP also causes loss of contact inhibition so that cells heap up in monolayer culture. LMP also causes Rat-1 or BALB/c-3T3 cells to lose their anchorage dependence so that they clone with a high efficiency in soft agar. Growth of BALB/c cells in soft agar correlates quantitatively with the extent of LMP expression. Rat-1 cells expressing LMP are tumorigenic in nude mice, whereas control Rat-1 cells are nontumorigenic.

LMP also alters the growth of non-EBV-infected Burkitt's-type tumor lymphoblasts when it is expressed at the appropriate level in such cells following gene transfer (Wang et al. 1988b). In two lymphoblast cell lines, LMP caused increased intracellular free calcium, cell clumping, increased villous projections, increased transferrin receptor, and LFA-1, ICAM-1, and LFA-3 expression. In one cell line, the LMP-converted cells exhibited increased acid production and increased TGF-β responsiveness. Despite the increased intracellular free calcium, calcium influx or efflux was unaffected by LMP expression. Interestingly, LMP expression does not simply cause increased plasma membrane translocation of adhesion molecules, but also induces higher levels of LFA-1 mRNA.

LMP induction of B-lymphocyte adhesion molecules is important because of at least two countervailing effects on tumor cell growth. First, homotypic B-lymphocyte adhesion (to other EBV-infected B lymphocytes) facilitates cell growth. Since proliferating B lymphocytes secrete autocrine growth factors that cross-feed each other, proliferation is heavily dependent on the effective cell concentration. Second, in vivo, the elimination of EBV-transformed B lymphocytes is important to host survival and therefore to the survival of latent virus. Increased conjugate formation with T cells as a consequence of EBV LMP induction of LFA-3 (and to a lesser extent, LFA-1) results in increased efficiency of immune T-cell surveillance and increased elimination of latently infected growth-transformed B lymphocytes.

Several lines of evidence suggest that the effects of LMP are in part mediated through linkage of the cell plasma membrane and the cell's cytoskeleton. First, in EBV-transformed lymphocytes or in non-EBV-infected Burkitt's lymphoma cells or continuous rodent fibroblasts in which LMP is expressed from heterologous promoters, LMP is, in part, concentrated in small patches at the cell periphery (Liebowitz et al. 1986, 1987). Live cell protease cleavage studies indicate that about one-third of the cell LMP is in the plasma membrane. A similar fraction of the cell's LMP resists detergent extraction, further indicating its association with the cytoskeleton. In B lymphocytes, newly translated LMP is not associated with the cytoskeleton. However, LMP is rapidly phosphorylated on serine and threonine residues. The phosphorylated LMP then associates with the cytoskeleton. These peripheral LMP patches colocalize with vimentin patches. Neither tubulin nor actin colocalizes with LMP in these cells. The peripheral, plasma membrane LMP patches are dependent on LMP rather than vimentin, since in non-EBV-infected Burkitt's tumor lymphoblasts without LMP, vimentin does not aggregate at the cell periphery until LMP is expressed following gene transfer. Expression of LMP in a Burkitt's tumor line that constitutively lacks vimentin still results in LMP patching (Liebowitz and Kieff 1989). However, vimentin can also determine LMP localization, since upon colcemid-induced vimentin relocalization, LMP relocalizes to the internal, perinuclear, vimentin rings and coils caused by colcemid treatment. The colocalization of LMP and vimentin is not dependent on any other EBV gene, since LMP and vimentin colocalize in Burkitt's lymphoma cells in which LMP is the only EBV gene. Surprisingly, vimentin expression is induced in B-lymphoma cells by EBV infection or by LMP expression following gene transfer (Birkenbach et al. 1989). The interaction between LMP and vimentin may be mediated through another plasma membrane cytoskeletal element, since expression of LMP in a Burkitt's tumor cell line that constitutively lacks vimentin results in LMP plasma membrane patches and induction of adhesion molecule expression.

A second line of evidence for the physiologic significance of the LMP–plasma membrane–cytoskeletal association arises from studies revealing the lack of effect of an amino-terminally deleted LMP in BALB/c rodent fibroblasts or in non-EBV-infected Burkitt's tumor cells in which LMP has profound effects (Wang et al. 1988a,b). The deletion mutant protein associates with cytoplasmic membranes but not with patches in the plasma membrane or with vimentin.

d. Model for EBV Induction of B-lymphocyte Transformation. The simplest hypothesis that incorporates these observations into a coherent model of B-cell transformation by EBV (Fig. 3) is that EBNA-2 causes enhanced B-lymphocyte proliferation by specifically *trans*-activating CD23 expression (and possibly also expression of an as yet unidentified autocrine B-cell growth factor[s]). CD23 mediates B-cell proliferation through its actions as a soluble autocrine B-cell growth factor or as a receptor for a low-molecular-weight B-cell growth factor (presumably also EBV induced). EBV LMP is a cooperating transforming protein. LMP aggregates in the B-lymphocyte plasma membrane (through an as yet unidentified link between the plasma membrane and vimentin) and acts to up-regulate

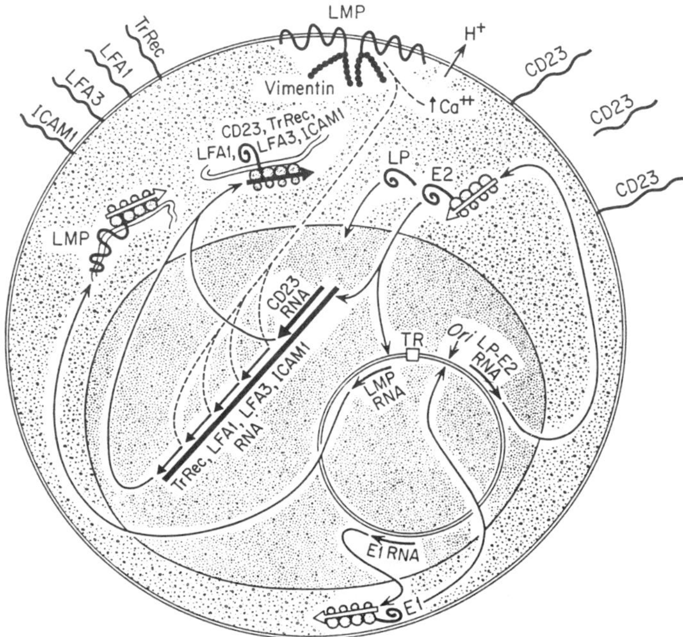

Figure 3 EBV gene effects in maintaining latent infection and B-lymphocyte growth transformation. EBV nuclear protein 1 binds to ori-P, maintaining the EBV episome. EBV nuclear protein 2 specifically *trans*-activates CD23 and not other B-cell activation markers. EBV LMP patches in the cell plasma membrane where it is associated with (and induces higher level expression of) vimentin. EBV LMP raises the lymphocyte intracellular free calcium and induces activation markers including transferrin receptor, LFA-3, LFA-1, and ICAM-1, and, in some cells, CD23. LMP also alters lymphoblast TGF-β responsiveness.

intracellular free calcium and a number of B-cell-specific and non-B-cell-specific activation markers. Pulse-chase experiments suggest that one function of the cytoskeletal associated LMP may be to stabilize the protein in the plasma membrane and lengthen its half-life (Liebowitz et al. 1987). Because of its unusual primary amino acid sequence, broad spectrum of effects, and plasma membrane association, LMP might be expected to act in membrane transport or through G proteins. However, attempts to demonstrate such associations have not been fruitful. Whether EBNA-2 and LMP are sufficient for lymphocyte growth transformation or whether other EBV proteins are also essential to this process is as yet uncertain.

3. Other Herpesvirus Oncogenes

MDV, Lucke herpesvirus, and HVS are three other herpesviruses that induce tumors with sufficient speed or efficiency that they are also likely to express one or more transforming genes. MDV or HVS tumor cells contain the entire virus genome as latent episomes (for reviews, see Kato and Hirai 1985; Calnek 1986). MDV and HVS tumor cells grow in continuous culture and express a restricted set of virus mRNAs. Only one protein has been identified in transformed cells (Nakajima et al. 1987). Like EBV, HVS encodes small nonpolyadenylated RNAs in transformed cells and in cells permissive for virus replication (Murthy et al. 1986).

An essential HVS transforming gene has been mapped to an open reading frame (Desrosiers et al. 1986). This open reading frame has some superficial similarity to EBV EBNA-2, in that spontaneous deletion of the open reading frame occurs and is the principal cause of naturally arising transformation-defective variants. Furthermore, as with EBNA-2, there are naturally occurring variant alleles at this locus that differ in their ability to initiate lymphocyte growth transformation. Unlike EBV, HVS can be grown to high titer in permissive continuous tissue culture cell lines (e.g., owl monkey kidney cells). Consequently, the HVS genome is susceptible to molecular genetic analysis. Prospective deletion mutant analyses confirm the importance of the open reading frame in cell transformation (Desrosiers et al. 1986). On the basis of predicted amino acid sequence, the open reading frame has no homology to previously described oncogenes (Murthy et al. 1989). The predicted amino acid sequence (without consideration of potential splicing) suggests that the protein encoded by the open reading frame would have a single potential transmembrane domain and a zinc finger consensus domain.

B. Herpes Simplex Cytomegalovirus and the "Hit and Run Hypothesis"

Because of the seroepidemiologic studies showing a correlation between cervical carcinoma and HSV-2 (but not HSV-1) antibody and a higher risk for cervical carcinoma among patients with HSV-2-specific antibody, HSV transforming activity has been evaluated in primary and continuous rodent fibroblasts and in experimental animal cervix infection. In studies using virus, the ability of virus to replicate and kill cells was abolished by UV light or by photo-inactivation. Hamster embryo fibroblasts infected with inactivated virus yielded a few "transformed" foci, one of which, after 21 tissue culture passages, was tumorigenic in weanling hamsters (Duff and Rapp 1971). The cells initially contained HSV-2-associated antigens, but these largely disappeared in the animal tumors. No HSV DNA or RNA could be found in late passage cells. Subsequent attempts to transform primary or continuous rodent fibroblast cells with restriction endonuclease fragments of HSV-2 or HSV-1 DNA identified specific fragments of each genome, which would give rise to transformed foci, but with very low efficiency. No HSV DNA, RNA, or protein could be reproducibly detected in the transformed foci. In mice, long-term, frequent, vaginal inoculation with live or inactivated HSV-1 or HSV-2 did not cause an increase in the cervical cancer incidence (Meignier et al. 1986). Similarly, with a few exceptions, HSV DNA, RNA, or proteins have been absent from human cervical cancer tissues. One hypothesis that would account for the seroepidemiologic and experimental transformation studies is that an HSV gene is only necessary for switching on transformation, or that only a very small piece of HSV DNA needs to integrate near and turn on a putative cell "oncogene." One set of experiments identified a small palindrome in human cytomegalovirus (CMV) DNA that seemed to possess transforming activity, albeit with a low efficiency. However, the persistence of the palindrome in transformed cell genomes could not be demonstrated, and the experiments have not been confirmed. An alternative hypothesis that would account for most of the seroepidemiologic data is that another virus, which is also spread by venereal transmission, is the etiologic agent of cervical cancer. In fact, human papillomaviruses HPV-16 and HPV-18 are venereally transmitted and have been found in over 90% of cervical cancers (Durst et al. 1983). Although more elaborate hypotheses could involve HSV-2 as a cocarcinogen in a transformation process in which HPV is the primary etiologic agent, the prevailing current hypothesis is that HPV may be a sufficient solo etiologic agent and that HSV has no direct oncogenic activity.

C. Herpesvirus *trans*-Activators and Transformation

HSV, pseudorabies virus, or CMV immediate early *trans*-activator genes can complement adenovirus E1A-deficient mutants in *trans*-activating early adenovirus gene expression and enabling E1A-deficient adenovirus to replicate (Tevethia et al. 1987). Since adenovirus E1A has immortalizing activity in primary rodent fibroblasts (Chapter 9), the ability of some herpesvirus immediate early genes to complement E1A suggests that herpesvirus immediate early regulatory genes could have immortalizing activity. CMV immediate early *trans*-activators are particularly good candidates for immortalizing activity, since CMV infection initially stimulates cell DNA synthesis. So far, however, attempts to demonstrate immortalizing activity with HSV or CMV DNA in fibroblast assays have been negative.

IV. SUMMARY

Herpesviruses are endemic in most animal species and have coevolved with their natural species. Although during virus replication the infected cell is killed, replication is not an invariant consequence of infection, and temperate persistence, in a latent state, occurs for each virus in some highly differentiated cell type(s). Some herpesviruses have incorporated or evolved genes that enhance the growth of latently infected differentiated cells and can cause these cells to be tumorigenic. At least one herpesvirus gene (EBV LMP) has a dominant transforming phenotype in rodent fibroblasts, as is characteristic of oncogenes. LMP has little sequence similarity to other genes and has unique effects in altering fibroblast or lymphoblast growth. Another herpesvirus "oncogene" (EBV EBNA-2) is a specific *trans*-activator in differentiated B lymphocytes. Thus, analysis of the biochemical basis for herpesvirus oncogenicity is likely to continue to uncover new aspects of differentiated and nondifferentiated cell growth control. The expression of herpesvirus genes within latently infected and growth-transformed cells not only causes cell proliferation, but also renders the cell susceptible to immune surveillance (Rickinson 1986). In normal hosts, there is a balance between the growth of latently infected cells and their immune destruction.

ACKNOWLEDGMENTS

Georg Bornkamm, Ron Desrosiers, Guy de The, Tony Epstein, Bernard Fleckenstein, Werner and Gertrude Henle, George and Eva Klein, Gilbert Lenoir, George Miller, Merle Mizell, Meihan Nonoyama, Joe Pagano, Gary Pearson, John Pope, Alan Rickinson, Bernard Roizman, Patricia Spear, Bill Sugden, Judy Tevethia, David Thorley-Lawson, Zeng Yi, Harald zur Hausen, and the coauthors of our primary publication have made important contributions to the work presented here. The U.S. Public Health Service (CA-47006) and, formerly, the American Cancer Society have been the principal supports of our research.

REFERENCES

Adams, J.M., A.W. Harris, C.A. Pinkert, L.M. Corcoran, W.S. Alexander, S. Cory, R.D. Palmiter, and R.L. Brinster. 1985. The c-*myc* oncogene driven by immunoglobulin enhancers induces lymphoid malignancy in transgenic mice. *Nature* **318:** 533–538.

Amen, P., N. Lewin, M. Nordstrom, and G. Klein. 1986. EBV-activation of human B-lymphocytes. *Curr. Top. Microbiol. Immunol.* **132:** 266–271.

Berger, R. and A. Bernheim. 1985. Cytogenetics of Burkitt's lymphoma-leukemia: A review. In *Burkitt's lymphoma* (ed. G. Lenoir et al.), pp. 65–80. IARC Publications, Lyon.

Birkenbach, M., D. Liebowitz, F. Wang, J. Sample, and E. Kieff. 1989. Epstein-Barr virus latent infection membrane protein increases vimentin expression in human B-cell lines. *J. Virol.* **63:** 4079–4084.

Bodescot, M. and M. Perricaudet. 1986. Epstein-Barr virus mRNAs produced by alternative splicing. *Nucleic Acids Res.* **14:** 7103–7114.

Brown, N., C. Lui, Y. Wang, and C. Garcia. 1988. B-cell lymphoproliferation and lymphomagenesis are associated with clonotypic intracellular terminal regions of the Epstein-Barr virus. *J. Virol.* **62:** 962–969.

Cairns, J., L. Flores-Romo, M.J. Millsum, G.R. Guy, S. Gillis, J.A. Ledbetter, and J. Gordon. 1988. Soluble CD23 is released by B lymphocytes cycling in response to interleukin 4 and anti-Bp50 (CDw40). *Eur. J. Immunol.* **18:** 349–353.

Calender, A., M. Billaud, J-P. Aubry, J. Banchereau, M. Vuillaume, and G.M. Lenoir. 1987. Epstein-Barr virus EBV induces expression of B-cell activation markers on *in vitro* infection of EBV-negative B-lymphoma cells. *Proc. Natl. Acad. Sci.* **84:** 8060–8064.

Calnek, B. 1986. Marek's disease: A model for herpes virus oncology. *CRC Crit. Rev. Microbiol.* **12:** 293–320.

Cleary, M., R. Dorfman, and J. Sklar. 1986. Failure in immunological control of the virus infection: Post transplant lymphomas. In *The Epstein-Barr virus: Recent advances* (ed. M.A. Epstein and B.G. Achong), pp. 164–181. William Heinemann Medical Books Ltd, London.

Dambaugh, T., K. Hennessy, S. Fennewald, and E. Kieff. 1986a. The genome and its expression in latent infection. In *The Epstein-Barr virus: Recent advances* (ed. M.A. Epstein and B.G. Achong), pp. 13–45. William Heinemann Medical Books Ltd, London.

Dambaugh, T., F. Wang, K. Hennessy, E. Woodland-Bushman, A. Rickinson, and E. Kieff. 1986b. Expression of the Epstein-Barr virus nuclear protein 2 in rodent cells. *J. Virol.* **59:** 453–462.

Desrosiers, R.C., D.P. Silva, L.M. Waldron, and N.L. Letvin. 1986. Nononcogenic deletion mutants of herpesvirus saimiri are defective for *in vitro* immortalization. *J. Virol.* **57:** 701–705.

de The, G. and Y. Zeng. 1986. Population screening for EBV markers: Toward improvement of nasopharyngeal carcinoma control. In *The Epstein-Barr virus: Recent advances* (ed. M.A. Epstein and B.G. Achong), pp. 237–249. William Heinemann Medical Books Ltd, London.

Duff, R. and F. Rapp. 1971. Oncogenic transformation of hamster cells after exposure to herpes simplex virus type 2. *Nature* **233:** 48–50.

Durst, M., L. Gissmann, H. Ikenberg, and zur Hausen, H. 1983. A papillomavirus DNA from a cervical carcinoma and its prevalence in cancer biopsy samples from different geographic regions. *Proc. Natl. Acad. Sci.* **80:** 3812–3815.

Glickman, J., J. Howe, and J. Steitz. 1988. Structural analysis of EBER-1 and EBER-2 ribonucleoprotein particles present in Epstein-Barr virus infected cells. *J. Virol.* **62:** 902–911.

Gordon, J., G. Guy, and L. Walker. 1985. Autocrine models of B-lymphocyte growth. I. Role of cell contact and soluble factors in T-independent B-cell responses. *Immunology* **56:** 329–335.

Hampar, B., A. Tanaka, M. Nonoyama, and J. Derge. 1974. Replication of the resident repressed EBV genome during early S phase of non-producer Raji cells. *Proc. Natl. Acad. Sci.* **71:** 631–633.

Heller, M., E. Flemington, E. Kieff, and P. Deininger. 1985. Repeat arrays in cellular DNA related to the Epstein-Barr virus IR3 repeat. *Mol. Cell. Biol.* **5:** 457–465.

Henle, W. and G. Henle. 1979. Seroepidemiology of the virus. In *The Epstein-Barr virus* (ed. M.A. Epstein and B.G. Achong), pp. 61–78. Springer-Verlag, Berlin.

Hennessy, K., S. Fennewald, M. Hummel, T. Cole, and E. Kieff. 1984. A membrane protein encoded by Epstein-Barr virus in latent growth-transforming infection. *Proc. Natl. Acad. Sci.* **81:** 7207–7211.

Kato, S., and K. Hirai. 1985. Marek's disease virus. *Adv. Virus Res.* **30:** 225–277.

Kishimoto, T. and T. Hirano. 1988. Molecular regulation of B lymphocyte response. *Annu. Rev. Immunol.* **6:** 485–512.

Klein, G. 1979. The relationship of the virus to nasopharyngeal carcinoma. In *The Epstein-Barr virus* (ed. M.A. Epstein and B.G. Achong), pp. 340–350. Springer-Verlag, Berlin.

Land, H., L.F. Parada, and R.A. Weinberg. 1983. Tumorigenic conversion of primary embryo fibroblasts requires at least two cooperating oncogenes. *Nature* **304:** 596–602.

Laux, G., M. Perricaudet, and P.J. Farrell. 1988. A spliced Epstein-Barr virus gene expressed in immortalized lymphocytes is created by circularization of the linear viral genome. *EMBO J.* **7:** 769–774.

Leder, A., P.K. Pattengale, A. Kuo, T.A. Stewart, and P. Leder. 1986. Consequences of widespread deregulation of the c-*myc* gene in transgenic mice: Multiple neoplasms and normal development. *Cell* **45:** 485–495.

Liebowitz, D. and E. Kieff. 1989. Epstein-Barr virus latent membrane protein: Induction of B-cell activation antigens and membrane patch formation does not require vimentin. *J. Virol.* **63:** 4051–4054.

Liebowitz, D., D. Wang, and E. Kieff. 1986. Orientation and patching of the latent infection membrane protein encoded by Epstein-Barr virus. *J. Virol.* **58:** 233–237.

Liebowitz, D., R. Kopan, E. Fuchs, J. Sample, and E. Kieff. 1987. An Epstein-Barr virus transforming protein associates with vimentin in lymphocytes. *Mol. Cell. Biol.* **7:** 2299–2308.

Lindahl, T., A. Adams, G. Bjursell, G.W. Bornkamm, G. Kaschka-Dierch, and U. Jehn. 1976. Covalently closed circular duplex DNA of Epstein-Barr virus in a human lymphoid cell line. *J. Mol. Biol.* **102:** 511–530.

Lombardi, L., E.W. Newcomb, and R. Dalla-Favera. 1987. Pathogenesis of Burkitt lymphoma: Expression of an activated c-*myc* oncogene causes the tumorigenic conversion of EBV-infected human B lymphoblasts. *Cell* **49:** 161–170.

Matsuo, T., M. Heller, L. Petti, E. O'Shiro, and E. Kieff. 1984. The entire Epstein-Barr virus genome integrates into human lymphocyte DNA. *Science* **226:** 1322–1325.

Meignier, B., B. Norrild, C. Thuning, J. Warren, N. Frenkel, A. Nahmias, F. Rapp, and B. Roizman. 1986. Failure to induce cervical cancer in mice by long-term, frequent vaginal exposure to live or inactivated herpes simplex virus. *Int. J. Cancer* **38:** 387–394.

Miller, G., J. Robinson, L. Heston, and M. Lipman. 1974. Differences between laboratory strains of Epstein-Barr virus based on immortalization, abortive infection, and interference. *Proc. Natl. Acad. Sci.* **71:** 4006–4010.

Mizell, M. 1985. Lucke frog carcinoma herpesvirus: Transmission and expression during early development. In *Advances in viral oncology* (ed. G. Klein), vol. 5, pp. 129–146. Raven Press, New York.

Murthy, S., J. Kamine, and R.C. Desrosiers. 1986. Viral-encoded small RNAs in herpes virus saimiri induced tumors. *EMBO J.* **5:** 1625–1632.

Murthy, S., J. Trimble, and R.C. Desrosiers. 1989. Deletion mutants of herpesvirus saimiri define an open reading frame necessary for transformation. *J. Virol.* **63:** 3307–3314.

Nakajima, K., K. Ikuta, M. Naito, S. Veda, S. Kato, and K. Hirai. 1987. Analysis of Marek's disease virus serotype-1 specific phosphorylated polypeptides in virus infected cells and Marek's disease lymphoblastoid cells. *J. Gen. Virol.* **68:** 1379–1389.

Pelicci, P.G., D.M. Knowles, Z.A. Arlin, R. Wieczorek, P. Luciw, D. Dina, C. Basilico, and R. Dalla-Favera. 1986. Multiple monoclonal B-cell expansion and c-*myc* oncogene rearrangements in acquired immune deficiency syndrome related lymphoproliferative disorders: Implications for lymphomagenesis. *J. Exp. Med.* **164:** 2049–2060.

Petti, L. and E. Kieff. 1988. A sixth Epstein-Barr virus nuclear protein (EBNA3B) is expressed in latently infected growth-transformed lymphocytes. *J. Virol.* **62:** 2173–2178.

Petti, L., J. Sample, F. Wang, and E. Kieff. 1988. A fifth Epstein-Barr virus nuclear protein is expressed in latently infected growth-transformed lymphocytes. *J. Virol.* **62:** 1330–1338.

Pope, J., M. Horne, and W. Scott. 1968. Transformation of fetal human leukocytes in vitro by filtrates of a human leukemic cell line containing herpes-like virus. *Int. J. Cancer* **3:** 857–866.

Raab-Traub, N. and K. Flynn. 1986. The structure of the termini of the EBV as a marker of clonal cellular proliferation. *Cell* **47:** 883–889.

Rawlins, D., G. Milman, S. Hayward, and G. Hayward. 1985. Sequence-specific DNA binding of the Epstein-Barr virus nuclear antigen EBNA-1 to clustered sites in the plasmid maintenance region. *Cell* **42:** 859–868.

Reisman, D., J. Yates, and B. Sugden. 1985. A putative origin of replication of plasmids derived from Epstein-Barr virus is composed of two *cis*-acting components. *Mol. Cell. Biol.* **5:** 1822–1832.

Rickinson, A. 1986. Cellular immunologic responses to the virus infection. In *The Epstein-Barr virus: Recent advances* (ed. M.A. Epstein and B.G. Achong), pp.75–125. William Heinemann Medical Books Ltd, London.

Rickinson, A., L. Young, and M. Rowe. 1987. Influence of the EBV nuclear antigen EBNA-2 in the growth phenotype of virus transformed B cells. *J. Virol.* **61:** 1310–1317.

Robinson, J.E., N. Brown, W. Andiman, K. Halliday, U. Francke, M.F. Robert, M.Andersson-Anvret, D. Horstmann, and G. Miller. 1980. Diffuse polyclonal B-cell lymphoma during primary infection with Epstein-Barr virus. *N. Engl. J. Med.* **302:** 1293–1297.

Roizman, B. and W. Batterson. 1985. Herpesviruses and their replication. In *Virology* (ed. B.N. Fields), pp. 497–526. Raven Press, New York.

Sample, J., D. Liebowitz, and E. Kieff. 1989. Two related Epstein-Barr virus membrane proteins are encoded by separate genes. *J. Virol.* **63:** 933–937.

Sample, J., M. Hummel, D. Braun, M. Birkenbach, and E. Kieff. 1986. Nucleotide sequences of mRNAs encoding Epstein-Barr virus nuclear proteins: A probable transcriptional initiation site. *Proc. Natl. Acad. Sci.* **83:** 5096–5100.

Shope, T.C., D. Dechairo, and G. Miller. 1973. Malignant lymphoma in cotton-top marmosets after inoculation with Epstein-Barr virus. *Proc. Natl. Acad. Sci.* **70:** 2487–2491.

Showe, L.C. and C.M. Croce. 1987. The role of chromosomal translocations in B- and T-cell neoplasia. *Annu. Rev. Immunol.* **5:** 253–277.

Skare, J., J. Farley, J. Strominger, K. Fresen, M. Cho, and H. zur Hausen. 1985. Transformation by Epstein-Barr virus requires DNA sequences in the region of *Bam*HI fragments Y and H. *J. Virol.* **55:** 286–297.

Sugden, B. and S. Metzenberg. 1982. Characterization of an antigen whose cell surface expression is induced by infection with Epstein-Barr virus. *J. Virol.* **46:** 800–807.

Swendeman, S. and D.A. Thorley-Lawson. 1987. The activation antigen BLAST-2, when shed, is an autocrine BCGF for normal and transformed B cells. *EMBO J.* **6:** 1637–1642.

Tevethia, M.J., D.J. Spector, K.M. Leisure, and M.F. Stinski. 1987. Participation of two human cytomegalovirus immediate early gene regions in transcriptional activation of adenovirus promoters. *Virology* **161:** 276–285.

Tosato, G. and R. Blaese. 1985. EBV infection and immunoregulation in man. *Adv. Immunol.* **37:** 99–149.

Tosato, G., K.B. Seamon, N.D. Goldman, P.B. Sehgal, L.T. May, G.C. Washington, K.D.

Jones, and S.E. Pike. 1988. Monocyte-derived human B-cell growth factor identified as interferon-B2 (BSF-2, IL-6). *Science* **239:** 502–504.

Trimble, J.J., S.C.S. Murthy, A. Bakker, R. Grassmann, and R.C. Desrosiers. 1988. A gene for dihydrofolate reductase in a herpesvirus. *Science* **239:** 1145–1147.

Volsky, D., T. Gross, F. Sinangil, C. Kuszynski, R. Bartzatt, T. Dambaugh, and E. Kieff. 1984. Expression of Epstein-Barr virus (EBV) DNA and cloned DNA fragments in human lymphocytes following Sendai virus envelope-mediated gene transfer. *Proc. Natl. Acad. Sci.* **81:** 5926–5930.

Wang, D., D. Liebowitz, and E. Kieff. 1985. An EBV membrane protein expressed in immortalized lymphocytes transforms established rodent cells. *Cell* **43:** 831–840.

———. 1988a. The truncated form of the Epstein-Barr virus latent infection membrane protein expressed in virus replication does not transform rodent fibroblasts. *J. Virol.* **62:** 2337–2346.

Wang, D., D. Liebowitz, F. Wang, C. Gregory, A. Rickinson, R. Larson, T. Springer, and E. Kieff. 1988b. Epstein-Barr virus latent infection membrane protein alters the human B-lymphocyte phenotype: Deletion of the amino terminus abolishes activity. *J. Virol.* **62:** 4173–4184.

Wang, F., L. Petti, D. Braun, S. Seung, and E. Kieff. 1987a. A bicistronic Epstein-Barr virus mRNA encodes two nuclear proteins in latently infected, growth-transformed lymphocytes. *J. Virol.* **61:** 945–954.

Wang, F., C.D. Gregory, M. Rowe, A.B. Rickinson, D. Wang, M. Birkenbach, H. Kikutani, T. Kishimoto, and E. Kieff. 1987b. Epstein-Barr virus nuclear antigen 2 specifically induces expression of the B-cell activation antigen CD23. *Proc. Natl. Acad. Sci.* **84:** 3452–3456.

Weisenberger, D. and D. Purtillo. 1986. Failure in immunologic control of the virus infection: fatal infectious mononucleosis. In *The Epstein-Barr virus: Recent advances* (ed. M.A. Epstein and B.G. Achong), pp. 127–161. William Heinemann Medical Books Ltd, London.

Zeng, Y. and G. de The. 1985. Nasopharyngeal carcinoma: Early detection and IGA-related pre-NPC condition. Achievements and prospectives. In *EBV and associated diseases* (ed. P. Levine et al.), pp. 151–163. Martinus Nijhoff, Boston.

zur Hausen, H., H. Schulte-Holthausen, G. Klein, W. Henle, G. Henle, P. Clifford, and L. Santesson. 1970. EBV DNA in biopsies of Burkitt tumors and anaplastic carcinomas of the nasopharynx. *Nature* **228:** 1056–1058.

11

Heritable Cancer and Tumor Suppressor Genes: A Tentative Connection

Eric J. Stanbridge
Department of Microbiology and Molecular Genetics
California College of Medicine
Irvine, California 92717

Webster K. Cavenee
Ludwig Institute for Cancer Research
Montreal, Quebec H3A 1A1 Canada

I. INTRODUCTION

In several of the foregoing chapters, the dominant expression and action of cellular oncogenes has been emphasized. Studies of these oncogenes have clearly indicated that they act as positive regulators of cell proliferation. In the early stages of the research on oncogenes, it was thought that activation of a single oncogene was sufficient for the neoplastic transformation of a normal cell. It rapidly became apparent that this was not the case, and further studies indicated the need for two or more cooperating oncogenes to be expressed for the neoplastic transformation of normal rodent cells to ensue. Further detailed analysis of oncogene-mediated transformation

Oncogenes and the Molecular Origins of Cancer.

revealed that other, as yet unidentified, genetic changes were required in addition to oncogene activation in order for cells to acquire tumor-forming properties. Data derived from somatic cell hybrid experiments together with cytogenetic and polymorphic allele analysis of human tumors have indicated that one frequent and often essential genetic alteration occurring during tumor development is the inactivation or loss of function of one or more genes. This phenomenon of loss of function suggests that these genes, when intact, play a negative regulatory role in the control of cell proliferation. In this chapter, we examine the evidence for negative regulatory elements and their possible role in the development of neoplasia.

II. SOMATIC CELL GENETICS OF TUMORIGENESIS

A. Tumor Suppression Is Demonstrated

Historically, the first attempts at a genetic analysis of malignancy utilized the technique of somatic cell hybridization. A simple question was asked: Upon fusion of a malignant cell with a normal cell, would the malignant or normal phenotype be expressed in the resulting hybrid cell? The technique of somatic cell fusion used to answer this question is presented schematically in Figure 1.

Early investigators in this field isolated hybrid cells derived from the fusion of mouse cells of low malignant potential with those of high malignant potential (Harris et al. 1969; Harris 1971). The intraspecific mouse cell hybrid populations derived from these fusions were as malignant as the highly malignant parent, thereby leading to the interpretation that malignancy behaves as a dominant trait vis-a-vis the normal growth phenotype. However, subsequent, more extensive studies of a large number of mouse somatic cell hybrids came to the opposite conclusion. In these later studies, investigators showed that when highly malignant mouse cells were fused with normal mouse embryo cells or mouse cells of low malignant potential, the resulting hybrids were transiently suppressed in their ability to form tumors. The interpretation from these later experiments—that malignancy behaves as a recessive trait in somatic cell hybrids— has been supported by the studies of many other investigators using mouse, rat, and hamster intraspecies somatic cell hybrids as well as interspecies rodent × human cell hybrids (Klinger 1982; Sager 1985). One notable exception to this generalization is seen when the malignant cells used in the hybridization have been transformed by oncogenic viruses (Croce 1984).

In retrospect, it is clear that a major determinant of hybrid cell phenotype is its chromosomal makeup (karyotype). The tetraploid (or greater) chromosomal array seen shortly after cell fusion is usually unstable, resulting in the loss of chromosomes originating with one or another parent during expansion of the hybrid cell clone. This karyotypic instability

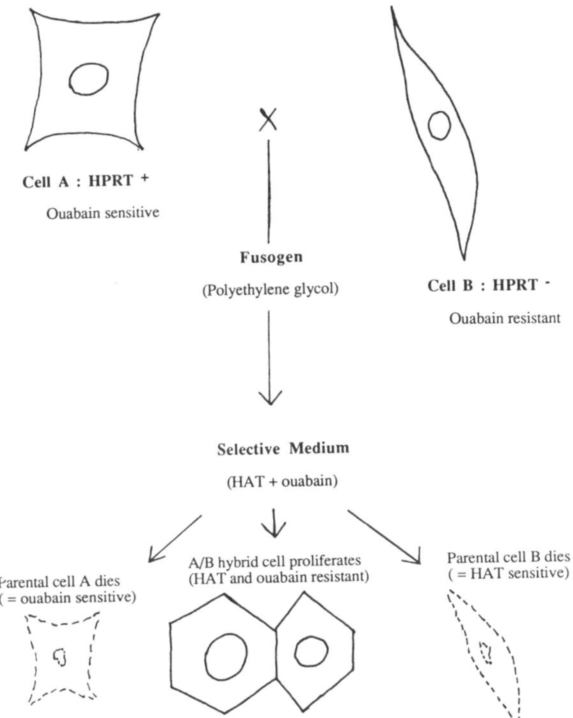

Figure 1 Schematic representation of somatic cell hybridization. Cell B is a double mutant. It is deficient for the enzyme hypoxanthine guanine phosphoribosyl transferase ($HPRT^-$) and therefore dies in medium containing hypoxanthine-aminopterin-thymidine (HAT). It is also resistant to the cytotoxic effects of ouabain. $HPRT^-$ is a recessive trait and ouabain resistance is a codominant trait, thus cell B is a "universal fuser." It can be fused to any cell that is wild type for these traits ($HPRT^+$, ouabain sensitive), and only the hybrid cell will proliferate in the selective medium.

greatly complicates an analysis that depends on understanding the respective genetic contributions of the two parents to the behavior of the hybrid cell. Thus, initially nontumorigenic hybrid cells were often seen to revert rapidly to a tumorigenic state, and this reversion could be correlated with the loss of substantial numbers of chromosomes. The chromosome losses may be random, as in the case of intraspecies rodent cell hybrids, or nonrandom, as in the case of human × rodent cell hybrids in which there is preferential loss of human chromosomes.

The problem of chromosomal instability was eventually overcome by using intraspecies human cell hybrids (Stanbridge 1976; Stanbridge et al. 1982). Extensive analyses of human carcinoma (HeLa) × human diploid fibroblast hybrid cells confirmed stable retention of both sets of parental chromosomes. At the same time, there was complete and stable suppression of tumor formation with tumorigenic segregants arising only rarely. Suppression of tumorigenicity has now been demonstrated in a variety of human malignant × human normal cell crosses, allowing us to conclude that tumor suppression is a fairly general result of introducing genetic information from normal cells into cancer cells. This allows the further conclusion that many types of tumors arise through loss of critical growth-regulating genes from their genomes.

B. Dissociation of Transformed and Tumorigenic Phenotypes by Cell Hybridization

Although tumor-forming ability is suppressed in malignant × normal hybrid cells, many continue to display certain phenotypes of transformation when grown in culture. It would seem that the normal genes operating in these hybrid cells are able to normalize some but not all of the traits of the malignant parent. This is in consonance with a model of tumor development that involves multiple genetic lesions in the tumor cell genome (see Chapter 12), only some of which are corrected by the normal genes expressed in the hybrids. Since these mutations are all presumably essential for tumorigenesis, the correction of any one of them following cell hybridization may suffice to cause the hybrid cell to lose its tumor-forming ability. It should also be noted in this context that some investigators have shown when studying certain malignant × normal cell fusions that all of their in vitro transformation phenotypes are suppressed, resulting in hybrid cells that behave as fully normal cells in culture and eventually senesce and die (Pereira-Smith and Smith 1983).

The availability of paired combinations of hybrid cells (one that behaves transformed in vitro but is nontumorigenic, the other transformed and tumorigenic) has made possible comparative analyses of these closely related cell types with the goal of identifying those in vitro cell phenotypes that correlate well with tumorigenicity in vivo. In both rodent and human cell culture systems, it was found that many in vitro traits that had previously been considered as reliable "markers of malignancy" continued to be expressed by the nontumorigenic hybrid cells (Stanbridge 1987). These included growth to high densities, growth in low serum concentrations, expression of a variety of antigenic and biochemical markers (e.g., placental alkaline phosphatase), and, surprisingly, ability to grow in soft agar, a phenotype hitherto thought to be tightly linked to tumorigenicity.

A few cell markers displayed by cells in culture have nonetheless been found to be specifically associated with the tumorigenic phenotype. One particularly interesting example is a 75-kD protein that is found on the membranes of HeLa cells and tumorigenic HeLa × fibroblast hybrids and is absent from nontumorigenic hybrids (Der and Stanbridge 1981). This provides the hope that yet other in vitro markers of tumorigenicity will be uncovered in the future.

C. Specific Chromosomes Associated with Control of Tumorigenic Expression

As mentioned above, the initial suppression of tumorigenicity seen after cell fusion is often followed by reexpression of this trait. Such changes are in accord with the notion that genetic information from the normal parent initially represses tumorigenic expression; when this information is lost from the hybrid cell (perhaps as a consequence of chromosomal nondisjunction at mitosis), this genetic control is removed, thereby leading to the reexpression of tumorigenicity.

This phenomenon provides an opportunity to associate the critical growth-regulating information with karyotypically identifiable chromosomes whose loss is repeatedly connected with reexpression of tumorigenicity. In this way, mouse chromosome 4 has been implicated in the control of malignant expression of a number of different mouse tumors (Evans et al. 1982), and human chromosome 11 in the control of the neoplastic expression of certain hamster × human hybrid cells (Klinger 1982). Cytogenetic analyses of intraspecies human cell hybrids implicate chromosome 11 in the control of tumorigenic expression of HeLa × normal fibroblast hybrids and chromosomes 1 and 4 in the control of HT1080 fibrosarcoma × normal fibroblast hybrids (Stanbridge et al. 1981; Benedict et al. 1984). In certain cases, the cytogenetic data have been reinforced by restriction fragment length polymorphism (RFLP) analyses using molecular probes that map to specific chromosomes (see below). In sum, it would seem that multiple cancer-controlling genes exist that map to several distinct chromosomes (Table 1).

Table 1 Chromosomes implicated in tumor suppression

Animal species	Chromosome number	Cancer cell suppressed
Mouse	4	a variety of malignant cells including carcinomas, sarcomas, and melanomas
Chinese hamster (CH)	3	CH fibrosarcoma cells
Syrian hamster (SH)	15	SH fibrosarcoma cells
Human	11	HeLa and Wilms' tumor cells
	13	osteosarcoma cells
	1 and/or 4	HT1080 fibrosarcoma cells

Chromosomes listed above have been implicated in tumor suppression on the basis of somatic cell hybrid or monochromosome transfer experiments.

D. Suppression by Single Chromosome Transfer

The suggestion that single chromosomes contain the genetic information sufficient to reverse neoplastic growth represented a welcome decrease in complexity from that which would prevail if genes on multiple chromosomes were required to act in concert to achieve this end. However, the evidence for such a role of single chromosomes was based only on the indirect evidence correlating chromosome loss with reversion to tumorigenicity. A more direct test of this model came from an ability to transfer single chromosomes individually from normal cells into cancer cells and to examine their effect on the tumor-forming properties of these recipients.

Such single chromosome transfer was made possible by the technique of microcell transfer (Fournier and Ruddle 1977; Saxon et al. 1985). The microcell procedure is schematically outlined in Figure 2. Briefly, proliferating cells are exposed to colcemid over a period of several days. The cells are initially blocked in metaphase, but a significant proportion escape the block and enter the G_1 phase of the cell cycle. However, because there is no mitotic spindle formation, the chromosomes condense as individual units, resulting in a multinucleate cell containing large numbers of micronuclei, each of which contains one or several chromosomes. Such cells are then enucleated with a combination of cytochalasin B and centrifugal force, resulting in a pellet of microcells. The microcells are then fused to the recipient cell of interest. The obvious difference between this strategy and whole-cell fusion is that only one or at most a few chromosomes are transferred from the donor cell to any recipient. It is important to note

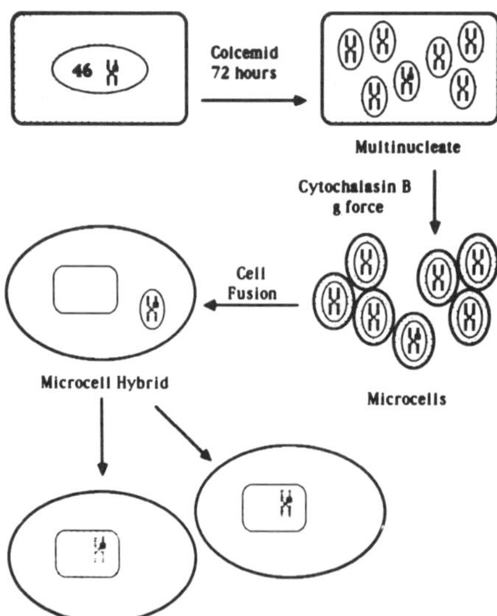

Figure 2 Schematic representation of microcell transfer. Details of the technique are presented in the text. The marked chromosome represents the chromosome that contains an integrated gene (e.g., the bacterial *neo* gene or *gpt* gene) that allows for dominant selection.

that, as with whole-cell fusions, the transferred chromosome is retained in succeeding generations as an intact structural unit.

A further refinement of this technique involves the use of dominant selectable marker genes that map to the donor chromosome of interest. Their association with this chromosome is accomplished by the physical integration of such markers (e.g., a neomycin-resistance gene) into chromosomal DNA following transfection or retroviral infection of donor cells. The presence of such a marker on the chromosome makes it possible to select for recipient cells that have acquired this particular donor cell chromosome. Using this technique, it has been possible to show that transfer of a normal human chromosome 11 into tumorigenic HeLa × fibroblast hybrids results in suppression of tumor-forming ability (Saxon et al. 1986). Transfer of a control chromosome, in this case the X chromosome, had no effect on tumorigenic behavior. As noted later, transfer of chromosome 11 into a Wilms' tumor cell line also resulted in suppression of tumorigenicity, whereas transfer of other chromosomes had no effect (Weissman et al. 1987). These results indicate that human chromosome 11 carries one or more genes expressing strong tumor-suppressing abilities.

E. Gene Transfer and Reversion of Transformation

A further goal of this avenue of research has been the determination of the molecular genetic basis of tumor suppression. The cloning of human "tumor suppressor" genes has been hampered by appropriate selection systems such as those that have proven so useful for the isolation of activated oncogenes. To illustrate this, one can point to the dominantly acting oncogenes that score positively in transfection-transformation assays such as the mouse NIH-3T3 system (see Chapter 5) and are readily detected by the multilayered foci of transformed cells that they induce on a background monolayer of contact-inhibited cells. Appropriate molecular genetic techniques have been available for cloning the transfected oncogene from the transformed cells. In contrast, when attempting to use comparable gene transfer techniques to clone genes that suppress tumorigenicity, one is confronted with an assay system in which one is looking for the rare transfected cell that is nontumorigenic growing amid a large background of similarly appearing, tumorigenic cells.

Despite these difficulties, reversion of transformation coupled with loss of tumorigenicity has been demonstrated in rodent cells into which DNA has been introduced by transfection. Unlike the human tumor cells discussed earlier, which derived from spontaneously arising tumors, the cells used in these particular experiments were transformed in vitro by insertion of well-defined oncogenes. Flat revertants were induced by transfection into transformed cells of cDNA libraries derived from normal human diploid fibroblasts. The transfected, revertant cells that lost their oncogene-induced phenotype grew in monolayer with the flat shape of normal cells and, unlike the transformants, failed to grow in medium containing low serum. Indeed, this latter property was utilized in the selection of flat revertants using [^{3}H]thymidine suicide incorporation techniques that selectively kill growing cells. Although these studies are in their early stages, at least two human cDNAs have been cloned that induce the flat revertant phenotype in sarcoma virus-transformed rodent cells (Schäfer et al. 1988; Noda et al. 1989).

In one of these cases, a gene termed K*rev-1* that reverts the *ras* oncogene-induced phenotype has been isolated by molecular cloning and found to encode a protein distantly related to the product of the *ras* oncogene (Kitayama et al. 1989). It would appear that overexpression of the normal K*rev-1* protein reverses *ras* oncogene action. This mechanism of reversion would seem to be distinct from that discussed previously, in that there is no evidence to date that the K*rev-1* gene is lost from cell genomes during tumor pathogenesis.

III. USE OF MOLECULAR GENETICS TO STUDY GENE LOSS DURING TUMOR PATHOGENESIS

The discussions in the previous sections established the principle that loss of genetic information is often critical for expression of the tumorigenic phenotype. In the cell hybrids and derived segregants described there, these changes in genetic makeup were achieved through the segregation of entire chromosomes. An inkling that chromosomal rearrangement may also underlie the genetic losses occurring during formation of human tumors came from the studies of Boveri early in this century. On the basis of his own observations of the development of sea urchin eggs and the studies of others who had found frequent nuclear and mitotic irregularities in carcinoma cells, Boveri (1914) posited that chromosomal abnormalities were the key cellular changes leading to the conversion of a normal cell into a malignant derivative. Data bearing on this hypothesis were acquired during subsequent decades through cytologic determination of chromosomal numbers and structures in many types of malignant cells. Such studies have uncovered a bewildering array of deviations from genetic normality. Nonetheless, careful analyses of chromosomal structure, including the microstructure revealed by chromosome banding patterns, have revealed specific chromosomal abnormalities associated at high frequency with particular malignant conditions. Examples of such abnormalities include chromosomal translocations, amplifications, and deletions.

In the context of the present discussion, the deletions are most pertinent. Such deletions, often involving only one or a small number of chromosome bands, may reflect the loss of millions of base pairs of DNA. These seemingly subtle changes in chromosomal constitution can cause the loss of one or several critical genes and, in so doing, achieve the same end result as the mechanisms that cause the loss of entire chromosomes, as discussed earlier. Although interstitial deletions have been seen in an impressive array of tumors (catalogued in Mitelman 1985), those found repeatedly in retinoblastomas and Wilms' tumors have proven particularly instructive. Indeed, in the case of retinoblastoma, they have led to the isolation of a single gene, the loss of which triggers tumor formation. The genetics of these tumors will be discussed in detail in the sections that follow.

A. Retinoblastoma

Cytogenetic indications that retinoblastomas are triggered by genetic loss came from the observations of Yunis and Ramsay (1978), who found a number of interstitial chromosomal deletions in retinoblastoma cells that shared the loss of the q14 band of chromosome 13. The repeated deletion of this band in a number of independently arising cases suggested the presence of a gene whose loss contributed to tumor formation cases.

In addition to these cytogenetic peculiarities, the disease of retinoblastoma has several other characteristics that set it apart from most malignancies and have attracted much scientific attention: The tumor derives directly from the cells of the embryonal neural retina and occurs only in young children up to the age of 5. Even more striking is its pattern of occurrence. Like most tumors, the majority of cases of retinoblastoma arise in a sporadic, random fashion in the population, suggestive of some stochastic triggering mechanism such as randomly occurring somatic mutations. However, as many as one third of retinoblastomas appear to arise from a genetic predisposition that is already determined at the moment of conception. The predisposition seen in these cases would seem to arise from a genetically defective gamete acquired from one or another parent. This defective gamete may have arisen during gametogenesis in the parent or may, alternatively, transmit a disease-predisposing allele that was already present in all cells of the parent, having previously caused that parent to suffer retinoblastoma in childhood. The form of disease that involves a predisposition already determined at conception is often called "heritable" retinoblastoma.

These phenomena surrounding retinoblastoma provoked several questions about the relationship between the cytogenetically identified chromosome 13 locus and the disease-predisposing alleles and about the genetic mechanisms connecting the sporadic and heritable forms of this disease. Knudson (1971) had addressed some of these issues by postulating that all types of retinoblastoma involve two separate mutations that are carried by all retinoblastoma tumor cells. In the case of sporadic retinoblastoma, he argued that both mutations occur somatically (i.e., postconception) in the same retinal precursor cell. In heritable retinoblastoma, in contrast, he proposed that one of the two mutations is already present at conception (and thus present subsequently in all cells of the developing retina), whereas the second occurs as a somatic event. This model explains the observed single focus of tumor formation seen in sporadic cases, since this tumor arises following the convergence of two rare genetic events on a single retinal target cell. Multiple tumor foci in both eyes are usually seen in heritable retinoblastoma, and these can be explained by the fact that one of the two mutations is already established in all retinal cells; in these cells, only a single mutation is required to complete the triggering process.

The other important issue concerned the relationship between the cytologically demonstrable 13q14 deletions and the genes that serve as targets in Knudson's model. This was addressed by studies of the gene encoding the enzyme esterase D, which maps very close to the cytologically identified 13q14 locus. By tracing the behavior of this gene, one could follow the fate of its closely linked neighbor, which was termed RB-1. The esterase D gene encodes two electrophoretically distinguishable enzyme forms. By following the genetic transmission of these esterase D alleles, it became clear that the disease-predisposing allele transmitted in familial cases of retinoblastoma was very closely linked to esterase D (Sparkes et al. 1983). This provided important evidence that the gene mapping to 13q14 and the gene conferring familial predisposition were indeed identical.

Still unanswered was the identity of the second target gene postulated by Knudson. Was it the second, surviving copy of the RB-1 locus at 13q14, or was it a fully unrelated gene mapping elsewhere in the genome? The use of linked genetic markers proved once again to be instructive. In addition to use of esterase D alleles, a more powerful and general genetic technique was developed to address this and related issues. This involved the use of Southern blotting analysis to detect RFLP markers that are scattered throughout the genome (Botstein et al. 1980). These markers derive from the presence or absence of restriction sites in chromosomal DNA; the sequences allowing or disallowing cleavage, being part of the chromosomal DNA structure, are transmitted as Mendelian alleles. Moreover, unlike the esterase D enzyme analyses (Godbout et al. 1983), the tests based on RFLP alleles are not affected by mechanisms that may turn on or shut off the expression of a gene and thus affect measurement of the presence or absence of an allele. In these particular experiments, RFLP markers mapping to chromosome 13 were used to trace the behavior of linked RB-1 alleles.

Conjoint use of both esterase D and these RFLP markers led to the conclusion that the second target gene postulated by Knudson was the second copy of the RB-1 locus (Cavenee et al. 1983). Although present in a heterozygous state in the normal cells of a patient predisposed to familial disease, these chromosome 13 markers were often found in a homozygous configuration in tumor cells as well as in primary surgical biopsies (Dryja et al. 1984). Such "reduction to homozygosity" (or "loss of heterozygosity") indicated the loss of one allele and its replacement by a duplicated copy of the surviving allele. In the case of retinoblastomas, the allele that emerged in duplicated form was invariably the defective RB-1 allele inherited from a genetically afflicted parent (Cavenee et al. 1985).

Taken together, this diverse collection of results converged on a simple conclusion: All retinoblastomas arise through loss of both functional RB-1 alleles. In heritable retinoblastoma, an individual is born with only a single intact RB-1 allele that is lost somatically in retinal cells that subsequently develop into tumor cell clones. In sporadic retinoblastoma, both alleles are lost somatically. Because children who are congenitally hemizygous for RB-1 are developmentally normal, it can be concluded that the null allele that they carry is phenotypically silent (i.e., recessive) during development. Moreover, because nullizygosity of RB-1 is seen in neoplastic cells, it appears that the RB-1 gene acts normally to negatively regulate cell growth, in analogy with genes discussed earlier in this chapter.

The mechanisms through which RB-1 alleles are reduced to homozygosity have been studied intensively by cancer geneticists. A number of distinct types of chromosomal rearrangements could serve to unmask an initially present recessive mutation through either the somatic reduction-to-homozygosity of the mutant allele or other mechanisms that serve to eliminate the wild-type allele (Cavenee et al. 1983). These are illustrated in Figure 3 and include the following chromosomal mechanisms (top to bottom): mitotic recombination between the chromosomal homologs with a breakpoint between the tumor locus and the centromere, which would result in heterozygosity at loci in the proximal region of the chromosome and homozygosity throughout the rest of the chromosome including the tumor locus; mitotic disjunction with loss of the wild-type chromosome, either without or with duplication of the mutant chromosome, resulting in homozygosity at all loci on the chromosome; mitotic or regional second events such as gene conversion, deletion, or point mutation. Like heritable retinoblastomas, the sporadic disease also arises frequently through the generation of homozygosity at the RB-1 locus, the difference being, in this instance, the involvement of two somatic events compared to the one germinal and one somatic event occurring in familial cases, in accord with Knudson's proposal.

Use of a series of chromosome-13-specific DNA probes (Lalande et al. 1986) has made it possible to isolate the RB-1 locus as a molecular clone (Friend et al. 1986; Fung et al. 1987; Lee et al. 1987a). The gene is unexpectedly large, being composed of more than 190 kilobases of DNA and at least 27 exons. Use of the DNA probes derived from various parts of this gene has revealed a number of distinct types of mutations that serve to inactivate the RB-1 locus either during gametogenesis or somatically. Large deletions involving thousands of base pairs of DNA are detected in

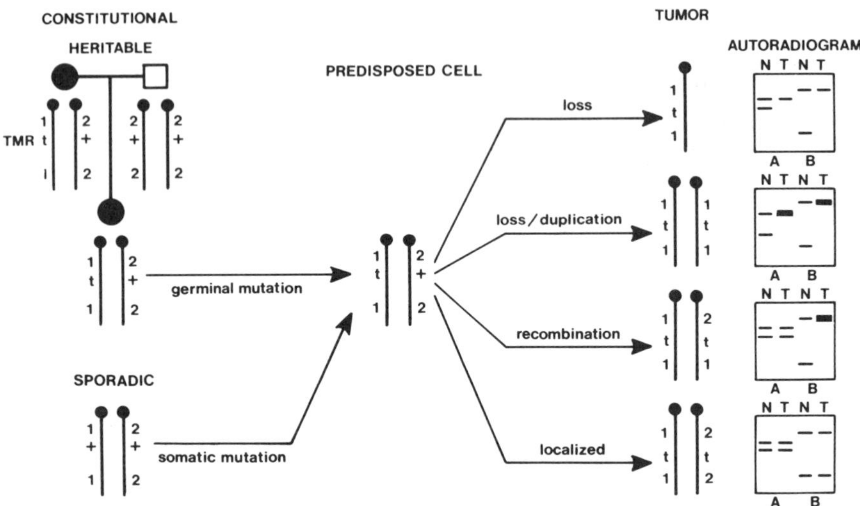

Figure 3 Chromosomal mechanisms that could effect homozygous losses of genetic information. (*Top left*) Inheritance of a chromosome 13 that carries a recessive defect at the tumor (TMR) locus designated "t" results in a child who is genotypically t/ + in all her cells. A retinoblastoma might develop by eliminating the dominant wild-type alleles at the TMR locus by one of the indicated mechanisms. (*Top right*) A recessive mutation occurring in a single retinal cell could also be unmasked by one of the same mechanisms. (*Far right*) The chromosomal mechanism involved in tumor formation can be discerned by comparing genotypes at loci nearer the centromere and the telomere of chromosome 13 in normal (N) and tumor (T) tissues; experimental predictions are shown at the far right. The use of marker loci in this way does not allow the detection or discrimination of the other regional mechanisms shown at bottom right.

10–30% of tumors by use of Southern blot analysis. Even more frequent are subtle changes in gene structure including point mutations that affect the posttranslational processing of the RB-1 primary transcript yielding misspliced mRNAs (e.g., Horowitz et al. 1989).

One proof of the identity of the cloned DNA with the RB-1 gene has been provided by a functional test in which the cloned wild-type DNA was introduced into retinoblastoma and osteosarcoma (see below) cells lacking intact copies of this gene (Huang et al. 1988). The growth of these cells slowed in vitro and they lost tumorigenicity in vivo. This reversion, in analogy with the cell hybridizations and microcell transfers described above, provides strong support for the idea that the tumor phenotype of these cells derives from loss of genetic information. Moreover, it indicates that loss of these particular sequences was a critical determinant of their tumorigenicity.

The RB-1 gene encodes a nuclear phosphoprotein of 105 kD mass that binds to DNA cellulose columns (Lee et al. 1987b). These properties might suggest that this protein is involved in some way in the regulation of transcription or DNA replication. The connections between these biochemical properties and the growth-regulating functions of this protein are at present obscure.

Use of DNA probes to analyze cellular DNAs and RNAs as well as antisera reactive with the 105 kilodalton RB protein (Lee et al. 1987b) has shown that this gene and its encoded products are altered in many more tumors than retinoblastomas. A number of sarcomas, notably osteosarcomas, have been found to carry inactive RB-1 alleles (Friend et al. 1987; Weichselbaum et al. 1988). This is consistent with the clinical observation that children who are cured of the heritable form of retinoblastoma have greatly increased risk for sarcomas later in life and, furthermore, that such osteosarcomas are frequently homozygous for the 13q14 region (Hansen et al. 1985). Of interest is the fact that most of the RB-1-negative sarcomas studied with the recently developed molecular probes involved individuals who had no history of retinoblastoma; accordingly, the lesions in their RB-1 alleles were purely of somatic origin, also consistent with genetic evidence (Hansen et al. 1985; Dryja et al. 1986).

Less expected has been the finding of defective RB-1 alleles in several other types of tumors, including small cell lung carcinomas (SCLC), bladder carcinomas, and mammary carcinomas (Harbour et al. 1988; Lee et al. 1988). Indeed, RB-1 inactivation is seen in virtually all SCLC tumors. This creates a puzzle in that these tumors, of purely somatic mutational origin, have not frequently been seen in individuals who carry a defective RB-1 allele from conception.

The RB-1 gene and, more specifically, its encoded protein may play a role in tumorigenic mechanisms that are quite distinct from those engendering these human tumors. This was made clear by the discovery in 1988 that the transforming mechanisms of several DNA tumor viruses may directly involve the RB-1-encoded protein, p105. Thus, the oncoproteins of the adenovirus E1A, SV40 large T (LT), and the human papillomavirus E7 genes were each found complexed with the RB-1 protein in virus-transformed cells or cell lysates (De Caprio et al. 1988; Whyte et al. 1988; Dyson et al. 1989). These complexes cannot be easily ascribed to aggregation artifacts, and in certain instances, they represent very tight protein-protein interactions. More importantly, mutations in these oncogenes that inactivate their respective transforming abilities simultaneously prevent their encoded oncoproteins from complexing with p105.

All this suggests that at least part of the transforming powers of these various viral oncoproteins derives directly from their abilities to bind p105 and alter its function. Since loss of p105 is implicated in the genesis of a variety of known human tumors, it is attractive to speculate that these viral oncoproteins mimic this state by inactivating any functional RB-1 protein present in target cells that they may infect. An alternative model would propose that the RB-1 protein plays a protective role in the activity of the viral oncoproteins or their cellular homologs.

B. Wilms' Tumor

The model that Wilms' tumor, a cancer of embryonal kidney stem cells, has a genetic component in its etiology has been strongly supported by direct examination of the chromosomes from normal and tumor cells of affected children. The first indication of the chromosomal localization of a locus playing a role in the genesis of nephroblastoma was provided by the identification of a constitutional (i.e., congenital) deletion of chromosome 11 band p13; this aberration has been subsequently observed in tumors of many other patients (Francke et al. 1979). These cases provide strong support for the involvement of a gene in the 11p13 region in the disease and also suggest the necessity for inactivation of this gene at some point in the process of tumor pathogenesis.

To determine whether genetic mechanisms similar to those described above for retinoblastoma play a role in the development of Wilms' tumor, DNA samples from normal and tumor tissues were analyzed for their array of RFLP alleles mapping to loci at various sites on chromosome 11 (Fearon et al. 1984; Koufos et al. 1984; Orkin et al. 1984; Reeve et al. 1984). The data showed loss of alleles in the majority of tumors. A likely explanation for these results based on previous work with retinoblastoma is that mitotic segregation events occurred during the process of tumorigenesis in kidney cells of genetically predisposed children such that one chromosome 11 homolog was lost and the remaining homolog was duplicated, resulting in a reduction to homozygosity. It can be inferred that the surviving 11p13 allele, now present in homozygous state, is a defective version of the Wilms' tumor gene.

If inactivation of both copies of the 11p13-associated Wilms' tumor gene underlies neoplastic growth of these kidney cells, then introduction of an intact copy of this gene into these cells should restore normal growth control. This has been tested recently by introducing a normal chromosome 11 into Wilms' tumor cells by the microcell transfer procedure described earlier. The resulting cells lost the ability to form tumors in nude mice; control experiments with introduction of other chromosomes into the tumor cells failed to affect their neoplastic properties (Weissman et al. 1987). Taken together, these data suggest that Wilms' tumor cells are homozygously defective for an 11p13 gene that functions as a suppressor of the neoplastic growth of kidney cells.

C. Renal Cell Carcinoma and Small Cell Lung Carcinoma

Renal cell carcinoma is a tumor of the precursors of the tubule cells in the kidney. The first evidence that renal cell carcinoma occurs subsequent to chromosomal rearrangement was provided by the karyotypic identification of a constitutional translocation between chromosomes 3 and 8 in a family with a high incidence of this tumor type (Cohen et al. 1979). Cytogenetic analyses of sporadic renal cell carcinomas have also uncovered chromosome 3 abnormalities manifested as deletions distal to 3p11. These findings are, of course, reminiscent of those seen with retinoblastoma and Wilms' tumor. A comparison of the germ-line and tumor genotypes at loci on chromosome 3p confirms and extends these impressions. In a small series of such studies, every renal cell carcinoma examined lost RFLP alleles at one or more such 3p loci without any generalized corresponding loss of alleles on other chromosomes (Zbar et al. 1987; Kovacs et al. 1988). Although heritable forms of these tumors were not examined, the specificity of the losses of heterozygosity and high frequency of such events suggests the involvement of predisposing recessive mutations in the etiology of this malignancy.

Small cell lung cancer (SCLC) has been associated with two distinct forms of genetic abnormalities. Amplification of members of the *myc* gene family has been observed in approximately 10% of cell lines obtained from untreated patients with SCLC and in 40% of cell lines obtained from treated patients (Little et al. 1983; Nau et al. 1985). The other genetic alteration is the consistent finding of deletion of chromosome 3p, although the cytogenetic analyses that developed this correlate were performed mostly on cultured cell lines (Whang-Peng et al. 1982).

A comparison of genotypes between constitutional and tumor cells from SCLC patients showed that each tumor examined had lost an RFLP allele at loci in the 3p14–23 region of the genome (Naylor et al. 1987; Yokota et al. 1987; Kok et al. 1988). Consistent with the cytogenetic findings and with results from other adult-onset tumors, these losses appeared to result in hemizygosity and thus appear to arise through intrachromosomal deletion. Whether these carcinomas arising from two distinct tissue lineages are caused by nullizygosity of the same locus is a most interesting question.

D. Colorectal Carcinoma

Colonic neoplasms provide an excellent system in which to investigate genetic alterations that contribute to the malignant condition. Neoplasms representing all stages of tumor progression can be readily identified histologically, from very small benign adenomas to large invasive carcinomas. Furthermore, colonic tumors occur in both familial and sporadic forms.

Extensive cytogenetic analyses of carcinomas of the large bowel have demonstrated consistent rearrangements of chromosome 17, including frequent deletions of its short arm (Muleris et al. 1985). This prompted investigators to study possible allele loss on chromosome 17p in colorectal cancers using RFLP probes specific for this chromosome. It was found that greater than 75% of tumor samples examined showed loss of chromosome

17p sequences in the region of 17p12; in some cases, the loss of one 17p RFLP allele appeared to be associated with the duplication of the retained allele, resulting in homozygosity of chromosome 17p sequences, whereas in others the allele loss seemed to be achieved through deletions (Vogelstein et al. 1988).

Yet other investigators found loss of RFLP alleles on chromosome 5q (5q21–22) in DNA extracted from carcinomas of sporadic colorectal carcinomas as well as from carcinomas of patients with familial adenomatous polyposis (FAP) (Bodmer et al. 1987; Leppert et al. 1987; Solomon et al. 1987). The frequency with which 5q allele loss is seen in these various colorectal carcinomas is as much as 40%. The adenocarcinomas exhibit the 5q or 17p allele loss or the combination of both losses (Law et al. 1988; Vogelstein et al. 1989). Most recently, significant loss of alleles on chromosome 18q has also been noted (Muleris et al. 1985; Law et al. 1988; Vogelstein et al. 1989). In addition to the loss of DNA sequences from chromosomes 5, 17, and 18, resulting in hemi- or homozygosity of relevant RFLP alleles, activation of the c-Ki-*ras* gene (usually by point mutation at codon 12) often occurs (Vogelstein et al. 1988). Unlike these allele losses, which are seen only in carcinomas, the activated *ras* gene is often found in the benign adenomas that are thought to be the premalignant precursors of the carcinomas. Consequently, multiple genetic alterations appear to occur during the progression of normal colonic cells to the malignant adenocarcinomas, with activation of *ras* genes being a relatively early event associated with benign hyperplasia and homozygous allele loss at one or more chromosomal loci being associated with the later stages of malignant development (see also Chapter 12).

E. Other Types of Malignancies

As described earlier, the process of reduction to homozygosity represents a favored mechanism for unmasking recessive null alleles, including the inactive versions of a number of tumor suppressor genes. Indeed, the very observation of frequent reductions to homozygosity of a chromosomal segment in a particular type of tumor presents a strong indication of the involvement of a gene acting like those that trigger retinoblastomas and Wilms' tumors. In the absence of cytogenetic data, the localization and identification of such a gene might be thought difficult or impossible. However, the power of RFLP analysis enables investigators to search through the entire genome of a tumor cell for regions that have lost heterozygosity, even without clues provided by cytogeneticists (Koufos et al. 1985). The thoroughness of such a search is limited only by the number of useful RFLP probes that have been mapped throughout the genome.

The initial successes of this RFLP strategy are summarized in Table 2. In most cases, the loci described in this way remain inferential. The next steps

Table 2 Tumors with evidence of specific loss of genetic information

Tumor type	Chromosomal region	Evidence
Neuroblastoma	1p; 14q	deletion, LOH[1]; LOH
Uveal melanoma	2	LOH
Renal cell carcinoma	3p	deletion, translocation, LOH
Lung adenocarcinoma	3p	deletion, LOH
Small cell lung carcinoma	3p; 13; 17	deletion, LOH; LOH, Rb gene alteration; LOH
Colorectal carcinoma	5q; 17p; 18	genetic linkage, deletion, LOH; LOH; LOH
Glioblastoma	10	loss, LOH
Breast carcinoma	11p; 13q	LOH; LOH, Rb gene alteration
Wilms' tumor	11p	deletion, LOH
Hepatoblastoma	11p	LOH, association with Wilms'
Adrenal carcinoma	11p	LOH, association with Wilms'
Rhabdomyosarcoma	11p15	LOH, association with Wilms'
Transitional cell bladder carcinoma	11p	LOH
Retinoblastoma (Rb)	13q14	deletion, translocation, genetic linkage, LOH
Osteosarcoma	13q14	association with retinoblastoma, LOH, Rb gene alteration
Astrocytoma	17p	LOH
Acoustic neurinoma	22	linkage to neurofibromatosis, LOH
Meningioma	22	linkage to neurofibromatosis, LOH

[1] LOH–Loss of constitutional heterozygosity in tumors.

will involve the association of each locus with a specific gene and the isolation of this gene through molecular cloning. Given existing techniques, the molecular cloning of these genes will likely prove difficult, although not impossible. The RFLP probes that define a chromosomal region may be millions of base pairs away from the gene of interest, and gene cloning by "chromosomal walking" techniques has proven exceedingly laborious. It is clear that new cloning strategies are required to expedite isolation of these genes.

F. *p53* and *erbA*

As described throughout this chapter, a diverse group of experimental strategies has been mustered to uncover genes that negatively regulate cell growth and contribute to cell transformation when inactivated. These genes, variously termed tumor suppressors, growth suppressors, emerogenes, and anti-oncogenes, form a large and apparently diverse group. The isolation of most of these, as discussed above, will prove very difficult. Unexpectedly, two new members of this group, *p53* and *erbA*, have been added by review of the activities of known genes. Both were classified as oncogenes for many years, but recent detailed examination of their structure and effects on cell physiology now points strongly to the anti-proliferative role of their normal alleles.

The *p53* gene was discovered through the ability of its encoded protein to complex with the SV40 large T (LT) antigen in virus-transformed cells (Lane and Crawford 1979; Linzer and Levine 1979). The p53 protein of the normal cell is metabolically unstable and accumulates to only very low steady-state levels; upon complexing with SV40 LT, turnover of p53 is virtually eliminated, and it accumulates to levels often 100-fold higher than normal (Oren et al. 1981). This was thought to underlie at least part of the transforming powers of SV40 LT: By causing accumulation of a cellular growth-promoting protein, the viral oncoprotein could deregulate and drive the growth of a virus-infected cell. This model was supported by other experiments in which a *p53* cDNA clone was converted into an oncogene when its expression was driven by a high-efficiency transcriptional promoter. Thus, a *p53* clone could immortalize primary cells and collaborate with a *ras* oncogene in their transformation (Eliyahu et al. 1984; Jenkins et al. 1984; Parada et al. 1984). Once again, overexpression of this gene (like overexpression of a cellular *myc* gene) elicited a neoplastic effect.

Fully unexpected was the discovery that each of the *p53* cDNAs used in these experiments, which were thought to encode wild-type p53 protein, carried point mutations in their reading frames. When bona fide wild-type *p53* cDNAs were used in such transfection experiments, they were found to be strongly growth-inhibitory (Finlay et al. 1989). An initial conclusion is that the normal *p53* gene acts to suppress cell growth and that certain of its mutant alleles act in an opposite fashion to promote proliferation. This conclusion has been strengthened by two more recent lines of work. One, at the biochemical level, has shown that some mutant p53 protein molecules are able to form complexes with wild-type p53 protein molecules with which they may coexist in the cell (Eliyahu et al. 1988; Rovinski and Benchimol 1988). In this way, the mutant protein may sequester the wild-type protein, thus releasing the cell from the anti-proliferative effects imposed by the wild-type protein. Indeed, SV40 LT may serve the same role when it complexes with p53 in the transformed cell.

A second line of work, in this instance genetic, has provided even more dramatic evidence. Study of certain tumor cell genomes has shown that they carry mutant *p53* genes or have lost them altogether. For example, one such study found *p53* genes inactivated in the genomes of a series of Friend leukemia virus-induced mouse tumors (Ben-David et al. 1988). Most powerful is the recent evidence indicating that the "tumor suppressor" locus on human chromosome 17 that is reduced to homozygosity in many colon carcinomas maps to the site of the cell's *p53* gene (Baker et al. 1989). This strongly indicates that the *p53* gene belongs to the group of recessive tumor genes discussed earlier.

To clarify and summarize, mutant versions of the *p53* gene can act in two genetic ways to promote growth. Subtle mutations in its reading frame can create a "dominant negative" *p53* allele that both inactivates its own antiproliferative function and, at the same time, enables it to counteract the functioning of the wild-type *p53* allele in the same cell. A second step involving elimination of this surviving wild-type allele (e.g., by reduction to homozygosity of the mutant allele) now creates a cell fully devoid of *p53* activity; in this latter way, the *p53* gene closely resembles the genes that trigger retinoblastomas and Wilms' tumors.

The second of these new members is the *erbA* oncogene that was first discovered in the genome of the avian erythroblastosis retrovirus together with the *erbB* oncogene. *erbA* is an altered version of the normal cellular receptor for triiodothyronine (thyroid hormone) (Sap et al. 1986); *erbB* is a mutated version of the normal cellular epidermal growth factor (EGF) receptor gene: These two oncogenes can collaborate to transform chicken erythroid precursor cells. The *erbB* oncogene forces the proliferation of these cells, but many differentiate to nonproliferating erythroid cells; *erbA* acts to block their differentiation, thereby trapping them in the pool of proliferating precursors (Kahn et al. 1986; see Chapter 12).

The *erbA* oncogene, like *p53*, is able to antagonize the function of its normal counterpart allele. The thyroid receptor protein encoded by its wild-type allele acts as a DNA-binding transcriptional factor. Having bound its ligand (thyroid hormone), the receptor acts to turn on expression of a bank of genes that allow the cell to differentiate and thus to enter a nonproliferating state. In this way, the normal receptor gene and protein operate to antagonize growth. The aberrantly structured protein encoded by the *erbA* oncogene is unable to induce this gene expression in the presence of ligand; at the same time, it competes effectively with the wild-type receptor for control sites on critical genes and prevents the normal receptor from mediating steps of differentiation (Damm et al. 1989; Sap et al. 1989). Thus, as in the case of *p53*, a mutant allele is acting in a dominant negative fashion to ablate wild-type function.

IV. FUNCTIONAL SIGNIFICANCE OF TUMOR SUPPRESSOR GENES

The functions of most of the candidate tumor suppressor genes described above are at present unknown. There are several reasonable and tantalizing possibilities that can be imagined, however. It is conceivable that the products of these loci interact with proto-oncogene and oncogene proteins in an antagonistic way. In fact, as described above, evidence in support of this idea has recently been obtained, since the retinoblastoma gene product has been shown to bind to the products of the transforming regions of adenovirus, SV40, and papillomavirus (DeCaprio et al. 1988; Whyte et al. 1988). Such data may indicate that these oncoproteins act to inactivate the Rb protein, in this way mimicking the loss of the protein as it occurs during formation of retinoblastomas. Tumor suppressor genes may also encode products required for the orderly progress of tissue differentiation and organismal development. Under this hypothesis, tumors might represent developmental arrests, and their analysis may therefore open new windows into such processes. It is also possible that these genes might encode products that enable cells to respond to signals causing inhibition of growth or induction of differentiation. We do not know yet whether the types of mutations that predispose family members to tumors occur in the same loci that serve as tumor suppressors in vitro. We also do not know whether such mutations are only active in initial stages of carcinogenesis or also play a role in the progressive attainment of malignancy that human tumors inevitably pass through.

Tumor suppressor genes may directly or indirectly influence the expression of the dominantly acting classes of oncogenes. In fact, as mentioned earlier, an alternative name has been used for this class of genes, namely, anti-oncogenes. Data derived from somatic cell hybrids and flat revertants provide evidence both for and against any such mechanism of action. In one experimental system, rat cells were transformed with Rous sarcoma virus (RSV), and these transformed cells were then fused with normal rat cells. The resulting hybrid cells retained the integrated RSV provirus but had a normal morphology, were nontumorigenic, and expressed little or no v-*src* protein. This is clearly suggestive of an anti-oncogene effect with significant down-regulation of the viral oncogene expression (Green and Wyke 1985).

A less compelling example has been noted with human HT1080 fibrosarcoma cells. These cells are pseudodiploid and contain one normal and one activated allele of N-*ras*. Nontumorigenic flat revertants have also been isolated that are now subtetraploid. In this system, the key difference between the tumorigenic and nontumorigenic states appears to be the threshold level of expression of the activated N-*ras* gene, irrespective of the level of expression of the normal allele, removing in effect the possibility of competitive levels of expression of normal versus activated alleles being the determining factor of cell phenotype (Paterson et al. 1987).

Many more examples exist that argue against a direct effect of tumor suppressor genes on oncogene expression. Several rodent cells transformed with sarcoma viruses have been fused with normal cells, resulting in hybrid cells that are nontumorigenic and yet express high levels of the viral oncogene (Craig and Sager 1985). The same has been found for flat revertants of sarcoma-virus-transformed cells. In a particularly illustrative case, the human EJ bladder carcinoma cell line, which contained an endogenous activated c-Ha-*ras* oncogene, was fused with normal human fibroblasts. The resulting hybrid cells were nontumorigenic, and tumorigenic segregants were derived from them. All hybrid cells, irrespective of their tumor-forming ability, expressed high levels of the mutant Ha-*ras* p21 protein (Geiser et al. 1986).

Thus, it would seem in many instances that tumor suppressor genes do not directly control expression of activated oncogenes (at least those that have been identified). Furthermore, these same studies also provide compelling evidence that expression of activated oncogenes may be necessary but is clearly not sufficient for neoplastic expression. Several other lines of experimental evidence not addressed here, including transgenic animals, are in keeping with this conclusion (see also Chapter 12).

V. SUMMARY

Loss of growth-regulating genes appears to play an important role in the genesis of most if not all human tumors. Such genes may be lost from the germ line, and their absence may predispose to tumor susceptibility. Even more frequently, losses of such genes and their functions would seem to occur through somatic mutations sustained in the genomes of evolving tumor cell clones. Although not yet proven, it would seem that many of these genes normally operate in a variety of ways to limit cell growth. The growth-constraining mechanism operating within the cell may be as diverse as the much-described mitogenic regulatory circuits of the cell. As such, the products of these growth-suppressing genes may act biochemically in diverse ways to ensure that cells do not proliferate beyond the limits dictated by normal development and tissue homeostasis.

Because randomly occurring mutations are far more effective in inactivating genes than in creating deregulated, hyperactive alleles, these tumor suppressor genes may well play a far more important role in tumor pathogenesis than the oncogenes, most of which act as dominant, deregulated versions of normal growth-promoting genes. Vindication of these models will be long in coming, since their study lags a decade behind the study of the oncogenes described elsewhere in this volume.

The lines of evidence discussed in this chapter taken together make a strong prima facie case for the frequent involvement in human cancer of recessive mutations in loci responsible for suppressing tumorigenesis. It is clear that a detailed understanding of the function of such loci has profound and exciting potential for therapeutic design. In addition, the ability to identify genetically predisposed individuals in a population may become possible, and this may in turn prove useful in making a variety of decisions, including those involving lifestyles and work choices. Already, the studies described here have provided clear explanations for the loci and genetic mechanism underlying many familial cancers. As the mapping and functional studies become more defined, it can be anticipated that much information concerning the locations, structure, and function of similarly acting loci will be forthcoming.

REFERENCES

Baker, S.J., E.R. Fearon, J.M. Nigro, S.R. Hamilton, A.C. Preisinger, J.M. Jessup, P. van Tuinen, D.H. Ledbetter, D.F. Barker, Y. Nakamura, R. White, and B. Vogelstein. 1989. Chromosome 17 deletion and p53 gene mutation in colorectal carcinomas. *Science* **244:** 217–221.

Ben-David, Y., V.R. Prideaux, V. Chow, S. Benchimol, and A. Bernstein. 1988. Inactivation of the p53 oncogene by internal deletion or retroviral integration in erythroleukemia cell lines induced by Friend leukemia virus. *Oncogene* **3:** 179–185.

Benedict, W.F., B.E. Weissman, C. Mark, and E.J. Stanbridge. 1984. Tumorigenicity of human HT1080 fibrosarcoma × normal fibroblast hybrids is chromosome dosage dependent. *Cancer Res.* **44:** 3471–3479.

Bodmer, W.F., C.J. Bailey, J. Bodmer, H.J.R. Bussey, A. Ellis, P. Gorman, F.C. Lucibello, V.A. Murday, S.H. Rider, P. Scambler, D. Sheer, E. Solomon, and N. Spurr. 1987. Localization of the gene for familial adenomatous polyposis on chromosome 5. *Nature* **328:** 614–616.

Botstein, D., R.L. White, M. Skolnick, and R.W. Davis. 1980. Construction of a genetic linkage map in man using restriction fragment length polymorphisms. *Am. J. Hum. Genet.* **32:** 314–331.

Boveri, T. 1914. *Zur frage der Erstehung maligner Tumoren.* Gustav Fischer, Jena.

Cavenee, W.K., M.F. Hansen, M. Nördenskjold, E. Kock, I. Maumenee, J.A. Squire, R.A. Phillips, and B.L. Gallie. 1985. Genetic origin of mutations predisposing to retinoblastoma. *Science* **228:** 501–503.

Cavenee, W.K., T.P. Dryja, R.A. Phillips, W.F. Benedict, R. Godbout, B.L. Gallie, A.L. Murphree, L.C. Strong, and R. White. 1983. Expression of recessive alleles by chromosomal mechanisms in retinoblastoma. *Nature* **305:** 779–784.

Cohen, A.J., F.P. Li, S. Berg, D.J. Marchetto, S. Tsai, S.C. Jacobs, and R.S. Brown. 1979. Hereditary renal cell carcinoma associated with a chromosomal translocation. *N. Engl. J. Med.* **301:** 592–595.

Craig, R.W. and R. Sager. 1985. Suppression of tumorigenicity in hybrids of normal and oncogene-transformed CHEF cells. *Proc. Natl. Acad. Sci.* **82:** 2062–2066.

Croce, C. M. 1984. Gene regulation in the expression of malignancy. *Cancer Surv.* **3:** 287–298.

Damm, K., C.C. Thompson, and R.M. Evans. 1989. Protein encoded by v-*erb*A functions as thyroid hormone receptor antagonist. *Nature* **339:** 593–597.

DeCaprio, J.A., J.W. Ludlow, J. Figge, J.-Y. Shew, C.-M. Huang, W.-H. Lee, E. Marsilio, E. Paucha, and D.M. Livingston. 1988. SV40 large tumor antigen forms a stable complex with the product of the retinoblastoma susceptibility locus. *Cell* **54:** 275–283.

Der, C.J. and E.J. Stanbridge. 1981. A tumor-specific membrane phosphoprotein marker in human cell hybrids. *Cell* **26:** 429–438.

Dryja, T.P., W.K. Cavenee, R.L. White, J.M. Rapoport, D.M. Alberts, and G.A.P. Bruns. 1984. Homozygosity of chromosome 13 in retinoblastoma. *N. Engl. J. Med.* **310:** 550–554.

Dryja, T.P., J.M. Rapoport, J. Epstein, A.M. Goorin, R. Weichselbaum, A. Koufos, and W. Cavenee. 1986. Chromosome 13 homozygosity in osteosarcoma without retinoblastoma. *Am. J. Hum. Genet.* **38:** 59–66.

Dyson, N., P.M. Howley, K. Münger, and E. Harlow. 1989. The human papilloma virus-16 E7 oncoprotein is able to bind to the retinoblastoma gene product. *Science* **243:** 934–937.

Eliyahu, D., A. Raz, P. Gruss, D. Givol, and M. Oren. 1984. Participation of p53 cellular tumour antigen in transformation of normal embryonic cells. *Nature* **312:** 646–649.

Eliyahu, D., N. Goldfinger, O. Pinhasi-Kimhi, G. Shaulsky, Y. Skurnik, N. Arai, V. Rotter, and M. Oren. 1988. Meth A fibrosarcoma cells express two transforming mutant p53 species. *Oncogene* **3:** 313–321.

Evans, E.P., M.D. Burtenshaw, B.B. Brown, R. Hennion, and H. Harris. 1982. The analysis of malignancy by cell fusion. IX. Reexamination and clarification of the cytogenetic problem. *J. Cell Sci.* **56:** 113–130.

Fearon, E.R., B. Vogelstein, and A.P. Feinberg. 1984. Somatic deletion and duplication of genes on chromosome 11 in Wilms' tumor. *Nature* **309:** 176–178.

Finlay, C.A., P.W. Hinds, and A.J. Levine. 1989. The p53 proto-oncogene can act as a suppressor of transformation. *Cell* **57:** 1083–1093.

Fournier, R.E.K. and F.H. Ruddle. 1977. Microcell-mediated transfer of murine chromosomes into mouse, Chinese hamster, and human somatic cells. *Proc. Natl. Acad. Sci.* **74:** 319–323.

Francke, U., L.B. Holmes, L. Atkins, and V.M. Riccardi. 1979. Aniridia-Wilms' tumor association: Evidence for specific deletions of 11p13. *Cytogenet. Cell Genet.* **24:** 185–190.

Friend, S.H., R. Bernards, S. Rogelj, R.A. Weinberg, J.M. Rapoport, D.M. Albert, and T.P. Dryja. 1986. A human DNA segment with properties of the gene that predisposes to retinoblastoma and osteosarcoma. *Nature* **323:** 643–646.

Friend, S.H., J.M. Horowitz, M.R. Gerber, X.F. Wang, E. Bogenmann, F.P. Li, and R.A. Weinberg. 1987. Deletions of a DNA sequence in retinoblastoma and mesenchymal tumors: Organization of the sequence and its encoded protein. *Proc. Natl. Acad. Sci.* **84:** 9059–9063.

Fung, Y.-K. T., A.L. Murphree, A. T'Ang, J. Qian, S.H. Hinrichs, and W.F. Benedict. 1987. Structural evidence for the authenticity of the human retinoblastoma gene. *Science* **236:** 1657–1662.

Geiser, A., C.J. Der, C.J. Marshall, and E.J. Stanbridge. 1986. Suppression of tumorigenicity with continued expression of the c-Ha-*ras* oncogene in EJ bladder carcinoma × human fibroblast hybrid cells. *Proc. Natl. Acad. Sci.* **83:** 5209–5213.

Godbout, R., T.P. Dryja, J. Squire, B.L. Gallie, and R.A. Phillips. 1983. Somatic inactivation of genes on chromosome 13 is a common event in retinoblastoma. *Nature* **304:** 451–453.

Green, A.R. and J.A. Wyke. 1985. Anti-oncogenes. A subset of regulatory genes involved in carcinogenesis? *Lancet* **II:** 475–477.

Hansen, M.F., A. Koufos, B.L. Gallie, R.A. Phillips, O. Fodstad, A. Brogger, T. Gedde-Dahl, and W.K. Cavenee. 1985. Osteosarcoma and retinoblastoma: A shared chromosomal mechanism revealing recessive predisposition. *Proc. Natl. Acad. Sci.* **82:** 6216–6220.

Harbour, J.W., S.L. Lai, J. Whang-Peng, A.F. Gazdar, J.D. Minna, and F.J. Kaye. 1988. Abnormalities in structure and expression of the human retinoblastoma gene in SCLC. *Science* **241:** 353–357.

Harris, H. 1971. Cell fusion and the analysis of malignancy: The Croonian lecture. *Proc. R. Soc. Lond. B. Biol. Sci.* **179:** 1–20.

Harris, H., O.J. Miller, G. Klein, P. Worst, and T. Tachibana. 1969. Suppression of malignancy by cell fusion. *Nature* **223:** 363–368.

Horowitz, J.M., D. Yandell, S.-H. Park, S. Canning, P. Whyte, K. Buchkovich, E. Harlow, R.A. Weinberg, and T.P. Dryja. 1989. Point mutational inactivation of the retinoblastoma antioncogene. *Science* **243:** 937–940.

Huang, H.-J.S., J.-K. Yee, P.L. Chen, R. Bookstein, T. Friedmann, E.Y.-H.P. Lee, and W.-H. Lee. 1988. Suppression of the neoplastic phenotype by replacement of the Rb gene in human cancer cells. *Science* **242:** 1563–1566.

Jenkins, J.R., K. Rudge, and G.A. Currie. 1984. Cellular immortalization by a cDNA clone encoding the transformation-associated phosphoprotein p53. *Nature* **312:** 651–654.

Kahn, P., L. Frykberg, C. Brady, I. Stanley, H. Beug, B. Vennström, and T. Graf. 1986. V-*erb*A cooperates with sarcoma oncogenes in leukemia cell transformation. *Cell* **45:** 349–356.

Kitayama, H., Y. Sugimoto, T. Matsuzaki, Y. Ikawa, and M. Noda. 1989. A *ras*-related gene with transformation suppressor activity. *Cell* **56:** 77–84.

Klinger, H.P. 1982. Suppression of tumorigenicity. *Cytogenet. Cell Genet.* **32:** 68–84.

Knudson, A.G. 1971. Mutation and cancer: Statistical study of retinoblastoma. *Proc. Natl. Acad. Sci.* **68:** 820–823.

Kok, K., J. Osinga, B. Carritt, M.B. Davis, A.H. van der Hout, A.Y. van der Veen, R.M. Landsvater, L.F.M.H. de Leiji, H.H. Berendsen, P.E. Postmus, S. Poppema, and C.H.C.M. Buys. 1988. Deletion of a DNA sequence of the chromosomal region 3p21 in all major types of lung cancer. *Nature* **330:** 578–581.

Koufos, A., M.F. Hansen, N.G. Copeland, N.A. Jenkins, B.C. Lampkin, and W.K. Cavenee. 1985. Loss of heterozygosity in three embryonal tumors suggests a common pathogenetic mechanism. *Nature* **316:** 330–334.

Koufos, A., M.F. Hansen, B.C. Lampkin, M.L. Workman, N.G. Copeland, N.A. Jenkins, and W.K. Cavenee. 1984. Loss of alleles at loci on human chromosome 11 during genesis of Wilms' tumor. *Nature* **309:** 170–172.

Kovacs, G., R. Eriandsson, F. Boldog, S. Ingvarrson, R. Muller-Brechlin, G. Klein, and J. Sumegi. 1988. Consistent chromosome 3p deletion and loss of heterozygosity in cell carcinoma. *Proc. Natl. Acad. Sci.* **85:** 1571–1575.

Lalande, M., T. Donlon, R.A. Petersen, R. Lieberfarb, S. Manter, and S.A. Latt. 1986. Molecular detection and differentiation of deletions in band 13q14 in human retinoblastoma. *Cancer Genet. Cytogenet.* **23:** 151–162.

Lane, D.P. and L.V. Crawford. 1979. T antigen is bound to a host protein in SV40-transformed cells. *Nature* **278:** 261–263.

Law, D.J., S. Olschwang, J.P. Monpezat, D. Lefrancois, D. Jagelman, N.J. Petrelli, and A.P. Feinberg. 1988. Concerted nonsyntenic allelic loss in human colorectal carcinoma. *Science* **241:** 961–965.

Lee, E.Y.-H.P., H. To, J.Y. Shew, R. Bookstein, P. Scully, and W.H. Lee. 1988. Inactivation of the retinoblastoma susceptibility gene in human breast cancers. *Science* **241:** 218–221.

Lee, W.-H., R. Bookstein, F. Hong, L.-H. Young, J.-Y. Shew, and E.Y.-H.P. Lee. 1987. Human retinoblastoma susceptibility gene: Cloning identification and sequence. *Science* **235:** 1394–1399.

Lee, W.H., J.-Y. Shew, F.D. Hong, T.W. Sery, L.A. Donoso, L.-J. Young, R. Bookstein, and E.Y.-H.P. Lee. 1987b. The retinoblastoma gene encodes a nuclear phosphoprotein associated with DNA binding activity. *Nature* **329:** 642–645.

Leppert, M., M. Dobbs, P. Scambler, P. O'Connell, Y. Nakamura, D. Stauffer, S. Woodward, R. Burt, J. Hughes, E. Gardner, M. Lathrop, J. Wasmuth, J.-M. Lalouel, and R. White. 1987. The gene for familial polyposis coli maps to the long arm of chromosome 5. *Science* **238:** 1411–1413.

Linzer, D.H. and A.J. Levine. 1979. Characterization of a 54K dalton cellular SV40 tumor antigen present in SV40-transformed cells and uninfected embryonal carcinoma cells. *Cell* **17:** 43–52.

Little, C.D., M.M. Nau, D.N. Carney, A.F. Gazdar, and J.D. Minna. 1983. Amplification and expression of the c-*myc* oncogene in human cancer cell lines. *Nature* **306:** 194–196.

Mitelman, F. 1985. Catalogue of chromosomal aberrations in cancer. Alan R. Liss, New York.

Muleris, M., R.J. Salmon, B. Zafrani, J. Girodet, and B. Dutrillaux. 1985. Consistent deficiencies of chromosome 18 and of the short arm of chromosome 17 in eleven cases of human large bowel cancer: A possible recessive determinism. *Ann. Genet.* **28:** 206–213.

Nau, M.M., B.J. Brooks. J. Battey, E. Sausville, A.F. Gazdar, I.R. Kirsch, O.W. McBride, V. Bertness, G.F. Hollis, and J.D. Minna. 1985. L-*myc*, a new *myc*-related gene amplified and expressed in human small cell lung cancer. *Nature* **318:** 69–73.

Naylor, S.L., B.E. Johnson, J.D. Minna, and A.Y. Sakaguchi. 1987. Loss of heterozygosity of chromosome 3p markers in small-cell lung cancer. *Nature* **329:** 451–454.

Noda, M., H. Kitayama, T. Matsuzaki, Y. Sugimoto, H. Okayama, R.H. Bassin, and Y. Ikawa. 1988. Detection of genes with a potential for suppressing the transformed phenotype associated with activated *ras* genes. *Proc. Natl. Acad. Sci.* **86:** 162–166.

Oren, M., W. Maltzman, and A.J. Levine. 1981. Post-translational regulation of the 54K cellular tumor antigen in normal and transformed cells. *Mol. Cell. Biol.* **1:** 101–110.

Orkin, S.H., D.S. Goldman, and S.E. Sallan. 1984. Development of homozygosity for chromosome 11p markers in Wilms' tumor. *Nature* **309:** 172–174.

Parada, L.F., H. Land, R.A. Weinberg, D. Wolf, and V. Rotter. 1984. Cooperation between gene encoding p53 tumour antigen and *ras* in cellular transformation. *Nature* **312:** 649–651.

Paterson, H., B. Reeves, R. Brown, A. Hall, M. Furth, J. Bos, P. Jones, and C. Marshall. 1987. Activated N-*ras* controls the transformed phenotype of HT1080 human fibrosarcoma cells. *Cell* **51:** 803-812.

Pereira-Smith, O.M. and J.R. Smith. 1983. Evidence for the recessive nature of cellular immortality. *Science* **221:** 964–966.

Reeve, A.E., P.J. Housiaux, R.J.M. Gardner, W.C. Chewings, R.M. Grindley, and L.J. Millow. 1984. Loss of a Harvey *ras* allele in sporadic Wilms' tumor. *Nature* **309:** 174–176.

Rovinski, B. and S. Benchimol. 1988. Immortalization of rat embryo fibroblasts by the cellular p53 oncogene. *Oncogene* **2:** 445–452.

Sager, R. 1985. Genetic suppression of tumor formation. *Adv. Cancer Res.* **44:** 43–68.

Sap, J., A. Muñoz, J. Schmitt, H. Stunnenberg, and B. Vennström. 1989. Repression of transcription mediated at a thyroid hormone response element by the v-*erb*A oncogene product. *Nature* **340:** 242–244.

Sap, J., A. Muñoz, K. Damm, Y. Goldberg, J. Ghysdael, A. Leutz, H. Beug, and B. Vennström. 1986. The c-*erb*A protein is a high-affinity receptor for thyroid hormone. *Nature* **324:** 635–640.

Saxon, P.J., E.S. Srivatsan, and E.J. Stanbridge. 1986. Introduction of human chromosome 11 via microcell transfer controls tumorigenic expression of HeLa cells. *EMBO J.* **5:** 3461–3466.

Saxon, P.J., E.S. Srivatsan, G.V. Leipzig, J.H. Sameshima, and E.J. Stanbridge. 1985. Selective transfer of individual human chromosomes to recipient cells. *Mol. Cell. Biol.* **5:** 140–146.

Schäfer, R. J. Iyer, E. Iten, and A.C. Nirkko. 1988. Partial reversion of transformed phenotypes in c-Ha-*ras* transfected, tumorigenic cells by transfer of a human gene. *Proc. Natl. Acad. Sci.* **85:** 1590–1594.

Solomon, E., R. Voss, V. Hall, W.F. Bodmer, J.R. Jass, A.J. Jeffreys, F.C. Lucibello, I. Patel, and S.H. Rider. 1987. Chromosome 5 allele loss in human colorectal carcinomas. *Nature* **328:** 616–619.

Sparkes, R.S., A.L. Murphree, R.W. Lingua, M.C. Sparkes, L.L. Field, S.J. Funderburk, and W.F. Benedict. 1983. Gene for hereditary retinoblastoma assigned to human chromosome 13 by linkage analysis to esterase D. *Science* **219:** 971–973.

Stanbridge, E.J. 1976. Suppression of malignancy in human cells. *Nature* **260:** 17–20.

———. 1987. Genetic regulation of tumorigenic expression in somatic cell hybrids. *Adv. Viral Oncol.* **6:** 83–101.

Stanbridge, E.J., R.R. Flandermeyer, D.W. Daniels, and W.A. Nelson-Rees. 1981. Specific chromosome loss associated with the expression of tumorigenicity in human cell hybrids. *Somatic Cell Mol. Genet.* **7:** 699–712.

Stanbridge, E.J., C.J. Der, C.J. Doersen, R.Y. Nishimi, D.M. Peehl, B.E. Weissman, and J. Wilkinson. 1982. Human cell hybrids: Analysis of transformation and tumorigenicity. *Science* **215:** 252–259.

Vogelstein, B., E.R. Fearon, S.E. Kern, S.R. Hamilton, A.C. Preisinger, Y. Nakamura, and R. White. 1989. Allotype of colorectal carcinomas. *Science* **244:** 207–211.

Vogelstein, B., E.R. Fearon, S.R. Hamilton, S.E. Kern, A.C. Preizinger, M. Leppert, Y. Nakamura, R. White, A.M.M. Smits, and J.L. Bos. 1988. Genetic alterations during colorectal tumor development. *N . Engl. J. Med.* **319:** 525–532.

Weichselbaum, R.R., M. Beckett, and A. Diamond. 1988. Some retinoblastomas, osteosarcomas and soft-tissue sarcomas may share a common etiology. *Proc. Natl. Acad. Sci.* **82:** 2106–2109.

Weissman, B.E., P.J. Saxon, S.R. Pasquale, G.R. Jones, A.G. Geiser, and E.J. Stanbridge. 1987. Introduction of a normal human chromosome 11 into a Wilms' tumor cell line controls its tumorigenic expression. *Science* **236:** 175–180.

Whang-Peng, J., C.S. Kao-Shan, E.C. Lee, P.A. Bunn, D.N. Carney, A.F. Gazdar, and J.D. Minna. 1982. Specific chromosome defect associated with human small-cell lung cancer: Deletion 3p(14-23). *Science* **215:** 181–182.

Whyte, P., K.J. Buchovich, J.M. Horowitz, S.H. Friend, M. Raybuck, R.A. Weinberg, and E. Harlow. 1988. Association between an oncogene and an antioncogene: The adenovirus E1A proteins bind to the retinoblastoma gene product. *Nature* **334:** 124–129.

Yokota, J.M. Wada, Y. Shimosato, M. Terada, and T. Sugimura. 1987. Loss of heterozygosity on chromosome 3, 13, and 17 in small-cell carcinoma and on chromosome 3 in adenocarcinoma of the lung. *Proc. Natl. Acad. Sci.* **84:** 9252–9256.

Yunis, J.J. and N. Ramsay. 1978. Retinoblastoma and subband deletion of chromosome 13. *Am. J. Dis. Child.* **132:** 161–163.

Zbar, B., H. Brauch, C. Talmadge, and M. Linehan. 1987. Loss of alleles at loci on the short arm of chromosome 3 in renal cell carcinoma. *Nature* **327:** 721–724.

12

Oncogenes and Multistep Carcinogenesis

Robert A. Weinberg
Whitehead Institute for Biomedical Research and
Department of Biology
Massachusetts Institute of Technology
Cambridge, Massachusetts 02142

I. INTRODUCTION

The tumors that arise spontaneously in humans and following chemical treatment of experimental animals are formed by a complex, multistep process. This has long been apparent to pathologists who classify tumors on the basis of invasiveness, loss of differentiated traits, and a host of cytological markers. In a number of instances, it has been apparent that tumors composed of benign, relatively differentiated cells represent precursors to more malignant tumors appearing later in the course of tumorigenesis.

Observations of this sort imply a process in which tumor cell populations evolve progressively from cells that deviate only minimally from normalcy toward cells having highly aggressive, invasive behavior (Foulds 1954; Nowell 1976, 1986; Farber 1984). Such change has formal similarities with models in which species change progressively through the processes of Darwinian evolution. According to such thinking, genetic and phenotypic variability in tumor cell populations makes possible the appearance of variants that display phenotypes conferring special growth advantage within a tissue or organism. As such cell clones expand to larger size, they spawn subclones that in turn have acquired yet other novel phenotypes that then drive their own preferential expansion and eventual dominance.

Oncogenes and the Molecular Origins of Cancer.

Tumor cell populations can thus be seen in constant flux, with new subpopulations continually replacing older ones by virtue of the display of one or another novel, advantageous phenotype.

The advantageous traits exhibited by tumor cell subclones might include increased growth rates, decreased dependency on growth factor stimulation, increased tolerance to anoxia, increased ability to evade immunological defenses, and increased invasive or metastatic ability. Although these changes are poorly understood, many investigators presume that changes in tumor cell genomes are responsible for generating such advantageous phenotypes. Indeed, cells in some types of tumors have unusually high genetic instability (Nicholson 1987). This is presumed to generate the rich diversity of subpopulations from which more malignant cell types are eventually selected.

These models of tumor progression separate the development of a tumor into distinct phases, each of which is initiated by a discrete and, in principle, definable genetic change. In many cases, the milestones demarcating each phase of tumor progression may be the acquisition of distinct cellular or viral oncogenes by an evolving tumor cell clone. As reported below, a number of animal and human models have been described in which the presence of specific oncogenes is indeed closely associated with an early or late stage of tumor progression.

II. MODELS OF TUMOR INITIATION AND PROMOTION IN RODENTS AND HUMANS

The best-documented example of multistep carcinogenesis stems from observations made almost 50 years ago that skin carcinomas can be induced reproducibly on the back of a mouse by topical application of a number of well-defined organic compounds. This mouse skin carcinogenesis model allowed the resolution of the skin tumorigenesis into at least three distinct phases termed initiation, promotion, and progression.

Initiation of skin carcinogenesis can be induced by a number of agents, including 7,12-dimethylbenzanthracene (DMBA) and *N*-methyl-*N*′-nitro-*N*-nitrosoguanidine (MNNG), which are applied in one dose or in a small number of successive doses. The immediate effects of such *initiators* are inapparent, in that the skin of a treated animal will appear normal. However, cells of an abnormal constitution have undoubtedly been created, since their existence is revealed following application of a second agent, the *promoter*. Repeated treatment of "initiated" skin with promoter leads to the appearance of precancerous outgrowths termed papillomas. Thus, the promoting agent serves to reveal the presence of dormant, initiated skin cells whose existence would otherwise have gone unnoticed. When applied alone or before treatment by an initiator, the promoter yields virtually no papillomas. One frequently used promoter is the phorbol ester TPA (12-*O*-tetradecanoyl phorbol-13-acetate).

Latent clones of initiated, promoter-responsive cells can survive in a mouse skin for as long as a year after a single exposure to an initiating agent (Van Duuren et al. 1975). This indicates that initiated cells have been marked in a stable way, perhaps by a specific genetic change. This idea is in consonance with the fact that many potent initiating agents are known to be strongly mutagenic. Promoting agents, in contrast, have weak or no mutagenic activity. This suggests that promoters induce nongenetic changes in an initiated cell that might involve the stimulation of certain growth regulatory circuits. Such changes apparently provide a preferential growth advantage to the initiated cells that enables them to expand into the large cell masses seen as papillomas. The growth of papillomas, at least in their earlier stages, is dependent on continual applications of promoter; when promoter is removed, the papillomas regress (Reddy and Fialkow 1987). It appears that the genetic changes induced by initiators collaborate with the epigenetic, reversible effects of promoters to create papillomas.

After prolonged application of promoting agents over a period of months, carcinomas may emerge spontaneously from the papillomas. These carcinomas deviate in two important ways from their papillomatous precursors: They have a distinctly malignant histology, and their growth is no longer dependent on continual stimulation by applied promoters. The acquired independence from promoter stimulation can be hastened greatly by applying mutagenic agents to the papillomatous skin (Hennings et al. 1983). This indicates that the progression of papillomas to carcinomas, like the earlier step of initiation, is driven by genetic change.

To sum up, the promoter serves to expand the clone of initiated cells to a size large enough that a second genetic event may happen in one or another cells of the expanded population (Armitage and Doll 1957). The two genetic changes, one occurring early, the other late in tumorigenesis, represent a minimal description of the genomic changes occurring during tumorigenesis. Some evidence suggests that other steps may intervene, including an intermediate step characterized by promoter-independent papillomas. Analogous observations have been made with chemically induced rat liver tumors (Potter 1984).

Almost all mouse papillomas resulting from initiation by DMBA carry Ha-*ras* oncogenes in their DNA. The presence of these oncogenes in the DNA of the papillomas suggests that their creation is an early event in skin tumorigenesis. This point is made directly by examining the mutations present in the *ras* oncogenes and responsible for their activation. In 90% of the DMBA-initiated tumors, a specific A → T mutation in codon 61 of the Ha-*ras* gene has been found. None of a dozen tumors initiated by MNNG carried this mutation (Quintanilla et al. 1986).

Because the specific mutations present in these tumors are dependent on the identity of the initiating carcinogen (DMBA or MNNG), it is highly likely that these lesions were created directly by interaction of these chemicals with Ha-*ras* DNA sequences in cells of the target organ. Such interaction must occur during the short period following introduction into the tissue when these carcinogens are chemically reactive. By this logic, the initiating event in DMBA-induced tumors corresponds precisely with the activation of a Ha-*ras* oncogene through mutation.

Other work on rat mammary carcinomas indicates that virtually all tumors initiated by a single treatment with nitrosomethyl urea (NMU) have a G $\rightarrow$ A transition mutation affecting the twelfth codon of the Ha-*ras* gene, whereas only one in four DMBA-initiated breast tumors has an activated Ha-*ras* oncogene (Sukumar et al. 1985; Zarbl et al. 1985). Once again, the identity of the initiating agent is reflected in the mutations found many months later in the malignant tumor. As before, the initiation event seems to correspond with the creation of oncogene-activating mutations.

In these skin and mammary tumor models, it appears that the essential and unique difference between normal and initiated cells is the presence of *ras* oncogenes. This point is made directly by recent experiments showing that infection of mouse skin by the Ha-*ras*-containing Harvey sarcoma virus creates cells that respond to TPA by yielding papillomas (Brown et al. 1986; Roop et al. 1986). In this instance, the initiated state can be mimicked by the experimental introduction of a specific oncogene into target cells.

These various animal models show that the Ha-*ras* oncogene allows initiated cells to be especially responsive to the growth-inducing effects of tumor promoters. The promoting agents may be the TPA used in the skin carcinogenesis or endogenous factors such as estrogen, which seems to serve an analogous role during mammary carcinogenesis. In both cases, it is unclear how the promoting agents and the *ras* oncogenes collaborate to produce expansion of initiated cell clones. Equally unclear is the nature of the secondary genetic changes that allow premalignant cells like papillomas to progress to carcinomas. Skin carcinomas have been found to carry amplified copy number of their Ha-*ras* oncogenes, but this change is not observed consistently. It appears that changes in other genes, involving other oncogenes and anti-oncogenes, must intervene to create full-blown carcinomas.

These rodent models of tumor evolution have analogies with several tumors found in humans. A study of six colon carcinomas found *ras* oncogenes in each. In five of these cases, examination of adjacent adenomatous polyps, the premalignant precursors of these carcinomas, found the identically mutated *ras* oncogenes there as well (Bos et al. 1987).

These adenomas have long been observed to have biological parallels with the rodent skin papillomas; the recent finding of these *ras* oncogenes indicates that similar molecular mechanisms are responsible for both types of premalignant growths.

Human myelodysplastic syndrome of the bone marrow is an indolent disease that may progress into a frank myeloid leukemia. Here again, benign or metaplastic cell clones appear to evolve into neoplastic cells that have lost virtually all growth regulation. These myelodysplastic cells also carry activated oncogenes of the *ras* type, once again suggesting that the activation of these oncogenes was a relatively early event in tumor formation (Hirai et al. 1987).

Although activation of *ras* oncogenes would appear to be the first event in the genesis of the chemically induced skin and mammary tumors of rodents, this may not be the case in the human tumors. For example, *ras* oncogenes were found in 58% of large but still premalignant colon adenomas. However, only 9% of small adenomas carried these activated oncogenes (Vogelstein et al. 1988). Such an observation suggests the following scenario: Unknown events initiate colon carcinogenesis by creating small adenomas; *ras* oncogene activation occurs during the subsequent evolution of these growths into larger adenomas; some of these larger adenomas then evolve into malignant carcinomas.

III. MODELS OF TUMOR PROGRESSION

The process of tumor progression refers to the later stages of tumor cell evolution. In some tumors, *ras* activation may occur during these later changes (Vousden and Marshall 1984). In one well-studied human patient, breast cancer effusions were studied at intervals during the progression of her disease. Cells present in the first two effusions lacked a *ras* oncogene, but cells of the third effusion carried an activated Ki-*ras* oncogene. Since the first effusion was collected at a relatively advanced, metastatic stage of disease, this suggests that activation of *ras* occurred even later during a subsequent progression of metastatic cells to an even more aggressive growth state (Liu et al. 1983).

Other human tumors, notably neuroblastomas and mammary carcinomas, have also yielded insight into later steps of tumor progression. In some childhood neuroblastomas, copies of the N-*myc* gene can be found amplified, in some cases up to 100-fold (Brodeur et al. 1984; Schwab et al. 1984). In some mammary carcinomas, copies of *neu* gene, also termed HER-2 and *erbB2*, are also found in multiple copies (Slamon et al. 1987). In the case of the childhood neuroblastomas, the degree of N-*myc* amplification has been found to be correlated with eventual clinical outcome: Tumors carrying many N-*myc* copies per cell are aggressive and respond poorly to therapy. A similar, although less-documented correlation between oncogene amplification and a prognosis of metastasis has been reported in the breast carcinomas.

The gene amplifications present in the human tumors seem to represent relatively late events in tumor progression. They are found in cell clones that were apparently tumorigenic even before oncogene amplification. Thus, these changes may allow slowly growing tumor cell clones to spawn highly malignant, aggressive offshoots. Such a model has been supported by introducing highly overexpressed N-*myc* genes into rat neuroblastomas that lacked significant N-*myc* amplification (Bernards et al. 1987). The resulting tumor cells subsequently grew much faster, yielding tumors having several hundredfold greater mass after several weeks of growth. They were also metastatic, whereas those lacking substantial N-*myc* expression were not. Analogous experiments undertaken with the normal human *neu/erbB2* gene show that amplified copies of this gene are potent in inducing transformation of mouse NIH-3T3 cells, underscoring the apparent causal role of this gene in tumor progression (Di Fiore et al. 1987).

Perhaps the most interesting phenotype of the N-*myc* oncogene overexpressors was the strong down-modulation of their class I histocompatability antigens. These antigens are essential for recognition of target cells by killer lymphocytes, and their loss may confer long-term advantage by making tumor cells invisible to components of the immune system. The absence of these antigens has also been observed in cells from childhood neuroblastomas.

Such examples of oncogene involvement in tumor progression, although illustrative, are hardly typical of all human tumors. To the extent that oncogenes are present, their causal role in one or another phase of tumor progression is usually obscure. In many tumors, other types of genetic elements may be involved in tumor progression. For example, as discussed later, colon carcinomas often show reductions to homozygosity of loci mapping to chromosomes 17 and 18. These are thought to indicate homozygous inactivation of tumor suppressor genes (also called anti-oncogenes) associated with these loci.

IV. USE OF TRANSGENIC MICE TO STUDY TUMORIGENESIS

The descriptions of tumor initiation and progression indicate that initiated cells display only a subset of the cancer phenotypes that will eventually be acquired by their malignant descendants. This suggests in turn that oncogenes like *ras*, implicated in the initiation of certain tumors, are able to induce only some of the traits displayed by a fully malignant cell. Support for this notion has come in recent years from experiments using transgenic mice. In these experiments, activated oncogenes are introduced into the germ line of a mouse strain. In animals of these strains, these oncogenes are acquired congenitally rather than arising de novo through somatic changes provoked by chemical carcinogens or viral infections. The cloned oncogenes chosen for germ-line insertion are placed under the control of tissue-specific promoters, ensuring their expression in a narrow range of tissues and at particular developmental stages. This strategy offers the prospect of orchestrating the critical steps of tumorigenesis in a precise and ordered way.

More than 20 distinct promoter/oncogene constructs have been used to generate transgenic mouse strains. During development, the congenitally acquired "transgenes" become widely if not ubiquitously expressed in all the cells of one or another type within a specific organ. Among the promoters used to date are mouse mammary tumor virus (MMTV), expressed largely in mammary epithelial cells; the elastase promoter, specific for the acinar cells of the pancreas; the insulin promoter, specific for the β cells of that organ; and an immunoglobulin promoter, specific for expression in cells of the B-lymphoid lineage. The oncogenes directed by these various promoters include the SV40 early region (specifying both small and large T antigens), Ha-*ras*, and *myc*.

Many of the mice carrying genetically transmitted oncogenes give evidence of tumors that occur with high frequency and on a tissue-specific basis. The specific type of tumor can usually be predicted by the nature of the promoter used to drive oncogene expression. Importantly, the tumors arising in almost all these transgenic mouse strains appear with a latency of several months after birth. When examined carefully, these tumors have often been found to be of monoclonal or oligoclonal origin, indicating that each tumor stems from a single cell or from a small number of ancestral cells. Thus, despite widespread oncogene expression in many cells of a tissue, only a few of these cells will undergo conversion to malignancy and then only with great delay (Stewart et al. 1984).

The lesson from this is dramatic and clear: A single oncogene like *ras* or *myc* is unable to malignantly transform the great majority of cells in which it is expressed. Although millions of cells in a tissue of a transgenic mouse may express an oncogene, most will remain quite normal; only a few will go on to generate a tumor mass. The expression of these single oncogenes may be necessary for tumorigenesis, but it is hardly sufficient. Other secondary changes, likely involving somatic mutational events, must intervene to trigger the clonal outgrowth of these oncogene-bearing cells. It is possible that these secondary events involve somatic activation of other oncogenes that complement the actions of the congenitally acquired oncogene.

V. MULTISTEP TRANSFORMATION OF CULTURED CELLS

The above descriptions of oncogene action in vivo underscore the complexity of the processes that create tumors in the environment of a tissue or organ. A thorough understanding of these processes will only come from studying the effects of oncogene action within individual cells. Accordingly, a number of investigators have turned to in vitro tissue culture models, attempting to introduce oncogenes into cells through virus infection or gene transfer (transfection).

Among the cell types used to analyze oncogene action, rodent fibroblasts have shown the greatest utility to date. Two types of these cells are used, either as cultures recently explanted from embryos or as cell lines that grow indefinitely in culture. When rodent embryo cells are placed in culture, they grow for 30–50 doublings before they enter a phase, termed senescence or crisis, in which virtually all the cells in the culture stop growing. The causes of this crisis and the associated limited life span in culture are poorly understood. The onset of crisis may indicate the workings of an endogenous clock that limits the doublings that a cell is allowed. An alternative explanation is provided by recent work suggesting that factors present in the serum of the culture medium actively promote cell crisis (Loo et al. 1987).

Emerging from the large population of cells in crisis may be a small number of cell clones that once again show strong and steady replicative potential. These clones can now be expanded and will have an unlimited number of doublings in culture. Such cell clones have undergone a process variously termed *establishment* or *immortalization*, and their descendants now constitute a cell line.

The nature of this spontaneous immortalization event is poorly understood. It occurs with different frequencies in different rodent cell types, and it has never been observed with avian cells in culture. The frequency of these usually rare events can be increased by treatment of rodent cells with mutagenic carcinogens, suggesting that immortalization in culture is the result of a genetic change (Newbold et al. 1982; Newbold and Overell 1983). The genes that permit spontaneous or chemically induced immortalization in culture have not been elucidated.

These immortalized cells will not form tumors in host animals; however, they should be considered premalignant in that they have undergone a change predisposing them to subsequent conversion to a tumorigenic state. Their continued passage in culture will often lead to the appearance of novel subclones that have ostensibly suffered a second change. These doubly altered cells often form dense foci in the midst of a less dense and uniform monolayer. Within these foci, the individual cells grow over one another—they have lost their *contact inhibition* that normally operates to prevent cultured cells from encroaching on the space of their neighbors. Cells picked from these foci will often show *anchorage independence* by forming colonies in soft agar suspension culture; such cells will often be tumorigenic. The appearance of these morphologically transformed, tumorigenic cells can also be hastened by the application of mutagens to already immortalized cells, suggesting that this second step in their in vitro evolution also has an underlying genetic basis. In several instances, the progression to tumorigenicity has been correlated with the appearance of an oncogene such as *ras* (Parada and Weinberg 1983).

This in vitro model recapitulates several aspects of tumor progression in vivo. It involves multiple, successive genetic changes in the cell genome, and in several cases, the tumorigenic cells display oncogenes that are also found in tumors arising in vivo. Nonetheless, the parallels with in vivo processes break down when examined in detail. As described above, in well-studied in vivo models, oncogenes such as *ras* often appear early in tumor cell evolution, whereas in cultured cells, *ras* activation may occur as a secondary event. In addition, the precise in vivo correlates of in vitro traits such as anchorage independence and immortalization are unclear. Indeed, it is possible that these two in vitro phenotypes have no precise counterparts in vivo but only represent experimentally convenient markers for physiologically related, yet distinct, in vivo processes.

VI. EFFECTS OF INTRODUCED ONCOGENES ON CELLS IN CULTURE

At least two distinct genetic changes would seem to intervene in tumorigenesis in vivo and in spontaneous transformation in vitro. Because the precise targets of these genetic changes are usually obscure, it would be valuable to reconstruct the stages of tumor progression using precisely defined genetic elements. Consequently, a number of experimenters have attempted to mimic one or both steps of tumor formation by introducing well-studied oncogenes into cultured cells. These experiments have provided insights into the distinctive workings of different oncogenes and the abilities of these genes to collaborate in tumorigenesis.

Early experiments of this sort involved the introduction of either the polyoma middle T (Rassoulzadegan et al. 1983) or Ha-*ras* (Newbold et al. 1982; Land et al. 1983; Newbold and Overell 1983) oncogenes into cells via transfection. The observed outcome was dependent on the cell type used to assay the effects of these genes. In dense monolayer cultures of primary embryo cells, these oncogenes had little if any effect on the behavior of the cell populations. In contrast, in monolayers of established cells, these oncogenes induced foci of morphologically altered cells. The cells from these foci were tumorigenic, whereas oncogene-bearing cells from the primary embryo cultures were not. Such results showed that cells that have undergone immortalization in culture also acquire a responsiveness to the transforming influences of these oncogenes. Unanswered, however, were reasons for the unsuccessful transformation of the nonimmortalized embryo cells by polyoma middle T or Ha-*ras*.

The apparent incomplete transformation of embryo fibroblasts by these oncogenes provoked a search for other agents, including other oncogenes, that would push this process to completion. In the case of polyoma middle T, the identity of the second agent was obvious: The intact polyomavirus genome is capable of inducing the full malignant transformation of rodent embryo fibroblasts, indicating that one of the other viral genes expressed in transformants must collaborate with the polyoma middle T gene in this process. In the case of *ras*, a possible collaborating oncogene was suggested by the finding that several human tumor cell types carried not only *ras* oncogenes, but also altered forms of the cellular *myc* gene as well.

The resulting experiments, involving cointroduction (cotransfection) of either polyoma middle T plus polyoma large T oncogenes or *ras* plus *myc* oncogenes, showed that two collaborating oncogenes could indeed complete the process of creating tumorigenic cells from fully normal embryo fibroblasts (Land et al. 1983; Rassoulzadegan et al. 1983). Other work performed at the same time revealed the abilities of *ras* to collaborate with the adenovirus E1A oncogene (Ruley 1983).

These findings established the principle that oncogenes are a functionally heterogeneous class of genes that act in distinct, complementary ways to change cell phenotype. Moreover, they suggested that growth regulation of the mammalian cell is organized in a way that single oncogenes, acting alone, are usually unable to transform a cell in a single step. This complexity of normal growth regulation may provide an important protective mechanism against spontaneously arising tumors by maintaining several barriers that impede the evolution of a cell from normalcy to full malignancy. However, as discussed later, under certain experimental conditions this requirement for multiple oncogenes is abrogated, and singly acting genes are indeed able to complete the process.

Numerous examples of such collaborating oncogenes have now been described. They stem from a variety of biological models, species, and tissue types. In aggregate, they reinforce the notion that the conversion to a tumorigenic phenotype is most readily achieved through the workings of at least two genetic elements, specifically oncogenes (Table 1). Examples of this are several retroviruses and DNA tumor viruses that carry multiple oncogenes in their genomes. Avian erythroblastosis virus (AEV) carries two distinct oncogenes, *erbA* and *erbB*, which collaborate to create erythroblastosis. *erbB*, which happens to be an altered form of the normal chicken gene encoding the epidermal growth factor receptor, is able to induce proliferation of erythroid stem cells, but these tend to differentiate spontaneously into red cells. *erbA*, derived from the gene specifying the normal triiodothyronine receptor, does little on its own; however, in the presence of *erbB*, it is able to block differentiation, trapping the *erbB* transformants in a stem cell state having unlimited proliferative potential (Frykberg et al. 1983). Interestingly, other oncogenes encoding cytoplasmic proteins, like v-*src*, v-*fps*, v-*sea*, and v-Ha-*ras* are able to replace *erbB* by cooperating with *erbA* in erythroid transformation (Kahn et al. 1986).

Table 1 Functional classification of cooperating oncogenes

in rat embryo fibroblasts	
Cytoplasmic oncogenes	Nuclear oncogenes
Ha-*ras*	*myc*
Ki-*ras*	N-*myc*
N-*ras*	L-*myc*
src	*p53*
polyoma middle T	adeno E1A
	polyoma large T
	SV40 large T
	papillomavirus E7
in avian bone marrow cells	
Cytoplasmic oncogenes	Nuclear oncogenes
erbB	*myc*
src	*myb*
fps	
mil	
Ha-*ras*	
ros	
yes	
sea	

Classification of oncogenes on the basis of their ability to collaborate in transformation. For example, a *ras* oncogene can collaborate with *myc,* p53, or adenovirus E1A to transform rat embryo fibroblasts.

Yet other retroviruses and DNA tumor viruses carry multiple oncogenes, further supporting the model that multiple cellular regulatory pathways must be activated for full transformation to ensue. The MH2 retrovirus carries both the *mil/raf* and *myc* oncogenes that collaborate to confer potent and rapid tumorigenicity (Graf et al. 1986). The adenovirus carries E1A and E1B oncogenes that show cooperative effects (van den Elsen et al. 1983). Papillomaviruses also carry multiple oncogenes (Howley and Schlegel 1987). The large T antigen of SV40 seems to incorporate multiple activities into one large, multifunctional polypeptide (Tooze 1981).

A repeating theme in many of these examples is that the collaborating oncogenes act at different cellular sites (Table 1). Oncogenes like *myc*, polyoma middle T, *myb*, p53, *erbA*, and *E7* have gene products in the nucleus and hence are often termed "nuclear oncogenes." The proteins specified by *ras*, polyoma middle T, *src*, *sea*, *fps*, and *erbB* are found in the cytoplasm, and the encoding sequences are often called "cytoplasmic oncogenes." Forms of the SV40 large T antigen are found at both locations. Strong synergy often results when a nuclear and a cytoplasmic oncogene are cointroduced into a cell. This has established the idea that at least two critical regulatory pathways must be perturbed in order for full malignant conversion to ensue. As discussed elsewhere in this volume, the oncogene proteins of the nucleus appear to be involved in regulation of gene expression, regulating either transcriptional or post-transcriptional processes. Oncogene proteins of the cytoplasm seem to perturb the levels of critical second-messenger molecules such as phosphatidylinositol metabolites. It would appear that deregulation of both the nuclear and cytoplasmic processes is often required for full transformation.

Study of the biological effects of oncogenes like E1A and *myc* showed that their effects on cells are, not unexpectedly, quite different from those of *ras* and polyoma middle T. Whereas oncogenes like *ras* induce growth factor secretion by transformed cells, those of the *myc* type have not been seen to do so. Instead, *myc* and related oncogenes may make cells more responsive to growth factors present in the surrounding medium, allowing cells to grow at lower serum concentrations. Such *myc* transformants can also grow at lower density in monolayer culture. In rodent embryo fibroblasts, *ras*-like oncogenes are potent in inducing anchorage independence, whereas *myc*-like oncogenes have only a relatively weak ability to do so. *myc* and E1A are adept at inducing immortalization in culture, whereas *ras* is weak in this function (Weinberg 1985). These aspects of collaborating oncogenes suggest that as cells acquire activated oncogenes during tumor progression, they acquire distinct sets of phenotypic changes that in aggregate constitute fully malignant behavior.

Recently, the actions of three of these nuclear oncogenes, each able to collaborate with a *ras* oncogene in transformation, have been tied to a common molecular mechanism. The proteins of the adenovirus E1A oncogene, the SV40 large T oncogene, and the papillomavirus E7 oncogene have all been seen to complex with a common target, the nuclear protein, p105, encoded by the cellular retinoblastoma gene (DeCaprio et al. 1988; Whyte et al. 1988; Dyson et al. 1989). This provides a unifying biochemical mechanism of action for these three structurally distinct oncoproteins. At the same time, it connects their actions to the workings of an anti-oncogene protein whose loss is also associated with the triggering of retinoblastomas (Chapter 11).

VII. LESSER COMPLEXITY: FULL TRANSFORMATION BY SINGLE ONCOGENES

The model of transformation by two collaborating oncogenes brings clarity and simplicity to a complex process. Although it is supported by a number of independent experimental results, there are examples of carcinogenesis that suggest either greater or lesser complexity. Not all oncogenes are readily classified as *ras*-like or *myc*-like, and some oncogenes have both immortalizing powers and an ability to induce anchorage independence. Such multiple functions exercised by a single oncogene might, under certain conditions, allow this oncogene to induce full cell transformation in a single step.

The most dramatic instances of such single-step carcinogenesis come from numerous, well-documented descriptions of tumorigenesis in vivo by rapidly oncogenic retroviruses that carry only a single oncogene (Bishop 1983). Examples of these include avian myelocytomatosis virus (carrying the *myc* oncogene), Abelson leukemia virus (*abl*), Harvey murine sarcoma virus (Ha-*ras*), and avian Rous sarcoma virus (*src*). In each case, a virus is able to enter an animal and induce tumors with such rapidity that it seems unlikely that additional cellular changes beyond the initial viral infection are required for tumorigenesis to occur.

A second type of apparent one-hit transformation occurs in vitro when a transforming retrovirus like Harvey sarcoma virus is introduced into an embryo fibroblast culture and then rapidly spreads throughout the cell population. In short order, the monolayer of cells becomes morphologically transformed en masse. Such cell populations are also tumorigenic (Land 1986).

Yet another example stems from the experiments in which oncogenes like *ras* are transfected into rat embryo fibroblasts. As described earlier, such transfections generally do not yield evidence of transformants in the monolayer. A variation of this experiment includes the cotransfection of a selectable marker gene together with the oncogene. Under such conditions, a number of doubly transfected cells arise. If these cultures are then exposed to selection by introduction of the appropriate selective agent, virtually the entire monolayer will be killed except the small number of cells that have acquired the marker gene and the cotransfected oncogene. These will now grow out and show clear signs of transformation (Land et al. 1983). The collection of such transformed colonies will rapidly cover the monolayer, and this mass population will form tumors upon introduction into a host animal. Once again, these cells carry only a single oncogene.

In all three examples, single oncogenes acting on their own appear able to effect full conversion to tumorigenicity. The involvement of rare secondary collaborating genetic changes seems unlikely, in light of the apparently large proportion of cells that undergo full transformation. These phenomena must be reconciled with observations discussed earlier suggesting a requirement for multiple, collaborating changes in a cell before it becomes tumorigenic.

One possible solution comes from the hypothesis that the environment of a cell represents a critical factor in its responsiveness to the influences of an oncogene that it may carry. Upon reexamination of these three cases, it becomes apparent that they share one aspect in common: In each instance, the cell that initially acquires a single oncogene is rapidly removed from close contact with neighboring normal cells. When an infectious retrovirus acts to introduce an oncogene into such a cell, the rapid secondary spread of viral progeny to adjacent cells recruits these neighbors into the pool of transformants and, by the same token, removes normal neighbors from the immediate surrounds of the initially infected cell. When selection is used to kill off untransfected cells in monolayer, their influence is once again removed.

These examples suggest that adjacent normal cells act to suppress the transformed phenotype of the single-oncogene-bearing cell. Such inhibitory effects of neighbors were already documented a quarter of a century ago (Stoker 1964). They may explain why secondary genetic events are usually required for tumorigenesis in vivo. These secondary changes, including secondarily acquired collaborating oncogenes, seem to allow the transformed cell to override growth-inhibitory influences exerted by neighbors. The action of tumor promoters also bears on these phenomena. Agents like TPA act to allow initiated cells bearing single oncogenes to proliferate despite the influences of their normal neighbors. Stated differently, tumor promoters create a physiological state that mimics in some of its aspects the phenotypes provided by a secondarily acquired, collaborating oncogene. Both the promoter and the second oncogene enable a cell to transcend barriers to growth created by neighboring normal cells.

It would appear that single oncogenes are able to induce the full range of tumor phenotypes under conditions involving virus spread or special experimental manipulation. Nonetheless, even in these circumstances, secondary collaborating changes are not fully excluded. Thus, the cohort of virus-transformed cells resulting from an infection by an acutely transforming retrovirus may grow so large that rare, secondary collaborating events may indeed occur in some transformants. Morever, it is unclear whether fully normal cultured cells transformed by single oncogenes are able to immediately send tumors in vivo. In any event, it is important to note that under conditions of nonviral carcinogenesis such as those leading to human tumors, multiple genetic changes appear to be essential in most if not all cases. Although still unproven, the poorly understood effects of neighboring cells may provide the explanation for reconciling these disparate phenomena.

VIII. GREATER COMPLEXITY: TRANSFORMATION REQUIRING MORE THAN TWO CELLULAR CHANGES

A diverse body of data suggests that carcinogenesis is more complex than the two-step process implied by much of the previous discussion. The age-dependent kinetics of human cancer onset are most consistent with a sequence of five or six independent, rate-limiting stochastic events (Peto 1977). The nature of these events is not revealed by such analysis. Thus, it is unclear which of these represent intrinsic changes of the tumor cell clone and which represent systemic changes in the host.

More direct evidence comes from recent manipulations of transgenic mice involving strains that carry either the *ras* or the *myc* oncogene, each gene being under the control of the same type of MMTV, mammary-specific promoter (Sinn et al. 1987). As described earlier, although such mice express one or the other oncogene constitutively in breast tissues, they give evidence of tumors only after many months' delay. By mating mice carrying a germ-line *myc* oncogene with those carrying a *ras* oncogene, one can obtain progeny that inherit both oncogenes. Since these two oncogenes are often able to collaborate to achieve full conversion to tumorigenicity, their joint constitutive expression in certain populations of breast cells might obviate the need for further somatic change. The outcome is otherwise. Although the oncogenes do act synergistically by speeding up the kinetics of tumor onset, the number of tumor cell clones is still small compared to the number of cells expressing both oncogenes. Such a result is most compatible with a requirement for the occurrence of at least one additional, rate-limiting step in the process of tumor formation. *ras* and *myc* seem necessary here but still not sufficient. Certain in vitro models support a similar view. In experiments with rodent fibroblasts and hematopoietic cells, *ras* and *myc* oncogenes do not suffice to induce full tumorigenic conversion. Subsequent shifts in karyotype seem to be correlated with the final progression of these cells to tumorigenicity (Oshimura et al. 1985; Vogt et al. 1986).

Yet another sign of greater complexity comes from study of rat REF52 cells. Although fully established as a cell line, they are not transformed to tumorigenicity by an introduced *ras* oncogene. They still require a second introduced collaborating oncogene like *myc* (Franza et al. 1986; Quinlan et al. 1988). This suggests that the genetic step conferring immortalization may be a precondition for transformation by *ras* but is not always sufficient. Thus, the responsiveness of certain established cells to transformation by oncogenes like *ras* is a trait that is distinct and separable from their immortalized state.

This theme is echoed by work on the adenovirus E1A oncogene showing that its ability to collaborate with a *ras* oncogene is separable from its ability to immortalize cells (Kuppuswamy et al. 1988). Three separate physiological changes may therefore be required for tumorigenicity. The first, induced directly by oncogenes like *ras*, involves phenotypes like loss of contact inhibition and acquisition of anchorage independence. The second change may be manifested as immortalization in culture. The third allows a cell to respond fully to the effects of oncogenes like *ras*. In certain cases, oncogenes like *myc* or E1A may be able to induce simultaneously at least two of these physiological changes required for full transformation.

IX. TOWARD A TOTAL DESCRIPTION OF MULTISTEP TUMORIGENESIS

Although nonviral tumorigenesis may depend on multiple genetic changes in the cell genome, it is hardly obvious that these changes invariably effect the conversion of proto-oncogenes into active oncogenes. Alterations of other types of genes may also be involved. Thus, multiple independently activated oncogenes have only been found in a very small number of human tumor cell genomes (Murray et al. 1983; Suarez et al. 1987). More frequently, a single oncogene is discovered, and the identity of all other genes participating in tumorigenesis remains obscure. Although this may reflect an inadequacy in the techniques used to detect activated oncogenes, it may also suggest that other types of genes are equally important in the tumorigenesis process.

Prominent in the array of other genetic elements implicated in tumorigenesis are the tumor-suppressing genes or anti-oncogenes, described in Chapter 11. The inactivation of such genes through germinal or somatic mutation may play a role as important as the processes that create active oncogenes. Indeed, the inactivation of an anti-oncogene may often supplant the requirement for activation of one or another oncogene, and the two types of genes may collaborate with one another in certain types of tumorigenesis. One indication of this comes from the work on the formation of colon carcinomas. As mentioned earlier, these studies demonstrate the frequent presence of *ras* oncogenes in premalignant adenomas, the apparent precursors to carcinoma cells; in addition, reduction to homozygosity of genes found on human chromosomes 17 and 18 is seen in the carcinomas (Vogelstein et al. 1988). These observations are consistent with *ras* oncogene activation occurring early in tumorigenesis followed by homozygous inactivation of chromosome 17/18 anti-oncogenes at a later stage in tumor progression (see also Chapter 11).

Oncogenes and anti-oncogenes need hardly represent the full range of genes involved in tumorigenesis. These two types of genes act to deregulate cell growth and related processes, including growth factor dependency. They can also affect responsiveness to differentiation-inducing signals, which in normal tissues lead to nonproliferating, highly differentiated cells. By blocking such differentiation, oncogenes can cause accumulation of large pools of proliferating undifferentiated cells, which in turn may spawn neoplastic cell clones. However, tumor cells often display a variety of distinctive traits that would not seem to be closely tied to deregulation of growth and differentiation. Prominent among these are the properties of immunoevasion, invasiveness, and metastasis.

Relatively little is known about the role of the immune system in defending against spontaneously arising tumors. Recognition and destruction of small nests of initiated cells may be an important barrier to tumor formation, but this is poorly documented. Such recognition and killing may be achieved by cytotoxic lymphocytes and related cell types (Wallich et al. 1985). In this case, the ability of a tumor cell to evade such immune activity may represent an important if not essential step in tumor formation. The involvement of specific genes conferring evasion from immune surveillance is poorly defined. One clue comes from previously mentioned studies of the adenovirus E1A and cellular N-*myc* oncogenes, which are able to force cells to down-modulate their class I histocompatibility antigens (Schrier et al. 1983; Bernards et al. 1987). In so doing, these cells lose cell-surface elements that are vital to recognition by certain types of killer lymphocytes. This escape from recognition may in turn permit the outgrowth of tumor cell clones.

The spread of tumor cells through the body, which often occurs as a late step in tumor progression itself, represents a complex process of multiple, distinct steps (Nicolson and Milas 1984). Included in these steps, which in aggregate are termed metastasis, are the invasion of cells from a primary tumor into adjacent, normal tissue; entrance into the circulatory system or lymphatics ("intravasation"); escape from these systems ("extravasation"); and implantation in appropriate target organs. Some of these steps may recapitulate processes involved in early embryogenesis. It is unclear whether all these processes may be induced by actions of single, pleiotropically acting genes, or whether several, functionally distinct genes need to intervene. In some cases, oncogenes like *ras* may be able to induce many of the steps of metastasis (Thorgeirsson et al. 1985; Pozzatti et al. 1986). In other tumors, other types of genes that specifically induce metastatic traits may become activated late in tumor progression.

Many of these tumor cell traits are difficult to study under the well-controlled conditions of in vitro culture. Accordingly, the genes associated with these in vivo phenotypes are still poorly understood. In addition, spontaneous tumors of a given type may achieve a phenotype through any one of a number of alternative genetic changes. Because of these factors, the nature of the molecular steps underlying many aspects of tumor progression remains obscure.

Oncogenes represent essential elements in tumorigenesis but only provide an incomplete description of it. Within the coming decade, a number of additional genetic elements essential to multistep carcinogenesis will be described. Such novel genes, acting in concert with the well-described oncogenes, offer the prospect of complete descriptions of tumorigenesis at the molecular level.

REFERENCES

Armitage, P. and R. Doll. 1957. A two-stage theory of carcinogenesis in relation to the age distribution of human cancer. *Br. J. Cancer* **11:** 161–169.

Bernards, R., S.K. Dessain, and R.A. Weinberg. 1987. N-*myc* amplification causes down-modulation of MHC Class 1 antigen expression in neuroblastoma. *Cell* **47:** 667–674.

Bishop, J.M. 1983. Cellular oncogenes and retroviruses. *Annu. Rev. Biochem.* **52:** 350–354.

Bos, J.L., E.R. Fearon, S.R. Hamilton, M. Verlaan-de Vries, J.H. van Boom, A. J. van der Eb, and B. Vogelstein. 1987. Prevalence of *ras* gene mutations in human colorectal cancers. *Nature* **327:** 293–297.

Brodeur, G.M., R.C. Seeger, M. Schwab, H.E. Varmus, and J.M. Bishop. 1984. Amplification of N-*myc* in untreated human neuroblastoma correlates with advanced disease stage. *Science* **224:** 1121–1124.

Brown, K., M. Quintanilla, M. Ramsden, I.B. Kerr, S. Young, and A. Balmain. 1986. v-*ras* genes from Harvey and Balb murine sarcoma viruses can act as initiators of two-stage mouse skin carcinogenesis. *Cell* **46:** 447–456.

De Caprio, J.A., J.W. Ludlow, J. Figge, J.-Y. Shew, C.-M. Huang, W.-H. Lee, E. Marsilio, E. Paucha, and D.M. Livingston. 1988. SV40 large tumor antigen forms a specific complex with the product of the retinoblastoma susceptibility gene. *Cell* **54:** 275–283.

Di Fiore, P.P., J.H. Pierce, M.H. Kraus, O. Segatto, C.R. King, and S.A. Aaronson. 1987. *erb*B-2 is a potent oncogene when expressed in NIH/3T3 cells. *Science* **237:** 178–182.

Dyson, N., P.M. Howley, K. Münger, and E. Harlow. 1989. The human papilloma virus-16 E7 oncoprotein is able to bind to the retinoblastoma gene product. *Science* **243:** 934–937.

Farber, E. 1984. Cellular biochemistry of the stepwise development of cancer with chemicals. *Cancer Res.* **44:** 5463–5474.

Foulds, L. 1954. Tumor progression. *Cancer Res.* **17:** 337–339.

Franza, B.R., K. Maruyama, J.I. Garrels, and H.E. Ruley. 1986. *In vitro* establishment is not a sufficient prerequisite for transformation by activated *ras* oncogenes. *Cell* **44:** 409–418.

Frykberg, L., S. Palmieri, H. Berg, T. Graf, M. J. Hayman, and B. Vennström. 1983. Transforming capacities of avian erythroblastosis virus mutants deleted in the *erb*A or *erb*B oncogenes. *Cell* **32:** 227–238.

Graf, T., F. von Weizsäcker, S. Grieser, J. Coll, D. Stehelin, T. Patschinsky, K. Bister, C. Bechade, G. Calothy, and A. Leutz. 1986. v-*mil* induces autocrine growth and enhanced tumorigenicity in v-*myc*-transformed avian macrophages. *Cell* **45:** 357–364.

Hennings, H., R. Shores, M.L. Wenk, E.F. Spangler, R. Tarone, and S.H. Yuspa. 1983. Malignant conversion of mouse skin tumours is increased by tumour initiators and unaffected by tumour promoters. *Nature* **304:** 67–69.

Hirai, H., Y. Kobayashi, H. Mano, K. Hagiwara, Y. Maru, M. Omine, H. Mizoguchi, J. Nishida, and F. Takaku. 1987. A point mutation at codon 13 of the N-*ras* oncogene in myelodysplastic syndrome. *Nature* **327:** 430–432.

Howley, P. M. and R. Schlegel. 1987. Papillomavirus transformation in the Papoviridae 2. In *The papillomaviruses* (ed. N. P. Salzman and P. M. Howley), pp. 141–166. Plenum Press, New York.

Kahn, P., L. Frykberg, C. Brady, I. Stanley, H. Berg, B. Vennström, and T. Graf. 1986. v-*erb* A cooperates with sarcoma oncogenes in leukemic cell transformation. *Cell* **45:** 349–356.

Kuppuswamy, M., T. Subramanian, and G. Chinnadurai. 1988. Separation of immortalization and T24-*ras* oncogene cooperative functions of adenovirus E1a. *Oncogene* **2:** 613–615.

Land, H. 1986. Oncogenes cooperate but how? In *Oncogenes and growth control* (ed. P. Kahn et al.), pp. 304–311. Springer Verlag, Heidelberg.

Land, H., L.F. Parada, and R.A. Weinberg. 1983. Tumorigenic conversion of primary embryo fibroblasts requires at least two cooperating oncogenes. *Nature* **304:** 596–602.

Liu, E., C. Dolbaum, G. Scott, C. Rochlitz, C. Benz, and H. S. Smith. 1988. Molecular lesions involved in the progression of a human breast cancer. *Oncogene* **3:** 323–327.

Loo, D.T., J.I. Fuquay, C.I. Rawson, and D.W. Barnes. 1987. Extended culture of mouse embryo cells without senescence: Inhibition by serum. *Science* **236:** 200–202.

Murray, M.J., J.M. Cunningham, L.F. Parada, F. Dautry, P. Lebovitz, and R.A. Weinberg. 1983. The HL-60 transforming sequence: A *ras* oncogene coexisting with altered *myc* genes in hematopoietic tumors. *Cell* **33:** 749–757.

Newbold, R.F. and R.W. Overell. 1983. Fibroblast immortality is a prerequisite for transformation by EJ c-Ha-*ras* oncogene. *Nature* **304:** 648–651.

Newbold, R.F., R.W. Overell, and J.R. Connell. 1982. Induction of immortality is an early event in malignant transformation of mammalian cells by carcinogens. *Nature* **299:** 633–635.

Nicholson, G.L. 1987. Tumor cell instability, diversification, and progression to the metastatic phenotype: from oncogene to oncofetal expression. *Cancer Res.* **47:** 1473–1487.

Nicolson, G.L. and L. Milas. eds. 1984. *Cancer invasion and metastasis: Biologic and therapeutic aspects.* Raven Press, New York.

Nowell, P.C. 1976. The clonal evolution of tumor cell populations. *Science* **194:** 23–28.

———. 1986. Mechanisms of tumor progression. *Cancer Res.* **46:** 2203–2207.

Oshimura, M., T. M. Gilmer, and J.C. Barrett. 1985. Nonrandom loss of chromosome 15 in Syrian hamster tumors induced by V-Ha-*ras* plus v-*myc* oncogenes. *Nature* **316:** 636–639.

Parada, L. F. and R. A. Weinberg. 1983. Presence of a Kirsten murine sarcoma virus *ras* oncogene in cells transformed by 3-methylcholanthrene. *Mol. Cell. Biol.* **3:** 2298–2301.

Peto, R. 1977. Epidemiology, multistage models, and short-term mutagenicity models. *Cold Spring Harbor Conf. Cell Proliferation* **4:** 1403–1428.

Potter, V.R. 1984. Use of two sequential applications of initiators in the production of hepatomas in the rat: An examination of the Solt-Farber protocol. *Cancer Res.* **44:** 2733–2736.

Pozzatti, R., R. Muschel, J. Williams, R. Padmanabhan, B. Howard, L. Liotta, and G. Khoury. 1986. Primary rat embryo cells transformed by one or two oncogenes show different metastatic potentials. *Science* **232:** 223–225.

Quinlan, M., P. Whyte, and T. Grodzicker. 1988. Growth factor induction by the adenovirus Type 5 E1A 12S protein is required for immortalization of primary epithelial cells. *Mol. Cell. Biol.* **8:** 3191–3203.

Quintanilla, M., K. Brown, M. Ramsden, and A. Balmain. 1986. Carcinogen-specific mutation and amplification of Ha-*ras* during mouse skin carcinogenesis. *Nature* **322:** 78–80.

Rassoulzadegan, M., Z. Nagashfar, A. Cowie, A. Carr, M. Grisoni, R. Kamen, and F. Cuzin. 1983. Expression of the large T protein of polyoma virus promotes the establishment in culture of "normal" rodent fibroblast cell lines. *Proc. Natl. Acad. Sci.* **80:** 4354–4358.

Reddy, A.L. and P.J. Fialkow. 1987. Sequential studies of skin tumorigenesis in PGK mosaic mice: The effect of repeated exposure to a carcinogen on regressed mouse skin papillomas. *Carcinogenesis* **8:** 1455–1459.

Roop, D.R., D.R. Lowy, P.E. Tambourin, J. Strickland, J.R. Harper, M. Balaschak, E.F. Spangler, and S.H. Yuspa. 1986. An activated Harvey *ras* oncogene produces benign tumours on mouse epidermal tissue. *Nature* **323:** 822–824.

Ruley, H.E. 1983. Adenovirus early region 1A enables viral and cellular transforming genes to transform primary cells in culture. *Nature* **304:** 602–606.

Schrier, P.I., R. Bernards, R.T.M.J. Vaessen, A. Houweling, and A.J. van der Eb. 1983. Expression of class I histocompatibility antigens switched off by highly oncogenic adenovirus 12 transformed rat cells. *Nature* **305:** 771–775.

Schwab, M., J. Ellison, M. Busch, W. Rosenau, H.E. Varmus, and J.M. Bishop. 1984. Enhanced expression of the human gene N-*myc* consequent to amplification of DNA may contribute to malignant progression of neuroblastoma. *Proc. Natl. Acad. Sci.* **81:** 4940–4944.

Sinn, E., W. Muller, P. Pattangale, I. Tepler, R. Wallace, and P. Leder. 1987. Coexpression of MMTV/v-Ha-*ras* and MMTV/c-*myc* genes in transgenic mice: Synergistic actions of oncogenes *in vivo*. *Cell* **49:** 465–475.

Slamon, D.J., G.M. Clark, S.G. Wong, W.J. Levin, A. Ullrich, and W.L. McGuire. 1987. Human breast cancer: Correlation of relapse and survival with amplification of HER-2/*neu* oncogene. *Science* **235:** 177–182.

Stewart, T.A., P.K. Pattengale, and P. Leder. 1984. Spontaneous mammary adenocarcinomas in transgenic mice that carry and express MTV/*myc* fusion genes. *Cell* **38:** 627–637.

Stoker, M.G.P. 1964. Regulation of growth and orientation in hamster cells transformed by polyoma virus. *Virology* **24:** 165–174.

Suarez, H.G., P.C. Nardeux, Y. Andeol, and A. Sarasin. 1987. Multiple activated oncogenes in human tumors. *Oncogene Res.* **1:** 201–207.

Sukumar, S., V. Notario, D. Martin-Zanca, and M. Barbacid. 1983. Induction of mammary carcinomas in rats by nitroso-methylurea involves malignant activation of H-*ras* 1 locus by single point mutations. *Nature* **306:** 658–661.

Thorgeirsson, U.P., T. Turpeenniemi-Hujanen, J.E. Williams, E.H. Westin, C.A. Heilman, J.E. Talmadge, and L.A. Liotta. 1985. NIH/3T3 cells transfected with human tumor DNA containing activated *ras* oncogenes express the metastatic phenotype in nude mice. *Mol. Cell. Biol.* **5:** 259–262.

Tooze, J. 1981. Molecular biology of tumor viruses, 2nd edition, revised: DNA tumor viruses. Cold Spring Harbor Laboratory, Cold Spring Harbor, New York.

Van Duuren, B.L., A. Sivak, C. Katz, I. Seidman, and S. Melchionine. 1975. The effect of aging and interval between primary and secondary treatment in two-stage carcinogenesis in mouse skin. *Cancer Res.* **35:** 502–505.

van den Elsen, P.J., A. Houweling, and A.J. van der Eb. 1983. Expression of region E1b of human adenovirus in the absence of region E1a is not sufficient for transformation. *Virology* **128:** 377–390.

Vogelstein, B., E.R. Fearon, S.R. Hamilton, S.E. Kern, B.A. Preisinger, M. Leppert, Y. Nakamura, R. White, A.M.M. Smits, and J.L. Bos. 1988. Genetic alterations during colorectal-tumor development. *N. Engl. J. Med.* **319:** 525–532.

Vogt, M., J. Lesley, J. Bogenberger, S. Volkman, and M. Haas. 1986. Coinfection with viruses carrying the v-Ha-*ras* and v-*myc* oncogenes leads to growth factor independence by an indirect mechanism. *Mol. Cell. Biol.* **6:** 3545-3549.

Vousden, K.H. and D.J. Marshall. 1984. Three different activated *ras* genes in mouse tumors: Evidence for oncogene activation during progression of a mouse lymphoma. *EMBO J.* **3:** 913–917.

Wallich, R., N. Bulbuc, G. J. Hämmerling, S. Katzav, S. Segal, and M. Feldman. 1985. Abrogation of metastatic properties of tumour cells by *de novo* expression of H-2K antigens following H-2 gene transfection. *Nature* **315:** 301–305.

Weinberg, R.A. 1985. The action of oncogenes in the cytoplasm and nucleus. *Science* **230:** 770–776.

Whyte, P., K.J. Buchkovich, J.M. Horowitz, S.H. Friend, J. Raybuck, R.A. Weinberg, and E. Harlow. 1988. Association between an oncogene and an anti-oncogene: The adenovirus E1A proteins bind to the retinoblastoma gene product. *Nature* **334:** 124–129.

Zarbl, H., S. Sukumar, A. Arthur, D. Martin-Zanca, and M. Barbacid. 1985. Direct mutagenesis of Ha-*ras* 1 oncogene by *N*-nitroso-*N*-methylurea during initiation of mammary carcinogenesis in rats. *Nature* **315:** 382–386.

13
Oncogenes and Clinical Cancer

J. Michael Bishop
George Williams Hooper Foundation
University of California
San Francisco, California 94143-0552

I. INTRODUCTION

Although observations on human cancer provided the earliest hints that genetic damage might underlie tumorigenesis (see Chapter 1), the first experimental access to genes that can cause cancer was gained with tumor viruses of birds and animals, and for some years, there was no assurance that these experimental models would provide insight into the genesis of human disease. Discovery of the proto-oncogenes from which retroviral

Oncogenes and the Molecular Origins of Cancer.

oncogenes arise made the mechanisms of viral tumorigenesis germane to human cancer and brought new questions to the fore. Might proto-oncogenes be damaged in human cancer cells, and if so, how might damage to these genes contribute to neoplastic growth? Answers have been sought primarily through two lines of enquiry: pursuit of the karyotypic abnormalities found in many human cancers and the use of functional assays to search for oncogenes in the DNA of human tumors. The provisional answers now in hand sustain the view that genetic damage is an important vehicle of tumorigenesis, demonstrate how some of the proto-oncogenes can be important targets for that damage, and in the long term, promise new approaches to the diagnosis and management of human cancer.

II. CHROMOSOMAL TRANSLOCATIONS AND INVERSIONS

In 1914, T. Boveri proposed that abnormalities of chromosomes might be a cause of cancer (Boveri 1929). More than 60 years passed before the prescience of Boveri's suggestion became evident. Now we know that human cancer cells can display a rich diversity of chromosomal abnormalities, and that at least some of these abnormalities are indeed involved in tumorigenesis. The abnormalities include the loss or gain of full chromosomes, focal ("interstitial") deletions within chromosomal arms, translocations between or inversions within chromosomes, and amplification of large domains in chromosomes, usually accompanied by translocation of the amplified region. Deletions within chromosomes and loss of chromosomes are typically recessive lesions that may deprive the cell of a vital function for the control of proliferation or differentiation (see Chapter 11). In contrast, translocation, inversion, focal amplification, and duplication of full chromosomes are potentially dominant lesions that may enhance and permute the activity of genes.

Chromosomal translocations and inversions appear to be the most common and diverse of the karyotypic abnormalities found in human cancer cells (Yunis 1986). Some of these abnormalities occur sporadically, without apparent relationship to the types of tumors in which they are found. Others are consistent features of specific malignancies; as a consequence, they are both useful as diagnostic criteria and suspected to have a role in tumorigenesis. Figure 1 illustrates a typical chromosomal translocation found in human leukemia cells.

The mechanism by which chromosomal translocations and inversions occur is not known, although there are hints that in B- and T-lymphocytes the genesis of these abnormalities may be mediated by the enzymatic machinery that normally rearranges immunoglobulin (Ig) and T-cell receptor genes (Tsujimoto et al. 1985a; Finger et al. 1986; Haluska et al.

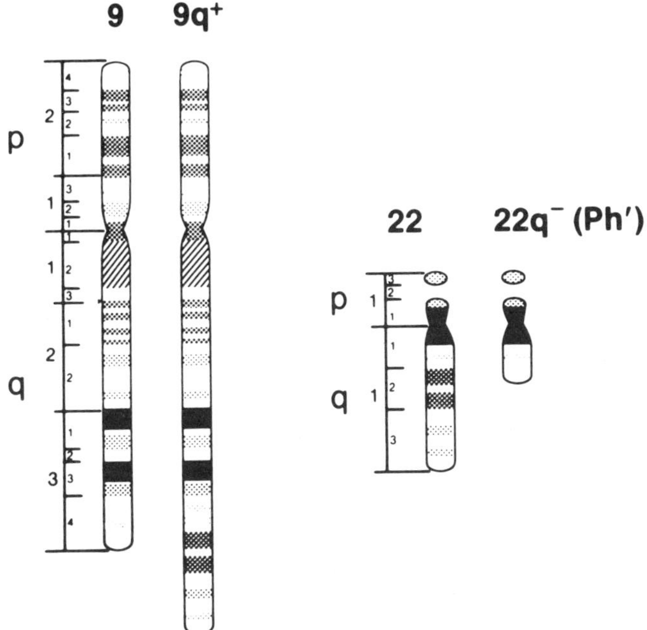

Figure 1 The translocation that creates the Philadelphia chromosome. During the genesis of human chronic myelogenous leukemia, a reciprocal translocation between chromosomes 9 and 22 creates abnormal versions of both chromosomes. The abnormality of chromosome 22 (a shortened version known as $22q^-$) was the first chromosomal translocation identified as a consistent feature of a human malignancy and was named the Philadelphia chromosome (designated by the convention Ph^1) in recognition of the city where the abnormality was discovered (Nowell and Hungerford 1961). The translocation that forms Ph^1 changes the structure of the proto-oncogene *ABL* and the activity of the gene product (see text).

1987). In contrast, great strides have been made in elucidating the molecular structure of translocations. In particular, it has been possible to characterize several of the "breakpoints" where translocation joins a region from one chromosome to the arm of another (Table 1). These explorations have led to the discovery that several of the previously known proto-oncogenes are affected by chromosomal translocations, have added new members to the roster of potential proto-oncogenes, and have revealed two functional disturbances caused by translocations: deregulation of gene expression and mutation of gene products. It now appears likely that the genetic damage produced by chromosomal translocations often contributes to tumorigenesis: The prescience of T. Boveri has been authenticated by the molecular cloning of DNA.

Table 1 Translocation of proto-oncogenes

Gene	Transduced[a]	Translocation	Reciprocal locus[b]
ABL	yes	(9; 22) (q34; q11)	*BCR*
ETS1	yes	(4; 11) (q21; q23)	?
		(9; 11) (p22; q23)	α/β-IFN
ETS2	yes	(8; 21) (q22; q22)	?
MYC	yes	(8; 14) (q24; q32)	Ig-H
		(2; 8) (p13; q24)	Ig-K
		(8; 22) (q24; q11)	Ig-λ
		(8; 14) (q24; q11)	TCR-δ
BCL1	no	(11; 14) (q13; q32)	Ig-H
BCL2	no	(14; 18) (q32; q21)	Ig-H
TCL1	no	inv(14) (q11.2) (q32.2)	TCR-α
TCL2	no	(11; 14) (p13; q11)	TCR-α
TCL3[c]	no	(7; 9) (q34; q34.3)	TCR-β
TCL3[c]	no	(10; 14) (q24; q11)	TCR-α

[a]Some of the translocated genes have been encountered also as proto-oncogenes transduced into retroviruses, others have not.

[b]Genes located at or in the vicinity of the reciprocal site for translocation. Abbreviations: (*BCR*) breakpoint cluster region gene; (IFN) interferon; (Ig) immunoglobulin; (H) heavy chain; (K) κ chain; (λ) λ chain; (TCR) T-cell receptor (Greek letters denote protein subunit).

[c]The designation *TCL3* has been assigned fortuitously to two different loci.

A. Translocation of *MYC* in Burkitt's Lymphoma

Burkitt's lymphoma (BL) is a malignancy of immature B cells whose characteristic features include consistent chromosomal translocations: most frequently (~80% of cases), t(8;14)(q24;q32); less commonly, either t(2;8)(p11;q24) or t(8;22)(q24;q11) (Yunis 1986; Haluska et al. 1987). The molecular characterization of these translocations (in concert with studies on analogous translocations in mouse plasmacytomas) provided the first insight into how chromosomal rearrangements might contribute to tumorigenesis.

Three clues informed efforts to explicate the molecular nature of the translocations in BL. First, chicken B-cell tumors induced by at least two strains of retroviruses originate from anomalous activation of the proto-oncogene *MYC*, prompting the notion that *MYC* might have a general role in the genesis of B-cell tumors (see Chapters 1 and 7). Second, the breakpoints of the three translocations found in BL all involve a chromosomal position (8q24) that proved to be the cytogenetic location of human *MYC* (Dalla-Favera et al. 1982a; Neel et al. 1982; Taub et al. 1982). Third, the distinctive positions of the breakpoints on chromosomes 2 (Malcolm et al. 1982), 14 (Croce et al. 1979; Kirsch et al. 1982), and 22 (Erikson et al. 1981) are all situated in the vicinity of immunoglobulin (Ig) genes (κ, heavy, and λ, respectively)—locales that are likely to be actively expressed in B cells. These clues led to the discovery that the translocation t(8;14) moves *MYC* to chromosome 14 and juxtaposes it to the Ig heavy-chain locus (Leder et al. 1983; Cory 1986; Haluska et al. 1987). The less frequent translocations t(2;8) and t(8;22) represent reciprocal exchanges between genes for Ig light chains and positions at various distances downstream from *MYC*; in these instances, the proto-oncogene remains at its native chromosomal location (Leder et al. 1983; Cory 1986; Haluska et al. 1987). Translocations involving *MYC* also occur in other forms of B-cell tumors (Care et al. 1986; Pelicci et al. 1986b; Sun et al. 1986; Guerrasio et al. 1987) and in T-cell malignancies, where the partner in the translocation is typically a gene that encodes a subunit of the T-cell receptor (Erikson et al. 1986; Mathieu-Mahul et al. 1986; Saglio et al. 1986; Shima et al. 1986).

The translocations of *MYC* in BL take four general forms, none of which alter the protein encoded by the gene, but each of which may alter the regulation of *MYC* expression (Cory 1986). In one form, *MYC* is joined to the heavy-chain locus within the first intron of the proto-oncogene. This configuration severs the coding domain of *MYC* from many of the elements that normally control its expression. In a second form of translocation to the heavy-chain locus, the breakpoint lies immediately upstream of *MYC*, disrupting domains that are thought to regulate transcription from the gene. Third, translocations involving the Ig light-chain genes do not relocate *MYC*, but some may occur sufficiently close to the proto-oncogene to affect its function. Fourth, the breakpoints of some translocations are quite distant from *MYC* and may affect either *MYC* itself or another proto-oncogene on chromosome 8, known provisionally as *PVT* (Graham and Adams 1986; Mengle-Gaw and Rabbitts 1987).

Numerous translocated forms of *MYC* in BL also contain point mutations. It is presumed (but not proven) that these mutations arise from the mechanisms that normally act to diversify Ig genes by somatic mutation in B cells. The significance of the mutations has not been established: Most are found in the 5′ noncoding domain carried by exon 1 of *MYC*, where they may interfere with regulation of the gene (Rabbitts et al. 1983; Cesarman et al. 1987; Szajnert et al. 1987); mutations have also been found in the coding domain of translocated *MYC*, but they are without known effect (Rabbitts et al. 1983; Murphy et al. 1986).

B. Pathogenesis of BL

Two forms of BL have been described (Ziegler 1981): endemic—the more prevalent form, found principally in equatorial Africa; and sporadic—relatively rare and worldwide in occurrence. The pathogenic mechanisms of both forms remain enigmas. Endemic BL has been attributed to a combination of factors, including infection with Epstein-Barr virus (EBV), the immunological stimulus of chronic malarial infection, and the malfunctioning of *MYC* elicited by translocation. In contrast, sporadic BL seems rarely (if ever) to involve infection with EBV; the translocations of *MYC* appear to be different from those found in endemic BL (Pelicci et al. 1986a); and other potential cofactors in etiology have not been identified.

The translocations that typify both forms of BL are thought to affect the function of *MYC*. Four major possibilities are in contention, all of them designed to explain how translocation could sustain or augment the expression of *MYC* and thus override the control of cellular proliferation. First, transcription of *MYC* may be released from its usual controls, causing constitutive expression of the gene at inappropriate times rather than in excessive quantities (Taub et al. 1984; Cesarman et al. 1987). Second, control regions provided by the adjacent Ig gene may drive the expression of *MYC* to levels that are higher than normal (Erikson et al. 1983a,b, 1986; Hayday et al. 1984). Third, damage inflicted on *MYC* by translocation may increase the stability of mRNA representing the gene; as a result, the abundance of the mRNA would increase and become less accessible to rapid modulation (Eick et al. 1985; Rabbitts et al. 1985). Fourth, truncation of *MYC* by loss of the first exon may enhance translation of the corresponding mRNA into protein (Battey et al. 1983; Saito et al. 1983; Darveau et al. 1985) (although this possibility has been challenged directly: see Butnick et al. 1985). At present, it appears unlikely that any one of these possible explanations applies to all the translocated alleles of *MYC*, and none of the explanations has been implicated decisively in tumorigenesis.

The role of *MYC* in the genesis of BL has received support from experimental data: Human lymphocytes transformed by EBV to established growth in cell culture become tumorigenic in animals only when they are engrafted with a vigorously expressed version of *MYC* (Lombardi et al. 1987), and transgenic mice carrying experimentally crafted facsimiles of translocated *MYC* in their germinal DNA develop lymphoid tumors (Adams et al. 1985). Efforts have also been made to implicate a gene known as *BLYM* in the genesis of BL (Diamond et al. 1983), but important reservations regarding this work have arisen (see below).

C. Philadelphia Chromosome of Chronic Myelogenous Leukemia

Chronic myelogenous leukemia (CML) is an inevitably fatal malignancy involving hematopoietic cells of various lineages (Fialkow 1984). The initial or chronic phase of the disease is an indolent leukemia that characteristically affects relatively mature myeloid cells. After a period of several years, the disease enters an acute phase or blast crisis, in which a rapidly advancing leukemia of immature hematopoietic cells (usually representing either the myeloid or lymphoid lineage) leads rapidly to death. Throughout both stages of CML, the leukemic cells are distinguished by an abnormality of chromosome 22 known as the Philadelphia chromosome (or Ph^1) that is formed by the reciprocal translocation 9;22(q34;q11)(Nowell and Hungerford 1961; Rowley 1973). Ph^1 occurs in more than 90% of individuals with CML, and the molecular lesion underlying the cytogenetic abnormality may be even more frequent. The discovery of Ph^1 represented the first description of a consistent association between a specific chromosomal abnormality and a particular form of malignancy.

D. Translocated *ABL* in Ph^1

As the mapping of proto-oncogenes to positions on human chromosomes proceeded, it became apparent that the formation of Ph^1 translocates two of these genes—*ABL* (9q34) and *SIS* (22q123-q131) (Dalla-Favera et al. 1982b; Heisterkamp et al. 1982; Swan et al. 1982). The translocation of *SIS* was dismissed as irrelevant to tumorigenesis because the gene is far removed from the breakpoint and is not expressed in the leukemic cells of CML (Gale and Canaani 1984). In contrast, the breakpoint interrupts *ABL* upstream of its second exon and joins it to chromosome 22, within a previously unrecognized gene known as *BCR* for breakpoint cluster region (Klein et al. 1982; Bartram et al. 1983; Heisterkamp et al. 1983, 1985; Groffen et al. 1984). The interruption of *ABL* occurs at positions that vary greatly from one tumor to another, over a region larger than 100 kbp

(Bernards et al. 1987), whereas the breakpoints on chromosome 22 always lie within a 5.8-kbp domain of *BCR* (Groffen et al. 1984).

The fusion between *BCR* and *ABL* is transcribed as a single gene to produce a chimeric mRNA (Collins et al. 1984; Shtivelman et al. 1985; Stam et al. 1985). The protein encoded by this mRNA combines an amino-terminal portion of the *BCR* product with the bulk of the protein encoded by *ABL*. The normal product of *ABL* is a protein tyrosine kinase (see Chapter 6). The hybrid protein encoded by the *BCR-ABL* fusion remains a protein tyrosine kinase, but the enzyme appears to be more active than its normal counterpart (Konopka et al. 1984; Konopka and Witte 1985; Ben-Neriah et al. 1986). The novel enzymatic properties of the *BCR-ABL* protein are attributed to replacement of the amino-terminal region of the normal *ABL* protein by the domain derived from *BCR*. It is not known why the replacement affects enzymatic activity, but a roughly analogous replacement by a portion of a viral structural protein occurs when *ABL* is transduced into the retroviral oncogene v-*abl* (Davis et al. 1985). It appears that *BCR* encodes a protein (Hariharan and Adams 1987), but nothing is known of its function.

At first glance, the translocation affecting *MYC* in BL and that affecting *ABL* in CML differ: The former causes deregulation of gene expression but spares the protein product of the gene, whereas the latter changes the structure of the gene product. However, the physiological consequences may be analogous—sustained and often increased quantities of the gene product in the case of translocated *MYC*, sustained and perhaps increased activity of the gene product in the case of translocated *ABL*.

E. Pathogenesis of CML

The leukemic cells of CML apparently arise from an abnormal (or transformed) stem cell that often remains pluripotent, capable of producing cells in more than one hematopoietic lineage (Fialkow 1980, 1984). The event that initiates transformation of the stem cell has not been identified, but translocation of *ABL* may not be responsible: Although the transformed stem cell sometimes gives rise to both leukemic and ostensibly normal cells, Ph^1 appears in the latter only rarely (Fialkow 1984). Translocation is nevertheless an early event in leukemogenesis because Ph^1 characteristically appears in all the leukemic cells of CML (Fialkow 1980).

On occasion, Ph^1 is found in ostensibly normal hematopoietic cells as well as in the leukemic cells of individuals with CML. This finding indicates that neither the initial transformation of a stem cell nor the subsequent translocation and malfunction of *ABL* suffice to elicit leukemic growth; additional events must occur before full malignancy is achieved. For example, mutations in *RAS* proto-oncogenes accompany Ph^1 in the leukemic cells of some individuals with CML (Hirai et al. 1985; Liu et al.

1988). The chimeric protein encoded by the *BCR-ABL* fusion appears to have pathogenic potential, however, because retroviral vectors carrying the hybrid gene can elicit abnormal growth of immature B lymphocytes in culture (McLaughlin et al. 1987).

It is likely that the progression of CML to the blast crisis also involves multiple pathogenic events. These events can include duplication of Ph^1, suggesting that an increased dose of translocated *ABL* exacerbates the malignant phenotype (Fialkow 1984); and mutational activation of oncogenes, such as *HRAS*, *NRAS*, and even novel oncogenes (Liu et al. 1988).

F. Translocations That May Affect Novel Proto-oncogenes in Human Tumors

Among the many different translocations found in human tumors, only a few have their breakpoints located near the cytogenetic positions of known proto-oncogenes (Yunis 1986). Therefore, it seemed reasonable to expect that molecular dissection in the vicinity of some breakpoints would uncover previously unrecognized proto-oncogenes. To initiate the dissection, however, it was necessary to have molecular markers situated at or near the breakpoints. Serendipity has provided such markers in a few instances, and their exploitation has been revealing (Table 1).

1. Novel Proto-oncogenes in B-cell Tumors

Several forms of human B-cell lymphomas and leukemias contain characteristic translocations between chromosomal position 14q32 and either 11q13 or 18q21. None of these locations harbors a known proto-oncogene. However, the position 14q32 is a familiar one because it participates in most of the translocations found in BL and represents the location of the Ig heavy-chain locus (see above). It was therefore possible to recognize and isolate the breakpoints of t(11;14) and t(14;18) by searching for abnormal rearrangements of heavy-chain genes. The isolated rearrangements revealed fusions between DNA derived from either chromosome 11 or chromosome 18 and the J region of the heavy-chain locus on chromosome 14 (for review, see Haluska et al. 1987).

It is presumed that the breakpoints on chromosomes 11 and 18 are located at or near previously unrecognized proto-oncogenes and that the translocations cause these genes to malfunction. The putative proto-oncogene located in the vicinity of 11q13 has been named *BCL1* but has not yet been found (Tsujimoto et al. 1984, 1985b). In contrast, a gene called *BCL2* has been identified on chromosome 18, close to the breakpoint of t(14;18) (Bakhshi et al. 1985; Cleary and Sklar 1985; Tsujimoto et al. 1985a; Cleary et al. 1986). The gene has been sequenced, and its protein products have been identified (Tsujimoto and Croce 1986; Tsujimoto et al. 1988). There is presently no clue as to what the function of *BCL2* might be, no indication of how translocation might affect the activity of the gene, and no direct evidence to implicate the translocated gene in tumorigenesis.

2. Novel Proto-oncogenes in T-cell Tumors

The genes that encode subunits of the T-cell receptor also provide access to potential proto-oncogenes by virtue of their proximity to the breakpoints of inversions and translocations in several kinds of T-cell malignancies (Croce et al. 1985; Erikson et al. 1985; Denny et al. 1986; Baer et al. 1988). Four examples have been explored in some detail, leading to the provisional definition of three or more new proto-oncogenes (Table 1). The pace of discovery has been so rapid that potential proto-oncogenes located on two different chromosomes were given the same name concurrently (*TCL3*) (Kagan et al. 1987; Reynolds et al. 1987). Nothing is known of how these genes act or how their actions are affected by translocation, and there is no direct evidence to identify any of the genes as authentic proto-oncogenes.

III. AMPLIFICATION OF PROTO-ONCOGENES IN CANCER CELLS

The presence of trisomies and even greater multiplicities of particular chromosomes in cancer cells raised the possibility that an excess of function for one or more genes might be involved in tumorigenesis. More tangible evidence of overactive genes in human tumors first emerged from a different quarter: the discovery of gene amplification. Both unicellular and metazoan organisms amplify regions of their DNA beyond the usual number of two in diploid cells (Schimke 1984; Stark and Wahl 1984). In some instances, the amplification is a scheduled and physiological event that meets a large demand for a specific gene product, such as can occur during embryogenesis. However, in mammalian cells, amplification appears always to be an abnormality; it underlies several forms of resistance to chemotherapeutic agents on the part of tumors, and it may play a role in some forms of tumorigenesis.

A. Gene Amplification in Mammalian Cells

Regions at which abnormal amplification occurs are scattered throughout the mammalian genome. The average frequency of amplification at any given locus on a chromosome is very low (perhaps once in every millionth cell division), but there are regions where amplification is relatively common and others where it may never occur (Wahl et al. 1984). Irrespective of its frequency, amplified DNA persists in proliferating cells only if a gene that it carries provides a selective advantage to the cells (see below).

Neither the cause nor the mechanism of gene amplification in mammalian cells is known (the issues are presently rife with controversy), but the abnormality has generally been found only in cells that are partially or fully malignant; whether it occurs in normal cells with any frequency remains uncertain (Stark 1986).

The unit of amplification in mammalian DNA is usually large (sometimes more than 1000 kbp) and is thought to represent part or all of a single replicon (the domain of DNA replicated by bidirectional synthesis from a single origin). As amplification continues, the reduplicated DNA grows large enough to be visible by microscopy as two karyotypic abnormalities (Fig. 2): double minute chromosomes (DMs), small and extranumerary chromosomes that are in reality pairs of giant episomes; and homogeneously staining regions (HSRs), adventitious domains within chromosomes that display no bands when stained (Schimke 1984; Stark and Wahl 1984). Both abnormalities comprise tandem arrays of amplified DNA, but their genesis remains controversial. One view holds that amplified DNA leaves the chromosome in a circular form while still submicroscopic in size, thereafter growing large enough to become visible as DMs (Von Hoff et al. 1988), and that HSRs arise in turn when DMs insert into chromosomes at diverse and possibly unselected positions; the amplified DNA of HSRs has usually been translocated from its original chromosomal position (Alitalo and Schwab 1986).

DMs multiply in concert with the remainder of chromosomal DNA, but they have no centromere and are sometimes not even paired structures

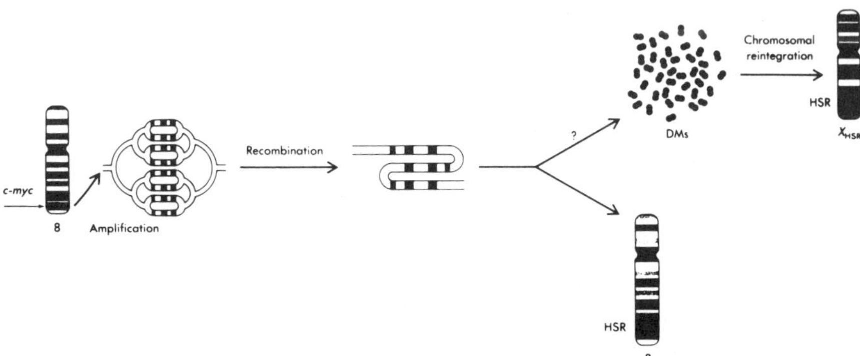

Figure 2 Amplification of DNA in vertebrate cells. Occasional amplification of DNA within vertebrate chromosomes gives rise to two karyotypic abnormalities, DMs and HSRs. The amplification is abnormal, but its mechanism is not known; the version shown here is only one of several possibilities. The figure also illustrates another common feature of gene amplification in cancer cells: the translocation of amplified DNA from one chromosome to another (amplified *MYC* from chromosome 8 to the X chromosome, in the example given).

(i.e., not double). They are thus distributed haphazardly when cells divide, and there is no guarantee that both daughter cells will receive at least one DM. As a result, cell lineages that no longer possess amplified DNA can develop quickly from cells in which the amplified DNA has been carried exclusively in DMs (Schimke 1984; Stark and Wahl 1984). In contrast, HSRs reside in chromosomes and are therefore a more stable constituent of the cell's genetic dowry. However, HSRs too can be lost, by mechanisms that remain mysterious. It follows that when DMs and HSRs survive extensive proliferation of the cells in which they are carried, they must embody a selective advantage for the cells.

An amplified gene gives rise to far more mRNA than usual, and production of the protein encoded by the gene is increased accordingly (Schimke 1984; Stark and Wahl 1984; Stark 1986). The increase in gene product is usually proportional to the magnitude of amplification, although there may be limits beyond which the machinery for transcription and translation cannot keep pace with amplification. There is presently no evidence that amplified genes are otherwise abnormal (although the matter is not easy to examine), so the phenotypic effects of gene amplification have been attributed to the mere abundance of gene product.

B. Amplification of Proto-oncogenes in Human Cancer Cells

In response to the notion that inordinate activity of proto-oncogenes may be involved in tumorigenesis, a large number of tumors and tumor cell lines have been screened for amplification or excessive expression of known proto-oncogenes. The screening has uncovered a variety of tumors in which one or another proto-oncogene is expressed abundantly because it resides within an amplified domain of DNA (Alitalo and Schwab 1986). Some of the tumors were examined without reference to their karyotype; others were singled out because they contained DMs or HSRs. It is not yet possible to estimate what fraction of human tumors contain amplified DNA, but the frequency of this abnormality probably exceeds previous expectations.

Amplification of proto-oncogenes in human tumors has been found in two patterns: as an occasional feature of diverse tumors or as a recurrent abnormality of specific proto-oncogenes in particular types of tumors (Table 2). Four proto-oncogenes first encountered in other contexts have since been recognized as consistent components of amplified DNA in specific tumors: *MYC* in carcinomas of the breast (Escot et al. 1986; Varley et al. 1987; Mariani-Costantini et al. 1988) and lung (Little et al. 1983; Johnson et al. 1987; Kiefer et al. 1987); *ERBB1* in squamous cell carcinomas (Yamamoto et al. 1986) and glioblastomas (Libermann et al. 1985; Wong et al. 1987); the closely linked *HSTF1* and *INT2* in carcinoma of the breast (Yoshida et al. 1988; Zhou et al. 1988); and *NEU* (also known

Table 2 Amplification of proto-oncogenes in human tumors

Gene	Transduced[a]	Characteristic tumors[b]
ERBB1	yes	squamous cell carcinomas glioblastomas
MYB	yes	no
MYC	yes	carcinoma of breast and lung
RAS	yes	no
GLI	no	glioblastomas[c]
NEU/ERBB2	no	carcinoma of breast, salivary glands, and stomach
LMYC	no	carcinoma of lung
NMYC	no	neuroblastoma and carcinoma of lung
INT2	no	carcinoma of breast

[a]Some of the amplified genes have been encountered also as proto-oncogenes transduced into retroviruses, others have not.
[b]Human tumors in which amplification has been encountered on multiple occasions.
[c]The frequency and prevalence of *GLI* amplification are not yet known.

as *ERBB2*) in carcinoma of the breast and other adenocarcinomas (Yokota et al. 1986, 1988; Slamon et al. 1987; van de Vijver et al. 1987, 1988). The consistency of these findings and the evidence that amplified DNA survives countless rounds of cellular proliferation only if it provides a selective advantage sustain the inference that the amplified genes (or genes linked to them in the amplified DNA) are not innocent bystanders but, instead, have played a role in tumorigenesis.

C. Uncovering Novel Proto-oncogenes in Amplified DNA

The early search for pathogenic loci in the amplified DNA of cancer cells focused on known proto-oncogenes because these had been implicated in tumorigenesis in other settings, but the pursuit led as well to previously unrecognized genes that expand the repertoire of proto-oncogenes.

1. NMYC

Efforts to detect *MYC* in the amplified DNA of human neuroblastoma cell lines led instead to the identification of a closely related gene presently called *NMYC* (for neuroblastoma *MYC*) (Kohl et al. 1983; Schwab et al. 1983). *NMYC* and *MYC* encode very similar proteins (see Chapter 6), but they differ entirely in the regions that control gene expression, suggesting that they have evolved to serve different purposes in the normal organism (Kohl et al. 1986; Stanton et al. 1986). Amplification of *NMYC* has also been reported in small cell carcinoma of the lung (Nau et al. 1986; Wong et al. 1986; Johnson et al. 1987) and retinoblastoma (Lee et al. 1984), although the significance of the latter finding has been disputed (Squire et al. 1986).

NMYC has never been encountered as an oncogene in a retrovirus, so no evidence of pathogenic potential antedated the discovery of the gene in human cells. The claim of *NMYC* to authenticity as a proto-oncogene therefore rests on other points of evidence: its close resemblance to an acknowledged proto-oncogene, *MYC* (Kohl et al. 1986; Stanton et al. 1986); the frequency and specificity of its amplification in human tumors (Schwab et al. 1983, 1984; Brodeur et al. 1984; Kohl et al. 1984); the fact that its amplification in neuroblastomas seems restricted to the more aggressive variants of tumor cells (Brodeur et al. 1984; Schwab et al. 1984; Seeger et al. 1985; Grady-Leopardi et al. 1986; Brodeur et al. 1987); and its ability to elicit neoplastic transformation when introduced into cultured cells as an abundantly expressed molecular clone (Schwab et al. 1985; Yancopoulos et al. 1985; Small et al. 1987), a property that affirms the gene's functional kinship with *MYC*.

Clues to the role of *NMYC* in the genesis of neuroblastoma have come from attention to diagnostic criteria. According to their severity, neuroblastomas are assigned to one of four major categories or stages (Evans et al. 1987): I and II, relatively localized and usually curable disease; and III and IV, more widespread and inevitably fatal disease. Amplification of *NMYC* has generally been found only in tumors of stages III and IV (Brodeur et al. 1984; Seeger et al. 1985), and within those tumors, only in the least differentiated (and presumably most malignant) cells (Schwab et al. 1984). These correlations raise the possibility that amplification of *NMYC* exacerbates the malignancy of neuroblastomas during tumor progression.

2. LMYC

A number of cell lines and primary specimens derived from carcinomas of the lung contain amplified DNA that includes one or another of three related genes (Nau et al. 1985, 1986; Wong et al. 1986; Johnson et al. 1987): *MYC*, *NMYC*, or a gene called *LMYC*—the last of these recognized by virtue of its kinship with *MYC* and its amplification in cells of lung cancers (Nau et al. 1985; Legouy et al. 1987; DePinho et al. 1988). The protein encoded by *LMYC* is very similar to the products of other *MYC* genes, but nothing is known of its function. The frequency at which the various *MYC* genes are amplified in carcinomas of the lung has not been determined decisively, but the presence of an amplified *MYC* gene in both the primary and metastatic lesions of several lung carcinomas has prompted the suggestion that amplification may be an early event in tumorigenesis (Wong et al. 1986).

3. *GLI*

The discovery of *NMYC* and *LMYC* occurred because these genes can cross-react with *MYC* when molecular hybridization is used to search for proto-oncogenes in amplified DNA. If the amplified DNA of a tumor does not contain a known proto-oncogene or related gene, however, other means must be found to identify a portion of the amplified domain that might be involved in tumorigenesis. Physical procedures have been developed for the isolation of amplified DNA from tumor cells, one of which has been used to identify a gene designated *GLI* that was amplified and expressed in at least two human glioblastomas (Kinzler et al. 1987, 1988). Although it would be premature to invoke *GLI* in the etiology of glioblastomas, identification of the gene dramatizes the prospects for expanding the roster of proto-oncogenes by further dissection of amplified DNA in tumor cells.

D. Anomalous Expression of Proto-oncogenes in the Absence of Gene Amplification or Chromosomal Translocation

It is conceivable that genetic lesions not visible to the cytogeneticist might evoke the anomalous expression of proto-oncogenes. For example, mutations that diminish the regulation of *MYC* and *LMYC* have been found in some specimens of small cell carcinoma of the lung (J. Minna, pers. comm.). However, most surveys of proto-oncogene expression in human tumors are difficult to interpret because the normal counterparts of tumor cells are not available for analysis, and definitions of anomalous expression thus become arbitrary. Expression of a proto-oncogene is not necessarily pathogenic: It is equally likely to represent a phenotypic property that has survived from the normal progenitor of the tumor cell or to reflect the proliferative activity of the tumor. These caveats have not deterred investigators from screening a wide variety of human tumors for the expression of diverse proto-oncogenes (e.g., see Slamon et al. 1984). Although the results may on occasion provide new approaches to the classification of tumors (Thiele et al. 1987) or the first hint of gene amplification (Alitalo and Schwab 1986), they have otherwise offered little insight into the etiology or mechanisms of tumorigenesis.

IV. ONCOGENES DETECTED BY GENE TRANSFER

The findings reviewed to this point demonstrate how cytogenetic and molecular analyses have uncovered genetic damage affiliated with particular forms of cancer. Functional tests have also been used to search for genes that might contribute to the neoplastic phenotype of human tumors. The search has succeeded beyond expectation by uncovering genetic damage in cancer cells that do not have visible abnormalities of chromosomes, by producing the first direct evidence that point mutations can figure in tumorigenesis, by adding to our repertoire of known proto-oncogenes, and by providing a means to explore the molecular genetics of chemical carcinogenesis. The details of these accomplishments have been described in Chapters 1, 5, and 12. Here, we review how the findings might bear on the pathogenesis and management of human cancer.

A. Transforming Genes in Human Cancer Cells

The oncogenes of tumor viruses are routinely detected by their ability to elicit neoplastic transformation of cells in culture. From this precedent, there arose the notion that tumor cells might also contain transforming genes. Gene transfer (transfection) was therefore used to test the DNA of tumor cells for the presence of genes that, when introduced into cells in culture, can elicit a transformed phenotype and the ability to form tumors in animals. The assay succeeded first with mouse cells transformed by a chemical carcinogen (Shih et al. 1979) but has now been applied to numerous lines of cancer cells and a growing number of tumor specimens (Weinberg 1982; Varmus 1984). Transforming activity can be detected in approximately 20% of all specimens tested, cell lines and original tumors alike, representing a large variety of human malignancies. Some types of tumors rarely if ever contain detectable transforming genes, whereas others do so with provocative consistency.

The great majority of the transforming genes detected by transfection with the DNA of human cancers are mutant alleles of the familiar proto-oncogenes *HRAS* and *KRAS*, or of a previously unrecognized member of the *RAS* family that was dubbed *NRAS* because it was first identified in a line of human neuroblastoma cells (see Chapter 4). All of the transforming alleles of *RAS* genes studied to date contain point mutations that change a single amino acid in the 21-kD *RAS* proteins, usually at residue 12, 13, or 61 (Barbacid 1987). The mutations are clearly responsible for the transforming activity of the genes. The limited variety of *RAS* mutations found in tumor cells presumably results from biological selection: Mutations that do not activate *RAS* proto-oncogenes to oncogenes would not be detected by gene-transfer assays and would appear in tumors only at random. The prevalence of mutant *RAS* genes among human tumors is still under study, but it is already clear that specific *RAS* mutations are relatively frequent features of some types of tumors, including *KRAS* in adenocarcinomas of the colon (Bos et al. 1987; Forrester et al. 1987; Yanez et al. 1987), lung (Rodenhuis et al. 1987), and pancreas (Almoguera et al. 1988), and *NRAS* in acute myelogenous leukemias (Bos et al. 1985; Farr et al. 1988; Janssen et al. 1988). The ranks of these consistencies may grow as the techniques for detecting point mutations in proto-oncogenes become more facile and the search for mutations is enlarged.

Gene transfer presently has no replacement as a means to detect previously unrecognized transforming genes in tumor cells. Once specific mutations have been found and characterized in a proto-oncogene, however, further examples of the same alleles can be sought by procedures that are less demanding and more readily applied on a large scale. These include the use of polymorphisms created in restriction sites by mutations (Barbacid 1987), molecular hybridization with oligonucleotides that will react only with a mutant allele (Bos et al. 1987), detection of mismatches between mutant and wild-type RNA by hydrolysis with RNase (Forrester et al. 1987), and the development of monoclonal antibodies that are specific for a mutant version of a gene product (Clark et al. 1985; Carney et al. 1986). These devices make it possible to screen large numbers of human tumors for previously described mutations in proto-oncogenes. Their use promises to revise our estimates of how prevalent mutant proto-oncogenes might be in human cancers.

B. Uncovering Novel Oncogenes with Gene Transfer

Mutations in *RAS* genes remain the most common form of genetic damage detected in tumor cells by gene transfer. The procedure has also detected other transforming genes, most of which have not been recognized before by any other means. The list of these new oncogenes is long and still growing (see Chapter 1). A representative few are described here, with the forewarning that many of these genes have transforming activity by virtue of physical rearrangements that occur artifactually during transfection assays. There is as yet no decisive evidence that transforming alleles of these genes occur in human tumors.

A transforming gene known originally as *HST* (but since rechristened *HSTF1*) was isolated first from a human gastric carcinoma and adjoining normal mucosa (Sakamoto et al. 1986; Yoshida et al. 1988). Transforming alleles of what may be the same gene have since been found by transfection with DNA from a variety of human cancers (summarized in Yoshida et al. 1987b); other than the various alleles of *RAS* genes, *HSTF1* has been the most commonly encountered transforming gene in human tumor DNAs. There is as yet no explanation for why the alleles of *HSTF1* have transforming activity, although sustained expression of the normal gene will also transform cells in culture (Yoshida et al. 1987a), and there is no evidence that the gene is abnormal in any of the tumors from which the transforming alleles have been isolated. The protein encoded by *HSTF1* resembles a fibroblast growth factor (Taira et al. 1987), but nothing else is known of its function.

Transformation assays with DNAs from two B-cell lymphomas have led to the isolation of a gene known as *DBL* (Eva and Aaronson 1985). The transforming activity of *DBL* has been attributed to rearrangements that damage the gene (Eva et al. 1987), but it now seems unlikely that these rearrangements were present in the original tumor cells. The product of *DBL* bears no resemblance to any previously described protein (Srivastava et al. 1986).

Transfections with DNA from at least two hepatocellular carcinomas have uncovered a transforming gene known as *LCA* (Ochiya et al. 1986). Neither the genetic lesion responsible for activation of *LCA* nor the frequency with which the oncogene may be encountered in liver cancer has been determined, and there is no other evidence to implicate the gene in tumorigenesis.

A presently unnamed transforming gene has been detected in a number of human papillary carcinomas of the thyroid, in both primary tumors and metastases (Fusco et al. 1987). Although the gene has yet to be isolated or characterized, it appears not to represent a previously known proto-oncogene, and transforming alleles of the gene may be a prevalent feature of papillary thyroid carcinomas.

A transforming gene known as *TRK* has been detected in one specimen of human colon carcinoma (Pulciani et al. 1982). The normal version of the gene encodes a transmembrane receptor with protein tyrosine kinase activity, but the allele found in the tumor was rearranged so that the extracellular portion of the receptor was replaced by a domain from nonmuscle tropomyosin (Martin-Zanca et al. 1986; Mitra et al. 1987). Although to date a transforming allele of *TRK* has been encountered only once as an inherent feature of a tumor, rearrangements that activate the transforming potential of the gene occur frequently during the course of experimental gene transfer and inevitably replace the portion of *TRK* that encodes the extracellular domain of the gene product (Kozma et al. 1988; Oskam et al. 1988). The nucleotide sequences constituting the replacement differ from one activated allele of *TRK* to another, although the variety of sequences that serve to activate the gene is not unlimited (Oskam et al. 1988). The proteins encoded by some of the activated alleles remain membrane proteins; others may be cytoplasmic. The findings with *TRK* dramatize the potential diversity of genetic damage that might activate oncogenes and raise the possibility that much of this diversity remains undetected.

C. False Alarms in the Search for Human Oncogenes by Gene Transfer

Considerable attention has been paid a gene known as *BLYM*, obtained first by gene transfer with DNA from chicken lymphomas (Goubin et al.

1983) and then isolated independently from BL (Diamond et al. 1983, 1984). The putative avian version of *BLYM* has since been shown to be a contaminant derived from repeated DNA in the mouse cells used for the gene-transfer assay (Rogers 1986). The *BLYM* isolated from BL is a unique gene in the human genome, but controversy surrounds its biological activity (Devine 1986), and there is no evidence that a mutant version of the gene is a consistent feature of BL. Few observers are presently willing to concede that *BLYM* is an authentic participant in the genesis of BL.

Similar doubts apply to a series of putative oncogenes detected in various forms of mouse and human leukemias (Lane et al. 1982). The original description of these genes attracted attention because of the claim that leukemias contain oncogenes specific for the hematopoietic lineages from which the malignancies arise. The claim remains suspect, for want of independent verification and characterization of the oncogenes.

D. Role of Transforming Genes in Tumorigenesis

The common belief that many carcinogens initiate tumorigenesis by mutating DNA has fostered the view that the point mutations in *RAS* genes can be early (if not the first) events in tumorigenesis. Results from experimental carcinogenesis have added credence to this view (see Chapter 12), and there are hints that the view may also apply to some human tumors. First, mutant *RAS* genes have been found in at least two benign disorders of humans from which malignant tumors arise: adenomatous polyps of the colon, which are frequent precursors to colon carcinoma (Bos et al. 1987), and myelodysplasia, which can evolve into acute myelogenous leukemia (AML) (Hirai et al. 1987; Liu et al. 1987; Padua et al. 1988). The mutant genes persist in the ensuing malignant tumors. Second, *RAS* mutations have been found in the normal as well as the leukemic cells of some individuals with AML, suggesting that the mutation arose early in the sequence of tumorigenesis and persisted in a common precursor for normal and leukemic cells (Farr et al. 1988).

Paradoxically, there is also evidence that mutations of *RAS* genes are *not* necessarily the initiating event in tumorigenesis. The evidence is of two sorts. First, in some individuals with AML, only a fraction of the leukemic cells contain a mutant allele of *NRAS* (Toksoz et al. 1987). Second, when cases of AML were examined during both the first presentation of the disease and a subsequent relapse from successful therapy, mutant alleles of *NRAS* were sometimes found in the initial disease but not in the relapse (Farr et al. 1988). It therefore appears that therapy eliminated leukemic cells bearing the *NRAS* mutations, but failed to ablate the transformed precursor from which the leukemia ultimately stems. Moreover, a few of the leukemias displayed two mutations of *NRAS* in separate alleles, apparently carried by different subclones of leukemic cells. These findings suggest that the *RAS* mutations arose subsequent to an initial (and still mysterious) transforming event and represent steps in the clonal evolution (or progression) of the leukemias.

No proto-oncogene has yet been implicated in the inheritance of naturally occurring cancers. The damage to proto-oncogenes found in cancer cells—be it chromosomal rearrangement, gene amplification, or point mutation—has been restricted to somatic tissue, usually to tumors alone. These findings are in accord with the view that cancers usually arise from genetic damage sustained in somatic cells, although inherited mutations can increase susceptibility to tumorigenesis. Alternatively, it is possible that the tumorigenic alleles of proto-oncogenes do not appear as congenital lesions because their presence precludes survival of the embryo.

V. ONCOGENES IN DIAGNOSIS AND PROGNOSIS

Diagnosis and prognosis are inextricably linked in the management of human cancer. The natural course of a tumor can be predicted only if the tumor has been properly identified, and the selection of therapeutic regimen depends similarly on accurate diagnosis. To the extent that specific forms of genetic damage are consistently associated with particular tumors, analysis of oncogenes may eventually improve the certainty with which individual cancers are identified, enhance the resolution of taxonomy, and influence strategies for therapy. Several examples are at hand to illustrate the prospects. They are provisional in nature, limited in scope, and partly speculative: Wider ranging and more conclusive inferences will be possible only when the catalog of genetic damage in human tumors is closer to completion.

1. The translocation between *ABL* and *BCR* in CML can be detected by molecular hybridization or by searching for the distinctive protein product of the fused genes. As a consequence, the diagnosis of CML can now be made with greater certainty, even when Ph^1 is not present in leukemic cells (Bartram et al. 1985).
2. Approximately 10% of individuals with acute lymphocytic leukemia (ALL) also have Ph^1 in their leukemic cells and have suffered a reciprocal translocation 9;22. The breakpoint of this translocation resides farther upstream in *BCR* than the breakpoint in CML (Croce et al. 1987; Hermans et al. 1987), and the resulting hybrid *BCR-ABL* protein is smaller than that of CML (Chan et al. 1987; Clark et al. 1987; Kloetzer et al. 1987; Walker et al. 1987). These findings can be used to distinguish ALL and CML when they might otherwise be confused with one another.
3. Provisional analyses indicate that the presence of amplified *NMYC* in human neuroblastomas identifies tumors with a particularly poor prog-

nosis (Brodeur et al. 1984, 1987). Amplification of *NMYC* has been said to have greater prognostic value for neuroblastoma than the clinical stage of the disease (Slamon 1987), and it may eventually guide the selection of therapeutic regimens for the tumor.

4. Myelodysplasia is a disorder of the bone marrow that gives rise to AML in approximately 30% of cases (Jacobs 1987). Mutant alleles of *KRAS* (Liu et al. 1987) and *NRAS* (Hirai et al. 1987; Padua et al. 1988) have been found in the bone marrow and peripheral blood cells of some individuals with myelodysplasia. In the limited number of cases examined to date, the presence of the mutations in *RAS* genes has correlated with poor prognosis in general (Padua et al. 1988) and progression to acute leukemia in particular (Hirai et al. 1987; Liu et al. 1987). These findings raise the possibility that the search for mutations in *RAS* genes will eventually offer a prognostic device for the management of individuals with myelodysplasia.
5. Several abnormalities have been associated tentatively with a poor prognosis for carcinoma of the breast: amplification of the protooncogenes *NEU*/*ERBB2* (Slamon et al. 1987; Varley et al. 1987; van de Vijver et al. 1987,1988), *MYC* (Varley et al. 1987), and *INT2* (Zhou et al. 1988); excessive expression of *HRAS* (Clair et al. 1987); and a deletion within the short arm of chromosome 11 (Ali et al. 1987). There is presently no reason to believe that these different lesions occur in the same subset of tumors, however, and no explanation as to why the lesions might be associated with a poor prognosis.
6. Amplification of one or another of the *myc* gene family (including *MYC, LMYC*, and *NMYC*) has been found in an appreciable fraction of cell lines established from small cell carcinomas of the lung (Little et al. 1983; Johnson et al. 1987; Kiefer et al. 1987). Provisional data suggest that amplification of genes in the *MYC* family may be associated with a variety of unfavorable circumstances, including aggressive and disseminated tumors, relapse following therapy, rapid tumor progression, and relatively short survival time (Johnson et al. 1987). In addition, a restriction site polymorphism of *LMYC* has been associated with the metastatic potential of lung cancer (Kawashima et al. 1988). It would be premature, however, to conclude that these findings embody reliable prognostic devices.
7. By using molecular techniques to search for the breakpoint of a chromosomal translocation, it is now possible to detect the presence of one leukemia cell among one million normal cells (Crescenzi et al. 1988). The procedure offers unprecedented sensitivity for the detection of leukemia cells in individuals who have completed a course of therapy and in bone marrow that is being evaluated for autologous transplantation.

VI. FOUNDATIONS FOR THERAPY

The desire to achieve more rational treatment of cancer has been a cardinal motivation for research into the mechanisms of carcinogenesis. The discovery of malfunctioning genes in human cancers raised hope that this desire might be fulfilled. The prospects still seem real but distant. The most immediate possibility is that analysis of oncogenes may soon influence the choice of therapy for at least a few types of tumors: Examples of this have been outlined above for myelodysplasia and neuroblastoma. What are the prospects for applying the burgeoning knowledge of oncogenes to the development of new therapeutic strategies?

Could damaged proto-oncogenes be repaired or removed? We presently have no means by which to do this, and the likelihood that it will be achieved in the foreseeable future seems small (Baltimore 1987). Plans for immediate strategies focus instead on the proteins encoded by oncogenes and their biochemical actions. The reasons for this are several. First, the products of oncogenes may offer specific targets for chemotherapy: In many instances, mutations have made the errant gene products unique to the cells of the tumor—a specificity not available to the great majority of current therapeutic regimens. Second, several of the oncogene products have biochemical actions that seem amenable to selective inhibition: Examples include the functions of *RAS* proteins (see Chapter 5) and the protein tyrosine kinase activity encoded by *ABL* and a number of other potentially important oncogenes (see Chapter 6). Third, in contrast to our ineptitude at genetic surgery, we have developed great facility for the design, production, and delivery of chemotherapeutic agents. Fourth, at least some products of oncogenes may be accessible to an immunological attack; for example, antibodies directed against the cell-surface product of *NEU*/*ERBB2* can block tumorigenesis by an oncogenic allele of the gene (Drebin et al. 1986).

Effective therapy against cancer founded on our knowledge of oncogenes will probably be slow to come. Elucidation of the mechanisms by which the gene products act is proceeding at a frustratingly slow pace. Design of therapy may require elaborate details of protein structure and function; no single therapy is likely to become a panacea. We must instead deal with a large variety of oncogenes, which can cooperate with and replace one another as tumors evolve.

VII. CONCLUSION

The notion that genetic changes are important in the genesis of cancer has met strenuous resistance over the years. The discovery of proto-oncogenes and the sorts of damage they display in cancer cells, along with the description of recessive mutations that transmit predispositions to cancer, has altered the balance in the debate. There is genetic damage in many if not all human cancers, and it embodies virtually every form that might have been anticipated.

The evidence for genetic origins of human cancer is not decisive: Molecular dissection of cancer cells is akin to archaeology—the past must be inferred from its remnants in the present. A full explanation of tumorigenesis seems far from view: Much of the genetic damage in cancer cells has yet to be explicated, and there is little experimental purchase on epigenetic phenomena that may also be required to produce a malignant cell. Nevertheless, the search for genetic damage in cancer cells and the elucidation of how that damage affects the biochemical functions of genes have become our present best hope to understand and thus to thwart the ravages of cancer.

REFERENCES

Adams, J.M., A.W. Harris, C.A. Pinkert, L.M. Corcoran, W.S. Alexander, S. Cory, R.D. Palmiter, and R.L. Brinster. 1985. The c-*myc* oncogene driven by immunoglobulin enhancers induces lymphoid malignancy in transgenic mice. *Nature* **318:** 533–538.

Ali, I.U., R. Lidereau, C. Theillet, and R. Callahan. 1987. Reduction to homozygosity of genes on chromosome 11 in human breast neoplasia. *Science* **238:** 185–188.

Alitalo, K. and M. Schwab. 1986. Oncogene amplification in tumor cells. *Adv. Cancer Res.* **47:** 235–281.

Almoguera, C., D. Shibata, K. Forrester, J. Martin, N. Arnheim, and M. Perucho. 1988. Most human carcinomas of the exocrine pancreas contain mutant c-K-*ras* genes. *Cell* **53:** 549–554.

Baer, R., A. Heppell, A.M.R. Taylor, P.H. Rabbitts, B. Boullier, and T.H. Rabbitts. 1988. The breakpoint of an inversion of chromosome 14 in a T-cell leukemia: Sequences downstream of the immunoglobulin heavy chain locus are implicated in tumorigenesis. *Proc. Natl. Acad. Sci.* **84:** 9069–9074.

Bakhshi, A., J.P. Jensen, P. Goldman, J.J. Wright, O.W. McBride, A.L. Epstein, and S.J. Korsmeyer. 1985. Cloning the chromosomal breakpoint of t(14;18) human lymphomas: Clustering around J_H on chromosome 14 and near a transcriptional unit on 18. *Cell* **41:** 899–906.

Baltimore, D. 1987. The impact of the discovery of oncogenes on cancer mortality rates will come slowly. *Cancer* **59:** 1985–1986.

Barbacid, M. 1987. *Ras* genes. *Annu. Rev. Biochem.* **56:** 779–827.

Bartram, C.R., E. Kleihauer, A. de Klein, G. Grosveld, J.R. Teyssier, N. Heisterkamp, and J. Groffen. 1985. C-*abl* and *bcr* are rearranged in a Ph^1-negative CML patient. *EMBO J.* **4:** 683–687.

Bartram, C. R., A. de Klein, A. Hagemeijer, T. van Agthoven, A. Geurts van Kessel, M.D. Bootsma, G. Grosveld, M.A. Ferguson-Smith, T. Davies, M. Stone, N. Heisterkamp, J.R. Stephenson, and J. Groffen. 1983. Translocation of c-*abl* oncogene correlates with the presence of a Philadelphia chromosome in chronic myelocytic leukaemia. *Nature* **306:** 277–280.

Battey, J., C. Moulding, R. Taub, W. Murphy, T. Stewart, H. Potter, G. Lenoir, and P. Leder. 1983. The human c-*myc* oncogene: Structural consequences of translocation into the IgH locus in Burkitt Lymphoma. *Cell* **34:** 779–787.

Ben-Neriah, Y., G.Q. Daley, A.-M. Mes-Masson, O.N. Witte, and D. Baltimore. 1986. The chronic myelogenous leukemia-specific P210 protein is the product of the *bcr/abl* hybrid gene. *Science* **233:** 212–215.

Bernards, A., C.M. Rubin, C.A. Westbrook, M. Paskind, and D. Baltimore. 1987. The first intron in the human c-*abl* gene is at least 200 kilobases long and is a target for translocations in chronic myelogenous leukemia. *Mol. Cell. Biol.* **7:** 3231–3236.

Bos, J.L., E.R. Fearon, S.R. Hamilton, M. Verlaan-de Vries, J.H. van Boom, A.J. van der Eb, and B. Vogelstein. 1987. Prevalence of *ras* gene mutations in human colorectal cancers. *Nature* **327:** 293–297.

Bos, J.L., D. Toksoz, C.J. Marshall, M. Verlaan-de Vries, G.H. Veeneman, A.J. van der Eb, J.H. van Boom, J.W.G. Janssen, and A.C. Steenvoorden. 1985. Amino-acid substitutions at codon 13 of the N-*ras* oncogene in human acute myeloid leukaemia. *Nature* **315:** 726–731.

Boveri, T. 1929. *The origin of malignant tumors.* Williams & Wilkins, Boston.

Brodeur, G.M., R.C. Seeger, M. Schwab, H.E. Varmus, and J.M. Bishop. 1984. Amplification of N-*myc* in untreated human neuroblastomas correlates with advanced disease stage. *Science* **224:** 1121–1124.

Brodeur, G.M., F.A. Hayes, A.A. Green, J.T. Casper, J. Wasson, S. Wallach, and R.C. Seeger. 1987. Consistent N-*myc* copy number in simultaneous or consecutive neuroblastoma samples from sixty individual patients. *Cancer Res.* **47:** 4248–4254.

Butnick, N.Z., C. Miyamoto, R. Chizzonite, B.R. Cullen, G. Ju, and A.M. Skalka. 1985. Regulation of the human c-*myc* gene: 5′ noncoding sequences do not affect translation. *Mol. Cell. Biol.* **5:** 3009–3016.

Care, A., L. Cianetti, A. Giampaolo, N.M. Sposi, V. Zappavigna, F. Mavilio, G. Alimena, S. Amadori, F. Madelli, and C. Peschle. 1986. Translocation of c-*myc* into the immunoglobulin heavy-chain locus in human acute B-cell leukemia. A molecular analysis. *EMBO. J.* **5:** 905–913.

Carney, W.P., D. Petit, P. Hamer, C.J. Der, T. Finkel, G.M. Cooper, M. Lefebvre, H. Mobtaker, R. Delellis, A.S. Tischler, Y. Dayal, H. Wolfe, and H. Rabin. 1986. Monoclonal antibody specific for an activated RAS protein. *Proc. Natl. Acad. Sci.* **83:** 7485–7890.

Cesarman, E., R. Dalla-Favera, D. Bentley, and M. Groudine. 1987. Mutations in the first exon are associated with altered transcription of c-*myc* in Burkitt lymphoma. *Science* **238:** 1272–1275.

Chan, L.C., K.K. Karhi, S.I. Rayter, N. Heisterkamp, S. Eridani, R. Powles, S.D. Lawler, J. Groffen, J.G. Foulkes, M.F. Greaves, and L.M. Wiedemann. 1987. A novel *abl* protein expressed in Philadelphia chromosome positive acute lymphoblastic leukaemia. *Nature* **325:** 635–637.

Clair, T., W.R. Miller, and Y.S. Cho-Chung. 1987. Prognostic significance of the expression of a *ras* protein with a molecular weight of 21,000 by human breast cancer. *Cancer Res.* **47:** 5290–5293.

Clark, R., G. Wong, N. Arnheim, D. Nitecki, and F. McCormick. 1985. Antibodies specific for amino acid 12 of the *ras* oncogene product inhibit GTP binding. *Proc. Natl. Acad. Sci.* **82:** 5280–5285.

Clark, S.S., J. McLaughlin, W.M. Crist, R. Champlin, and O.N. Witte. 1987. Unique forms of the *abl* tyrosine kinase distinguish Ph^1-positive CM from Ph^1-positive ALL. *Science* **235:** 85–88.

Cleary, M.L. and J. Sklar. 1985. Nucleotide sequence of a t(14;18) chromosomal breakpoint in follicular lymphoma and demonstration of a breakpoint-cluster region near a transcriptionally active locus on chromosome 18. *Proc. Natl. Acad. Sci.* **82:** 7439–7444.

Cleary, M.L., S.D. Smith, and J. Sklar. 1986. Cloning and structural analysis of cDNAs for *bcl*-2 and a hybrid *bcl*-2/immunoglobulin transcript resulting from the t(14;18) translocation. *Cell* **47:** 19–28.

Collins, S.J., I. Kubonishi, I. Miyoshi, and M.T. Groudine. 1984. Altered transcription of the c-*abl* oncogene in K-562 and other chronic myelogenous leukemia cells. *Science* **225:** 72–74.

Cory, S. Activation of cellular oncogenes in hemopoietic cells by chromosome translocation. 1986. *Adv. Cancer Res.* **47:** 189–239.

Crescenzi, M., M. Seto, G.P. Herzig, P.D. Weiss, R.C. Griffith, and S.J. Korsmeyer. 1988. Thermostable DNA polymerase chain amplification of t(14;18) chromosome breakpoints and detection of minimal residual disease. *Proc. Natl. Acad. Sci.* **85:** 4869–4873.

Croce, C.M., K. Huebner, M. Isolbe, E. Fainstain, B. Lifshitz, E. Shtivelman, and E. Canaani. 1987. Mapping of four distinct *BCR*-related loci to chromosome region 22q11: Order of *BCR* loci relative to chronic myelogenous leukemia and acute lymphoblastic leukemia breakpoints. *Proc. Natl. Acad. Sci.* **84:** 7174–7179.

Croce, C.M., M. Shander, J. Martinis, L. Cicurel, G.G. D'Anconaj, T.W. Dolby, and H. Koprowski. 1979. Chromosomal location of the genes for human immunoglobulin heavy chains. *Proc. Natl. Acad. Sci.* **76:** 3416–3419.

Croce, C.M., M. Isobe, A. Palumbo, J. Puck, J. Ming, D. Tweardy, J. Erikson, M. Davis, and G. Rovera. 1985. Gene for α-chain of human T-cell receptor: Location on chromosome 14 region involved in T-cell neoplasms. *Science* **227:** 1044–1047.

Dalla-Favera, R., R.C. Gallo, A. Giallongo, and C.M. Croce. 1982a. Chromosomal localization of the human homolog (c-*sis*) of the simian sarcoma virus *onc* gene. *Science* **218:** 686-688.

Dalla-Favera, R., M. Bregni, J. Erikson, D. Patterson, R.C. Gallo, and C.M. Croce. 1982b. Human c-*myc* onc gene is located on the region of chromosome-8 that is translocated in Burkitt lymphoma cells. *Proc. Natl. Acad. Sci.* **79:** 7824–7827.

Darveau, A., J. Pelletier, and N. Sonenberg. 1985. Differential efficiencies of *in vitro* translation of mouse c-*myc* transcripts differing in the 5′ untranslated region. *Proc. Natl. Acad. Sci.* **82:** 2315–2319.

Davis, R.L., J.B. Konopka, and O.N. Witte. 1985. Activation of the c-*abl* oncogene by viral transduction or chromosomal translocation generates altered c-*abl* proteins with similar *in vitro* kinase properties. *Mol. Cell. Biol.* **5:** 204–213.

Denny, C.T., Y. Yoshikai, T.W. Mak, S.D. Smith, G.F. Hollis, and I.R. Kirsch. 1986. A chromosome 14 inversion in a T-cell lymphoma is caused by site-specific recombination between immuno-globulin and T-cell receptor loci. *Nature* **320:** 549–552.

DePinho, R.A., K.S. Hatton, A. Tesfaye, G.D. Yancopoulos, and F.W. Alt. 1988. The human *myc* gene family: Structure and activity of L-*myc* and an L-*myc* pseudogene. *Gene Dev.* **1:** 1311–1327.

Devine, J.M. 1986. Mechanism of activation of *HuBlym*-1 gene unresolved. *Nature* **321:** 437–439.

Diamond, A., J.M. Devine, and G.M. Cooper. 1984. Nucleotide sequence of a human *Blym* transforming gene activated in a Burkitt's lymphoma. *Science* **225:** 516–519.

Diamond, A., G.M. Cooper, J. Ritz, and M.-A. Lane. 1983. Identification and molecular cloning of the human Blym transforming gene activated in Burkitt's lymphomas. *Nature* **305:** 112–116.

Drebin, J.A., V.C. Link, R.A. Weinberg, and M.I. Greene. 1986. Inhibition of tumor growth by a monoclonal antibody reactive with an oncogene encoded tumor antigen. *Proc. Natl. Acad. Sci.* **83:** 9129–9134.

Eick, D., M. Piechaczyk, B. Henglein, J.-M. Blanchard, B. Traub, E. Kofler, S. Wiest, G.M. Lenoir, and G.W. Bornkamm. 1985. Aberrant c-*myc* RNAs of Burkitt's lymphoma cells have longer half-lives. *EMBO J.* **4:** 3717–3727.

Erikson, J., J. Martinis, and C.M. Croce. 1981. Assignment of the genes for human γ immunoglobulin chains to chromosome 22. *Nature* **294:** 173–175.

Erikson, J., A. ar-Rushdi, H.L. Drwinga, P.C. Nowell, and C.M. Croce. 1983a. Transcriptional activation of the translocated c-*myc* oncogene in Burkitt lymphoma. *Proc. Natl. Acad. Sci.* **80:** 820–824.

Erikson, J., D.L. Williams, J. Finan, P.C. Nowell, and C.M. Croce. 1985. Locus of the α-chain of the T-cell receptor is split by chromosome translocation in T-cell leukemias. *Science* **229:** 784–786.

Erikson, J., K. Nishikura, A. ar-Rushdi, J. Finan, B. Emanuel, G. Lenoir, P.C. Nowell, and C.M. Croce. 1983b. Translocation of an immunoglobulin κ locus to a region 3′ of an unrearranged c-*myc* oncogene enhances c-*myc* transcription. *Proc. Natl. Acad. Sci.* **80:** 7581–7585.

Erikson, J., L. Finger, L. Sun, A. ar-Rushdi, K. Nishikura, J. Minowada, J. Finan, B.S. Emanuel, P.C. Nowell, and C.M. Croce. 1986. Deregulation of c-*myc* by translocation of the α-locus of the T-cell receptor in T-cell leukemias. *Science* **232:** 884–886.

Escot, C., C. Theillet, R. Lidereau, F. Spyratos, M.-H. Champeme, J. Gest, and R. Callahan. 1986. Genetic alteration of the c-*myc* protooncogene (*MYC*) in human primary breast carcinomas. *Proc. Natl. Acad. Sci.* **83:** 4834–4838.

Eva, A. and S. A. Aaronson. 1985. Isolation of a new human oncogene from a diffuse B-cell lymphoma. *Nature* **316:** 273–275.

Eva, A., G. Vecchio, M. Diamond, S.R. Tronick, D. Ron, G.M. Cooper, and S.A. Aaronson. 1987. Independently activated *dbl* oncogenes exhibit similar yet distinct structural alterations. *Oncogenes* **1:** 355–361.

Evans, A.E., G.J. D'Angio, K. Propert, J. Anderson, and H.-W.L. Hann. 1987. Prognostic factors in neuroblastoma. *Cancer* **59:** 1853–1860.

Farr, C.J., R.K. Saiki, H.A. Erlich, F. McCormick, and C.J. Marshall. 1988. Analysis of *ras* gene mutations in acute myeloid leukemia using the polymerase chain reaction and oligonucleotide probes. *Proc. Natl. Acad. Sci.* **85:** 1629–1633.

Fialkow, P.J. 1980. Clonal and stem cell origin of blood cell neoplasms. In *Contemporary hematology/oncology* (ed. J. Lobue et al.), p.1. Plenum Press, New York.

———. 1984. Clonal evolution of human myeloid leukemias. *UCLA Symp. Mol. Cell. Biol.* **17:** 215–226.

Finger, L.R., R.C. Harvey, R.C.A. Moore, L.C. Showe, and C.M. Croce. 1986. A common mechanism of chromosomal translocation in T- and B-cell neoplasia. *Science* **234:** 982–985.

Forrester, K., C. Almoguera, K. Han, W.E. Grizzle, and M. Perucho. 1987. Detection of high incidence of K-*ras* oncogenes during human colon tumorigenesis. *Nature* **327:** 298–303.

Fusco, A., M. Grieco, M. Santoro, M.T. Berlingieri, S. Pilotti, M.A. Pierotti, G.D. Porta, and G. Vecchio. 1987. A new oncogene in human thyroid papillary carcinomas and their lymph-nodal metastases. *Nature* **328:** 170–172.

Gale, R.P. and E. Canaani. 1984. An 8-kilobase *abl* RNA transcript in chronic myelogenous leukemia. *Proc. Natl. Acad. Sci.* **81:** 5648–5652.

Goubin, G., D.S. Goldman, J. Luce, P.E. Neiman, and G.M. Cooper. 1983. Molecular cloning and nucleotide sequence of a transforming gene detected by transfection of chicken B-cell lymphoma DNA. *Nature* **302:** 114–118.

Grady-Leopardi, E.F., M. Schwab, A.R. Ablin, and W. Rosenau, 1986. Detection of N-*myc* oncogene expression in human neuroblastoma by *in situ* hybridization and blot analysis: Relationship to clinical outcome. *Cancer Res.* **46:** 3196–3199.

Graham, M. and J.M. Adams. 1986. Chromosome 8 breakpoint far 3′ of the c-*myc* oncogene in a Burkitt's lymphoma 2;8 variant translocation is equivalent to the murine *pvt*-1 locus. *EMBO J.* **5:** 2845–2853.

Groffen, J., J.R. Stephenson, N. Heisterkamp, A. de Klein, C.R. Bartram, and G. Grosveld. 1984. Philadelphia chromosomal breakpoints are clustered within a limited region, bcr, on chromosome 22. *Cell* **36:** 93–99.

Guerrasio, A., G.C. Avanzi, L. Pegoraro, X. Estivill, A. Serra, M.C. Giubellino, M.T. Fierro, A. Novarino, R. Foa, and G. Saglio. 1987. Rearrangement of the c-*myc* oncogene with heavy-chain immunoglobulin enhancer in tumor DNA from an acute lymphoblastic leukemia patient. *J. Natl. Cancer Inst.* **78:** 845–853.

Haluska, F.G., Y. Tsujimoto, and C.M. Croce. 1987. Oncogene activation by chromosome translocation in human malignancy. *Annu. Rev. Genet.* **21:** 321–338.

Hariharan, I.K. and J.M. Adams. 1987. cDNA sequence for human *bcr*, the gene that translocates to the *abl* oncogene in chronic myeloid leukaemia. *EMBO J.* **6:** 115–121.

Hayday, A.C., S.D. Gillies, H. Saito, C. Wood, K. Wiman, W.S. Hayward, and S. Tonegawa. 1984. Activation of a translocated human c-*myc* gene by an enhancer in the immunoglobulin heavy-chain locus. *Nature* **307:** 334–340.

Heisterkamp, N., K. Stam, J. Groffen, A. de Klein, and G. Grosveld. 1985. Structural organization of the *bcr* gene and its role in the Ph^1 translocation. *Nature* **315:** 758–761.

Heisterkamp, N., J.R. Stephenson, J. Groffen, P.F. Hansen, A. de Klein, C.R. Bartram, and G. Grosveld. 1983. Localization of the c-*abl* oncogene adjacent to a translocation break point in chronic myelocytic leukaemia. *Nature* **306:** 239–242.

Heisterkamp, N., J. Groffen, J.R. Stephenson, N.K. Spurr, P.N. Goodfellow, E. Solomon, B. Carret, and W.F. Bodmer. 1982. Chromosomal localization of human cellular homologues of two viral oncogenes (c-*fes* and c-*abl*). *Nature* **299:** 747–750.

Hermans, A., N. Heisterkamp, M. von Lindern, S. van Baal, D. Meijer, D. van der Plas, L.M. Wiedemann, J. Groffen, D. Bootsma, and G. Grosveld. 1987. Unique fusion of *bcr* and c-*abl* genes in Philadelphia chromosome positive acute lymphoblastic leukemia. *Cell* **51:** 33–40.

Hirai, H., Y. Kobayashi, H. Mano, K. Hagiwara, Y. Maru, M. Omine, H. Mizoguchi, J. Nishida, and F. Takaku. 1987. A point mutation at codon 13 of the N-*ras* oncogene in myelodysplastic syndrome. *Nature* **327:** 430–432.

Hirai, H., S. Tanaka, M. Azuma, Y. Anraku, Y. Kobayashi, M. Fujisawa, T. Okabe, A. Urabe, and F. Takaku. 1985. Transforming genes in human leukemia cells. *Blood* **66:** 1371–1378.

Jacobs, A. 1987. Human preleukemia: Do we have a model? *Brit. J. Cancer* **55:** 1–5.

Janssen, J.W.G., A.C.M. Steenvoorden, J. Lyons, B. Anger, J.U. Bohle, J.L. Bos, H. Seliger, and C.R. Bartram. 1988. *RAS* gene mutations in acute and chronic myelocytic leukemias, chronic myeloproliferative disorders, and myelodysplastic syndromes. *Proc. Natl. Acad. Sci.* **84:** 9228–9233.

Johnson, B.E., D.C. Ihde, R.W. Makuch, A.F. Gazdar, D.N. Carney, H. Oie, E. Russell, M.M. Nau, and J.D. Minna. 1987. *myc* family oncogene amplification in tumor cell lines established from small cell lung cancer patients and its relationship to clinical status and course. *J. Clin. Invest.* **79:** 1629–1634.

Kagan, J., J. Finan, J. Letofsky, E.C. Besa, P.C. Nowell, and C.M. Croce. 1987. α-chain locus of the T-cell antigen receptor is involved in the t(10;14) chromosome translocation of T-cell acute lymphocytic leukemia. *Proc. Natl. Acad. Sci.* **84:** 4543–4547.

Kawashima, K., H. Shikama, K. Imoto, M. Izawa, T. Naruke, K. Okabayashi, and S. Nishimura. 1988. Close correlation between restriction fragment length polymorphism of the L-*MYC* gene and metastasis of human lung cancer to the lymph nodes and other organs. *Proc. Natl. Acad. Sci.* **85:** 2353–2356.

Kiefer, P.E., G. Bepler, M. Kubasch, and K. Havemann. 1987. Amplification and expression of protooncogenes in human small cell lung cancer cell lines. *Cancer Res.* **47:** 6236–6242.

Kinzler, K.W., J.M. Ruppert, S.H. Bigner, and B. Vogelstein. 1988. The *GLI* gene is a member of the Kruppel family of zinc finger proteins. *Nature* **332:** 371–374.

Kinzler, K.W., S.H. Bigner, D.D. Bigner, J.M. Trent, M.L. Law, S.J. O'Brien, A.J. Wong, and B. Vogelstein. 1987. Identification of an amplified, highly expressed gene in a human glioma. *Science* **236:** 70–73.

Kirsch, I.R., C.C. Morton, K. Nakahara, and P. Leder. 1982. Human immunoglobulin heavy chain genes map to a region of translocations in malignant B lymphocytes. *Science* **216:** 301–303.

Klein, A.D., A.G. Van Kessel, G. Grosveld, C.R. Bartram, A. Hagemeijer, D. Bootsma, N.K. Spurr, N. Heisterkamp, K. Groffen, and J.R. Stephenson. 1982. A cellular oncogene is translocated to the Philadelphia chromosome in chronic myelocytic leukaemia. *Nature* **300:** 765–767.

Kloetzer, W.S., M. Talpas, J.M. Trujillo, M. Blick, M. Beran, and J.U. Gutterman. 1987. A novel c-*abl* protein in Philadelphia-positive acute lymphoblastic leukaemia. *Nature* **325:** 631–635.

Kohl, N.E., C.E. Gee, and F.W. Alt. 1984. Activated expression of the N-*myc* gene in human neuroblastomas and related tumors. *Science* **226:** 1335–1337.

Kohl, N.E., N. Kanda, R.R. Schreck, G. Bruns, S.A. Latt, F. Gilbert, and F.W. Alt. 1983. Transposition and amplification of oncogene-related sequences in human neuroblastomas. *Cell* **35:** 359–367.

Kohl, N.E., E. Legouy, R.A. DePinho, P.D. Nisen, R.K. Smith, C.E. Gee, and F.W. Alt. 1986. Human N-*myc* is closely related in organization and nucleotide sequence to c-*myc*. *Nature* **319:** 73–77.

Konopka, J.B., and O.N. Witte. 1985. Detection of c-*abl* tyrosine kinase activity *in vitro* permits direct comparison of normal and altered *abl* gene products. *Mol. Cell. Biol.* **5:** 3116–3123.

Konopka, J.B., S.M. Watanabe, and O.N. Witte. 1984. An alteration of the human c-*abl* protein in K562 leukemia cells unmasks associated tyrosine kinase activity. *Cell* **37:** 1035–1042.

Kozma, S.E, S.M.S. Redmond, F. Xiao-Chang, S.M. Saurer, B. Groner, and N.E. Hynes. 1988. Activation of the receptor kinase domain of the *trk* oncogene by recombination with two different cellular sequences. *EMBO J.* **7:** 147–155.

Lane, M.-A., A. Sainten, and G.M. Cooper. 1982. Stage-specific transforming genes of human and mouse B- and T-lymphocyte neoplasms. *Cell* **28:** 873–880.

Leder, P., J. Battey, G. Lenoir, C. Moulding, W. Murphy, H. Potter, T. Stewart, and R. Taub. 1983. Translocations among antibody genes in human cancer. *Science* **222:** 765–770.

Lee, W.-H., A.L. Murphree, and W.F. Benedict. 1984. Expression and amplification of the N-*myc* gene in primary retinoblastoma. *Nature* **309:** 458–460.

Legouy, E., R. DePinho, K. Zimmerman, R. Collum, G. Yancopoulos, L. Mitscok, R. Kriz, and F.W. Alt. 1987. Structure and expression of the murine L-*myc* gene. *EMBO J.* **6:** 3359–3367.

Libermann, T.A., H.R. Nusbaum, N. Razon, R. Kris, I. Lax, H. Soreq, N. Whittle, M.D. Waterfield, A. Ullrich, and J. Schlessinger. 1985. Amplification, enhanced expression and possible rearrangement of EGF receptor gene in primary human brain tumours of glial origin. *Nature* **313:** 144–147.

Little, C.D., M.M. Nau, D.N. Carney, A.F. Gazdar, and J.D. Minna. 1983. Amplification and expression of the c-*myc* oncogene in human lung cancer cell lines. *Nature* **306:** 194–196.

Liu, E., B. Hjelle, and J.M. Bishop. 1988. Transforming genes in chronic myelogenous leukemia. *Proc. Natl. Acad. Sci.* **85:** 1952–1956.

Liu, E., B. Hjelle, R. Morgan, F. Hecht, and J.M. Bishop. 1987. Mutations of the Kirsten-*ras* proto-oncogene in human preleukaemia. *Nature* **330:** 186–188.

Lombardi, L., E.W. Newcomb, and R. Dalla-Favera. 1987. Pathogenesis of Burkitt lymphoma: Expression of an activated c-*myc* oncogene causes the tumorigenic conversion of EBV-infected human B lymphoblasts. *Cell* **49:** 161–170.

Malcolm, S., P. Barton, C. Murphy, M.A. Ferguson-Smith, D.L. Bentley, and T.H. Rabbitts. 1982. Localization of human immunoglobulin κ light chain variable region genes to the short arm of chromosome 2 by *in situ* hybridization. *Proc. Natl. Acad. Sci.* **74:** 4957–4961.

Mariani-Costantini, R., C. Escot, C. Theillet, A. Gentile, G. Merlo, R. Lidereau, and R. Callahan. 1988. *In situ* c-*myc* expression and genomic status of the c-*myc* locus in infiltrating ductal carcinomas of the breast. *Cancer Res.* **48:** 199–205.

Martin-Zanca, D., S.H. Hughes, and M. Barbacid. 1986. A human oncogene formed by the fusion of truncated tropomyosin and protein tyrosine kinase sequences. *Nature* **319:** 743–748.

Mathieu-Mahul, D., F. Sigaux, C. Zhu, A. Bernheim, M. Mauchauffe, M.-T. Daniel, R. Berger, and C.-J. Larsen. 1986. A t(8;14)(q24;q11) translocation in a T-cell leukemia (L1-ALL) with c-*myc* and TCR-α chain locus rearrangements. *Int. J. Cancer* **38:** 835–841.

McLaughlin, J., E. Chianese, and O.N. Witte. 1987. *In vitro* transformation of immature hematopoietic cells by the P210 *BCR/ABL* oncogene product of the Philadelphia chromosome. *Proc. Natl. Acad. Sci.* **84:** 6558–6563.

Mengle-Gaw, L. and T.H. Rabbitts. 1987. A human chromosome 8 region with abnormalities in B cell, HTLV-I^{+} T cell and c-*myc* amplified tumours. *EMBO J.* **6:** 1959–1567.

Mitra, G., D. Martin-Zanca, and M. Barbacid. 1987. Identification and biochemical characterization of $p70^{TRK}$, product of the human *TRK* oncogene. *Proc. Natl. Acad. Sci.* **84:** 6707–6712.

Murphy, W., J. Sarid, R. Taub, T. Vasicek, J. Battey, G. Lenoir, and P. Leder. 1986. A translocated human c-*myc* oncogene is altered in a conserved coding sequence. *Proc. Natl. Acad. Sci.* **83:** 2939–2944.

Nau, M.M., B.J. Brooks, Jr., D.N. Carney, A.F. Gazdar, J.F. Battey, E.A. Sausville, and J.D. Minna. 1986. Human small-cell lung cancers show amplification and expression of the N-*myc* gene. *Proc. Natl. Acad. Sci.* **83:** 1092–1097.

Nau, M. M., B.J. Brooks, J. Battey, E. Sausville, A.F. Gazdear, I.R. Kirsch, O.W. McBride, V. Bertness, G.F. Hollis, and J. D. Minna. 1985. L-*myc*, a new *myc*-related gene amplified and expressed in human small cell lung cancer. *Nature* **318:** 69–73.

Neel, B.G., S.C. Jhanwar, R.S.K. Chaganti, and W.S. Hayward. 1982. Two human c-*onc* genes are located on the long arm of chromosome-8. *Proc. Natl. Acad. Sci.* **79:** 7842–7846.

Nowell, P.C., and D.A. Hungerford. 1961. Chromosome studies in human leukemia. II. Chronic granulocytic leukemia. *J. Natl. Cancer Inst.* **27:** 1013–1035.

Ochiya, T., A. Fujiyama, S. Fukushige, I. Htada, and K. Matsubara. 1986. Molecular cloning of an oncogene from a human hepatocellular carcinoma. *Proc. Natl. Acad. Sci.* **83:** 4993–4997.

Oskam, R., F. Coulier, M. Ernst, D. Martin-Zanca, and M. Barbacid. 1988. Frequent generation of oncogenes by in vitro recombination of *TRK* protooncogene sequences. *Proc. Natl. Acad. Sci.* **85:** 2964–2969.

Padua, R.A., G. Carter, D. Hughes, J. Gow, C.J. Farr, D. Oscier, F. McCormick, S. Smith, and A. Jacobs. 1988. N-*ras* mutation in myelodysplasia detected by amplification. Oligonucleotide hybridization and transformation. *Leukemia* **2:** 503–510.

Pelicci, P.-G., D.M. Knowles II, I. Magrath, and R. Dalla-Favera. 1986a. Chromosomal breakpoints and structural alterations of the c-*myc* locus differ in endemic and sporadic forms of Burkitt lymphoma. *Proc. Natl. Acad. Sci.* **83:** 2984–2988.

Pelicci, P.-G., D.M. Knowles II, Z.A. Arlin, R. Wieczorek, P. Luciw, D. Dina, C. Basilico, and R. Dalla-Favera. 1986b. Multiple monoclonal B cell expansions and c-*myc* oncogene rearrangements in acquired immune deficiency syndrome-related lymphoproliferative disorders. Implications for lymphomagenesis. *J. Exp. Med.* **164:** 2049–2061.

Pulciani, S., E. Santos, A.V. Lauver, L.K. Long, S.A. Aaronson, and M. Barbacid. 1982. Oncogenes in solid human tumors. *Nature* **300:** 539–542.

Rabbitts, P.H., A. Forster, M.A. Stinson, and T.H. Rabbitts. 1985. Truncation of exon 1 from the c-*myc* gene results in prolonged c-*myc* mRNA stability. *EMBO J.* **4:** 3727–3735.

Rabbitts, T.H., P.H. Hamlyn, and R. Baer. 1983. Altered nucleotide sequences of a translocated c-*myc* gene in Burkitt lymphoma. *Nature* **306:** 760–765.

Reynolds, T.C., S.D. Smith, and J. Sklar. 1987. Analysis of DNA surrounding the breakpoint of chromosomal translocations involving the β T cell receptor gene in human lymphoblastic neoplasms. *Cell* **50:** 107–117.

Rodenhuis, S., M.L. van de Wetering, W.J. Mooi, S.G. Evers, N. van Zandwijk, and J.L. Bos. 1987. Mutational activation of the K-*ras* oncogene. A possible pathogenetic factor in adenocarcinoma of the lung. *New Engl. J. Med.* **317:** 929–936.

Rogers, J. 1986. Relationship of *Blym* genes to repeated sequences. *Nature* **320:** 579.

Rowley, J.B. 1973. A new consistent chromosomal abnormality in chronic myelogenous leukaemia identified by quinacrine fluorescence and Giemsa staining. *Nature* **243:** 290–293.

Saglio, G., B.S. Emanuel, A. Guerrasio, M.C. Giubellino, A. Serra, P. Lusso, G.R. Cambrin, U. Mazza, F. Malavasi, L. Pegoraro, and R. Foa. 1986. 3′ c-*myc* rearrangement in a human leukemic T-cell line. *Cancer Res.* **46:** 1413–1418.

Saito, H., A.C. Hayday, K. Wiman, W.S. Hayward, and S. Tonegawa. 1983. Activation of the c-*myc* gene by translocation: A model for translational control. *Proc. Natl. Acad. Sci.* **80:** 7476–7480.

Sakamoto, H., M. Mori, M. Taira, T. Yoshida, S. Matsukawa, K. Shimizu, M. Sekiguchi, M. Terada, and T. Sugimura. 1986. Transforming gene from human stomach cancers and a noncancerous portion of stomach mucosa. *Proc. Natl. Acad. Sci.* **83:** 3997–4002.

Schimke, R.T. 1984. Gene amplification in cultured animal cells. *Cell* **37:** 705–713.

Schwab, M., H.E. Varmus, and J.M. Bishop. 1985. Human N-*myc* gene contributes to neoplastic transformation of mammalian cells in culture. *Nature* **316:** 160–162.

Schwab, M., J. Ellison, M. Busch, W. Rosenau, H.E. Varmus, and J.M. Bishop. 1984. Enhanced expression of the human gene N-*myc* consequent to amplification of DNA may contribute to malignant progression of neuroblastoma. *Proc. Natl. Acad. Sci.* **81:** 4940–4945.

Schwab, M., K. Alitalo, K.-H. Klempnauer, H.E. Varmus, J.M. Bishop, F. Gilbert, G. Brodeur, M. Goldstein, and J. Trent. 1983. Amplified DNA with limited homology to *myc* cellular oncogene is shared by human neuroblastoma cell lines and a neuroblastoma tumour. *Nature* **305:** 245–247.

Seeger, R.C., G.M. Brodeur, H. Sather, A. Dalton, S.E. Siegel, K.Y. Wong, and D. Hammond. 1985. Association of multiple copies of the N-*myc* oncogene with rapid progression of neuroblastomas. *New Engl. J. Med.* **313:** 1111–1116.

Shih, C., B.Z. Shilo, M.P. Goldfarb, A. Dannenberg, and R.A. Weinberg. 1979. Passage of phenotypes of chemically transformed cells via transfection of DNA and chromatin. *Proc. Natl. Acad. Sci.* **76:** 5714–5718.

Shima, E.A., M.M. Le Beau, T.W. McKeithan, J. Minowada, L.W. Showe, T.W. Mak, M.D. Minden, J.D. Rowley, and M.O. Diaz. 1986. Gene encoding the α chain of the T-cell receptor is moved immediately downstream of c-*myc* in a chromosomal 8;14 translocation in a cell line from a human T-cell leukemia. *Proc. Natl. Acad. Sci.* **83:** 3439–3444.

Shtivelman, E., B. Lifshitz, R.P. Gale, and E. Canaani. 1985. Fused transcript of *abl* and *bcr* genes in chronic myelogenous leukaemia. *Nature* **315:** 550–554.

Slamon, D.J. 1987. Proto-oncogenes and human cancers. *New Engl. J. Med.* **317:** 955–957.

Slamon, D.J., J.B. deKernion, I.M. Verma, and M.J. Cline. 1984. Expression of cellular oncogenes in human malignancies. *Science* **224:** 256–262.

Slamon, D.J., G.M. Clark, S.G. Wong, W.J. Levin, A. Ullrich, and W.L. McGuire. 1987. Human breast cancer: Correlation of relapse and survival with amplification of the HER-2/*neu* oncogene. *Science* **235:** 177–182.

Small, M.B., N. Hay, M. Schwab, and J.M. Bishop. 1987. Neoplastic transformation by the human gene N-*myc*. *Mol. Cell. Biol.* **7:** 1638–1645.

Squire, J., A.D. Goddard, M. Canton, A. Becker, R.A. Phillips, and B.L. Gallie. 1986. Tumour induction by the retinoblastoma mutation is independent of N-*myc* expression. *Nature* **322:** 555–557.

Srivastava, S.K., R.H.P. Wheelock, S.A. Aaronson, and A. Eva. 1986. Identification of the protein encoded by the human diffuse B-cell lymphoma (*dbl*) oncogene. *Proc. Natl. Acad. Sci.* **83:** 8868–8873.

Stam, K., N. Heisterkamp, G. Grosveld, A. de Klein, R.S. Verma, M. Coleman, H. Dosik, and J. Groffen. 1985. Evidence of a new chimeric *bcr/c-abl* mRNA in patients with chronic myelocytic leukemia and the Philadelphia chromosome. *New Engl. J. Med.* **313:** 1429–1433.

Stanton, L.W., M. Schwab, and J.M. Bishop. 1986. Nucleotide sequence of the human N-*myc* gene. *Proc. Natl. Acad. Sci.* **83:** 1772–1777.

Stark, G.R. 1986. DNA amplification in drug resistant cells and in tumours. *Cancer Surv.* **5:** 1–25.

Stark, G.R. and G.M. Wahl. 1984. Gene amplification. *Ann. Rev. Biochem.* **53:** 447–493.

Sun, L.K., L.C. Showe, and C.M. Croce. 1986. Analysis of the 3′ flanking region of the human c-*myc* gene in lymphomas with the t(8;22) and t(2;8) chromosomal translocations. *Nucleic Acids Res.* **14:** 4037–4051.

Swan, D.G., O.W. McBride, K.C. Robbins, D.A. Keithley, E.P. Reddy, and S.A. Aaronson. 1982. Chromosomal mapping of the simian sarcoma virus *onc* gene analogue in human cells. *Proc. Natl. Acad. Sci.* **79:** 4691–4695.

Szajnert, M.-F., S. Saule, G.W. Bornkamm, H. Wajcman, G.M. Lenoir, and J.-C. Kaplan. 1987. Clustered somatic mutations in and around first exon of non-rearranged c-*myc* in Burkitt lymphoma with t(8;22) translocation. *Nucleic Acids Res.* **15:** 4553–4567.

Taira, M., T. Yoshida, K. Miyagawa, H. Sakamoto, M. Terada, and T. Sugimura. 1987. cDNA sequence of human transforming gene *hst* and identification of the coding sequence required for transforming activity. *Proc. Natl. Acad. Sci.* **84:** 2980–2985.

Taub, R., C. Moulding, J. Battey, W. Murphy, T. Vasicek, G.M. Lenoir, and P. Leder. 1984. Activation and somatic mutation of the translocated c-*myc* gene in Burkitt lymphoma cells. *Cell* **36:** 339–348.

Taub, R., C. Kirsch, G. Morton, D. Lenoir, S. Swan, S. Tronick, S. Aaronson, and P. Leder. 1982. Translocation of the c-*myc* gene into the immunoglobulin heavy chain locus in human Burkitt lymphoma and murine plasmacytoma cells. *Proc. Natl. Acad. Sci.* **79:** 7837–7841.

Thiele, C.J., C. McKeon, T.J. Triche, R.A. Ross, C.P. Reynolds, and M.A. Israel. 1987. Differential protooncogene expression characterizes histopathologically indistinguishable tumors of the peripheral nervous system. *J. Clin. Invest.* **80:** 804–811.

Toksoz, D., C.J. Farr, and C.J. Marshall. 1987. *ras* gene activation in a minor proportion of the blast population in acute myeloid leukemia. *Oncogene* **1:** 409–415.

Tsujimoto, Y., J. Yunis, L. Onorato-Showe, J. Erikson, P.C. Nowell, and C.M. Croce. 1984. Molecular cloning of the chromosomal breakpoint of B-cell lymphomas and leukemias with the t(11;14) chromosome translocation. *Science* **224:** 1403–1406.

Tsujimoto, Y. and C.M. Croce. 1986. Analysis of the structure, transcripts, and protein products of *bcl*-2, the gene involved in human follicular lymphoma. *Proc. Natl. Acad. Sci.* **83:** 5214–5218.

Tsujimoto, Y., N. Ikegaki, and C.M. Croce. 1988. Characterization of the protein product of *bcl*-2, the gene involved in human follicular lymphoma. *Oncogene* **2:** 3–9.

Tsujimoto, Y., J. Gorham, J. Cossman, E. Jaffe, and C.M. Croce. 1985a. The t(14;18) chromosome translocations involved in B-cell neoplasms result from mistakes in VDJ joining. *Science* **229:** 1390–1393.

Tsujimoto, Y., E. Jaffe, J. Cossman, J. Gorham, P.C. Nowell, and C.M. Croce. 1985b. Clustering of breakpoints on chromosome 11 in human B-cell neoplasms with the t(11;14) chromosome translocation. *Nature* **315:** 340–343.

van de Vijver, M.J., W.J. Mooi, P. Wisman, J.L. Peterse, and R. Nusse. 1988. Immunohistochemical detection of the *neu* protein in tissue sections of human breast tumors with amplified *neu* DNA. *Oncogene* **2:** 175–179.

van de Vijver, M., R. van de Bersselaar, P. Devilee, C. Cornelisse, J. Peterse, and R. Nusse. 1987. Amplification of the *neu* (c-*erb*B-2) oncogene in human mammary tumors is relatively frequent and is often accompanied by amplification of the linked c-*erb*A oncogene. *Mol. Cell. Biol.* **7:** 2019–2023.

Varley, J.M., J.E. Swallow, W.J. Brammar, J.L. Whittaker, and R.A. Walker. 1987. Alterations to either c-*erb*B-2 (*neu*) or c-*myc* proto-oncogenes in breast carcinomas correlate with poor short-term prognosis. *Oncogene* **1:** 423–431.

Varmus, H.E. 1984. The molecular genetics of cellular oncogenes. *Annu. Rev. Genet.* **18:** 553–612.

Von Hoff, D.D., D.R. Needham-VanDevanter, J. Yucel, B.E. Windle, and G.M. Wahl. 1988. Amplified human *MYC* oncogenes localized to replicating submicroscopic circular DNA molecules. *Proc. Natl. Acad. Sci.* **85:** 4804–4808.

Wahl, G.M., B.M. de Saint Vincent, and M.L. DeRose. 1984. Effect of chromosomal position on amplification of transfected genes in animal cells. *Nature* **307:** 516–520.

Walker, L.C., T.S. Ganesan, S. Dhut, B. Gibbons, T.A. Lister, J. Rothbard, and B.D. Young. 1987. Novel chimaeric protein expressed in Philadelphia positive acute lymphoblastic leukaemia. *Nature* **329:** 851–853.

Weinberg, R.A. 1982. Oncogenes of spontaneous and chemically induced tumors. *Adv. Cancer Res.* **36:** 149–163.

Wong, A.J., S.H. Bigner, D.D. Bigner, K.W. Kinzler, S.R. Hamilton, and B. Vogelstein. 1987. Increased expression of the epidermal growth factor receptor gene in malignant gliomas is invariably associated with gene amplification. *Proc. Natl. Acad. Sci.* **84:** 6899–6903.

Wong, A.J., J.M. Ruppert, J. Eggleston, S.R. Hamilton, S.B. Baylin, and B. Vogelstein. 1986. Gene amplification of c-*myc* and N-*myc* in small cell carcinoma of the lung. *Science* **233:** 461–464.

Yamamoto, T., N. Kamata, H. Kawano, S. Shimizu, T. Kuroki, K. Toyoshima, K. Riukimaru, N. Nomura, R. Ishizaki, I. Pastan, S. Gamou, and N. Shimizu. 1986. High incidence of amplification of the epidermal growth factor receptor gene in human squamous carcinoma cell lines. *Cancer Res.* **46:** 414–416.

Yancopoulos, G.D., P.D. Nisen, A. Tesfaye, N.E. Kohl, M.P. Goldfarb, and F.W. Alt. 1985. N-*myc* can cooperate with *ras* to transform normal cells in culture. *Proc. Natl. Acad. Sci.* **82:** 5455–5459.

Yanez, L., J. Groffen, and D.M. Valenzueal. 1987. c-K-*ras* mutations in human carcinomas occur preferentially in codon 12. *Oncogene* **1:** 315–319.

Yokota, J., K. Toyoshima, T. Sugimura, T. Yamamoto, M. Terada, H. Battifora, and M.J. Cline. 1986. Amplification of c-*erb*B-2 oncogene in human adenocarcinomas *in vivo*. *Lancet* **I:** 765–766.

Yokota, J., T. Yamamoto, N. Miyajima, K. Toyoshima, N. Nomura, H. Sakamoto, T. Yoshida, M. Terada, and T. Sugimura. 1988. Genetic alterations of the c-*erb*B-2 oncogene occur frequently in tubular adenocarcinoma of the stomach and are often accompanied by amplification of the v-*erb*A homologue. *Oncogene* **2:** 283–287.

Yoshida, M.C., M. Wada, H. Satoh, T. Yoshida, H. Sakamoto, K. Miyagawa, J. Yokota, T. Koda, M. Kakinuma, T. Sugimura, and M. Terada. 1988. Human *HST1* (*HSTF1*) gene maps to chromosome band 11q13 and coamplifies with the *INT*2 gene in human cancer. *Proc. Natl. Acad. Sci.* **85:** 4861–4864.

Yoshida, T., H. Sakamoto, K. Miyagawa, P.F.R. Little, M. Terada, and T. Sugimura. 1987a. Genomic clone of *hst* with transforming activity from a patient with acute leukemia. *Biochem. Biophys. Res. Commun.* **14:** 1019–1025.

Yoshida, T., K. Miyagawa, H. Odagiri, H. Sakamoto, P.F.R. Little, M. Terada, and T. Sugimura. 1987b. Genomic sequence of *hst*, a transforming gene encoding a protein homologous to fibroblast growth factors and the *int*-2-encoded protein. *Proc. Natl. Acad. Sci.* **84:** 7305–7310.

Yunis, J.J. 1986. Chromosomal rearrangements, genes, and fragile sites in cancer: Clinical and biologic implications. In *Important advances in oncology 1986* (ed. V.T. De Vita, Jr. et al.), pp. 93–128. J.B. Lippincott, Philadelphia.

Zhou, D.J., G. Casey, and M.J. Cline. 1988. Amplification of human *int*-2 in breast cancers and squamous carcinomas. *Oncogene* **2:** 279–282.

Ziegler, J.L. 1981. Burkitt's Lymphoma. *New Engl. J. Med.* **305:** 735–745.

Subject Index